Basic ICD-10-CM and ICD-10-PCS Coding Exercises

Seventh Edition

Lou Ann Schraffenberger, MBA, RHIA, CCS, CCS-P, FAHIMA
Michelle Dionisio, MA, MSc, RHIA, CCS

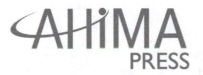

AHIMA PRESS

ISBN **978-1-58426-706-5**

AHIMA Product No. AC210518

AHIMA Staff:
Megan Grennan, Managing Editor
Kimberly Hooker, Production Development Editor
James Pinnick, Senior Director of Publications
Rachel Schratz, MA, Assistant Editor

Cover image: ©iStock: Studio-Pro

References used for ICD-10-CM coding in this book are from the ICD-10-CM Official Guidelines for Coding and Reporting taken from the 2020 updated version.

For more information, including updates, about AHIMA Press publications, **visit http://www .ahima.org/education/press.**

American Health Information Management Association
233 North Michigan Avenue, 21st Floor
Chicago, Illinois 60601-5809

ahima.org

Contents

About the Authors v

Preface vii

Acknowledgments ix

Online Resources xi

Chapter 1   Certain Infectious and Parasitic Diseases 1

Chapter 2   Neoplasms 11

Chapter 3   Diseases of Blood and Blood-forming Organs and Certain
Disorders Involving the Immune Mechanism 23

Chapter 4   Endocrine, Nutritional, and Metabolic Diseases 31

Chapter 5   Mental, Behavioral, and Neurodevelopmental Disorders 41

Chapter 6   Diseases of the Nervous System 51

Chapter 7   Diseases of the Eye and Adnexa 61

Chapter 8   Diseases of the Ear and Mastoid Process 69

Chapter 9   Diseases of the Circulatory System 77

Chapter 10   Diseases of the Respiratory System 91

Chapter 11   Diseases of the Digestive System 103

Chapter 12   Diseases of the Skin and Subcutaneous Tissue 117

Chapter 13   Diseases of the Musculoskeletal System and Connective Tissue 127

Chapter 14   Diseases of the Genitourinary System 137

Chapter 15   Pregnancy, Childbirth, and the Puerperium 147

Chapter 16   Certain Conditions Originating in the Perinatal Period 157

Chapter 17   Congenital Malformations, Deformations, and Chromosomal
              Abnormalities 165

Chapter 18   Symptoms, Signs, and Abnormal Clinical and Laboratory
              Findings, Not Elsewhere Classified 175

Chapter 19A   Injuries, Effects of Foreign Body, Burns and Corrosions, and Frostbite 183

Chapter 19B   Poisoning by, Adverse Effects, Underdosing, Toxic Effects
              of Substances, Other Effects of External Causes, Certain Early
              Complications of Trauma and Complications of Surgical
              and Medical Care 195

Chapter 20   External Causes of Morbidity. 205

Chapter 21   Factors Influencing Health Status and Contact with Health Services 211

Chapter 22   Advanced Coding Scenarios for *Basic ICD-10-CM
              and ICD-10-PCS Coding Exercises* 219

Answer Key. 239

About the Authors

Lou Ann Schraffenberger, MBA, RHIA, CCS, CCS-P, FAHIMA, is retired from Advocate Aurora Health as the manager of clinical data in their Center for Health Information Services based in Downers Grove, Illinois. Prior to her most recent position, Ms. Schraffenberger served as director of hospital health record departments, director of the Professional Practice Division of the American Health Information Management Association (AHIMA), and as a faculty member at the University of Illinois at Chicago and Moraine Valley Community College. Ms. Schraffenberger is an AHIMA-approved ICD-10-CM/PCS trainer. In 1997, Ms. Schraffenberger received the first AHIMA Volunteer Award, and in 2008 she received the AHIMA Legacy Award in recognition of her coding textbooks published by AHIMA. Ms. Schraffenberger graduated from the University of Illinois at the Medical Center with a bachelor's degree in health information management and received her MBA from the Loyola University Chicago's Chicago Quinlan School of Business.

Michelle Dionisio, MA, MSc, RHIA, CCS, is a coder at Atlantic Health System in New Jersey and an instructor in the Health Information Management program at the Rutgers University School of Health Professions, where she teaches courses on coding. She completed her postbaccalaureate studies in health information management at Rutgers and achieved her RHIA and CCS certifications. She also served as technical editor for the 2019 and 2020 updates of AHIMA's *Clinical Coding Workout* book.

Preface

Basic ICD-10-CM and ICD-10-PCS Coding Exercises, Seventh Edition, helps you develop the coding skills necessary to be an effective and efficient coding professional. This text can be used as a companion to AHIMA's *Basic ICD-10-CM and ICD-10-PCS Coding*, 2020, or as a stand-alone resource for coding practice. Each chapter offers exercises in the form of short case studies and operative descriptions of real-life patient encounters in healthcare. These exercises are designed to provide students and professionals with further ICD-10-CM and ICD-10-PCS coding practice opportunities.

The case studies provide students with the opportunity to code clinical information, rather than coding one- or two-line diagnostic and procedural statements. Whether the case study describes an inpatient hospital admission or an outpatient visit, the reader must determine the appropriate diagnoses and procedure codes to be assigned and in the appropriate sequence. For inpatient hospital admissions, the principal diagnosis should be listed first; for outpatient encounters, the main reason for the visit should be the first-listed diagnosis code. Students must decide what information to include as secondary diagnoses based on the clinical information presented and the coding guidelines.

Not every case study will require secondary diagnoses or a principal or first-listed diagnosis. Not every inpatient case study will require a procedure code(s). This is true in the real world as well; the coder must develop strong problem-solving coding skills to correctly decide what clinical information should be coded.

The exercises in *Basic ICD-10-CM and ICD-10-PCS Coding Exercises*, Seventh Edition, were coded with the FY 2020 release of ICD-10-CM diagnosis codes and the ICD-10-PCS procedure codes. The FY 2020 release of ICD-10-CM files and Official Guidelines for Coding and Reporting are available for access at https://www.cdc.gov/nchs/icd/icd10cm.htm. For the procedure codes, one can access the ICD-10-PCS 2020 files at https://www.cms.gov/Medicare/Coding/ICD10/2020-ICD-10-PCS.html. Every effort has been made to include the most current coding information.

Clinical Coding Workout: Practice Exercises for Skill Development, also published by AHIMA, is another excellent resource that provides beginning to advanced coding practice. The case studies in the book help new coders become adept at sorting through detail to prioritize and code diagnoses, skills that will be essential in their coding profession.

Acknowledgments

AHIMA Press and the authors would like to thank **Stacey Murphy, MPA, RHIA, CPC,** AHIMA-approved ICD-10-CM/PCS trainer, for her technical review of this edition.

Online Resources

For Instructors

Instructor materials for this book are provided only to approved educators. Materials include the **full answer key**. Please visit http://www.ahima.org/publications/educators.aspx for further instruction. If you have any questions regarding the instructor materials, please contact AHIMA Customer Relations at (800) 335-5535 or submit a customer support request at https://my.ahima.org/messages.

Chapter 1

Certain Infectious and Parasitic Diseases

Coding Scenarios for *Basic ICD-10-CM and ICD-10-PCS Coding Exercises*

The following case studies are organized following the sequence of the chapters in the ICD-10-CM Tabular List of Diseases and Injuries as published on the Centers for Disease Control and Prevention National Center for Health Statistics website (http://www.cdc.gov/nchs /icd/icd10cm.htm). The objective of this book is to provide the student with detailed clinical information to code, rather than one- or two-line diagnosis and procedure statements.

ICD-10-CM diagnosis codes are to be assigned to both the inpatient hospital admission and the outpatient visit case studies. In this book, the ICD-10-PCS procedure codes are to be assigned only to the inpatient hospital admission cases. In actual practice, outpatient cases are assigned CPT/HCPCS codes. The ICD-10-PCS codes are only required for inpatient procedures. In the answer key for the exercises, the Alphabetic Index entry is listed after the code to indicate the main terms and subterms used to locate the code that must be verified in the ICD-10-CM Tabular List or in the ICD-10-PCS Code Tables prior to assigning the code.

1

A 22-year-old female presented to the Family Practice Clinic after being told she should see her physician because her partner had recently been treated for nongonococcal urethritis. The woman did not have any complaints other than some vague pelvic discomfort and vaginal discharge that she did not consider serious. A physical examination, pelvic examination, and Papanicolaou test (Pap smear) were performed. Based on her history and physical findings, the patient was diagnosed with acute chlamydial cervicitis and given a prescription for two weeks of antibiotic oral medications and an appointment for a follow-up examination in three weeks.

First-Listed Diagnosis: _____

Secondary Diagnoses: _____

2

A male patient, known to have acquired immune deficiency syndrome (AIDS), was admitted with a fever, shortness of breath, and a dry cough. The symptoms had been increasing in severity over the past several days. A chest x-ray showed extensive pulmonary infiltrates. A sputum culture was obtained, and the diagnosis of pneumocystic pneumonia was made based on the microscopic examination. The patient was told that his pneumonia was a result of having AIDS. During his hospital stay, he developed oral candidiasis, which was treated along with the pneumonia using a combination of medications administered intravenously and orally. The patient was discharged with an appointment to the HIV outpatient clinic in 1 month.

Principal Diagnosis: _____

Secondary Diagnoses: _____

Principal Procedure: _____

Secondary Procedure(s): _____

3

A 38-year-old male with known chronic viral hepatitis resulting from hepatitis B is seen in the outpatient infectious disease clinic to be evaluated for therapy. The patient also has cirrhosis of the liver with suspected early stages of liver failure. His liver disease continues to be monitored. The patient is a known heroin addict in remission and has been taking methadone faithfully on a long-term basis through a program at this university medical center. All of these factors were considered when a combination of antiviral agent interferon-alpha plus lamivudine treatment was chosen and will be initiated at his next visit, scheduled in 1 week.

First-Listed Diagnosis: _____

Secondary Diagnoses: _____

4

An 85-year-old female who lived alone was found in her bed semiconscious during a visiting nurse well-being check. The nurse immediately called the rescue squad to transport the patient to the nearest emergency department (ED). The patient was able to tell the first-responders that she had been sick for a week with a fast heartbeat, fever, chills, and difficulty breathing. She had been in bed for three days and was unable to get out of bed to answer the phone or the door. When she was taken to the ED, her vital signs were markedly abnormal with a temperature of over 39 degrees Celsius, a heart rate of 100, and a respiratory rate of 22/min. She was admitted to the intensive care unit (ICU), with an admitting diagnosis of "sepsis" and was treated with antibiotics administered intravenously, stat. Within one day of admission, the infectious disease consulting physician described her condition as severe sepsis with resulting respiratory failure. Despite aggressive measures, after admission the patient required endotracheal intubation and mechanical ventilation for 36 hours to treat acute respiratory failure. The physicians sought to identify the underlying source of infection as well as to provide hemodynamic and respiratory support and were successful in avoiding septic shock in this patient. The patient's attending physician provided the diagnoses of severe gram-negative sepsis due to *Escherichia coli* (*E. coli*) with acute respiratory failure.

Principal Diagnosis: _____

Secondary Diagnoses: _____

Principal Procedure: _____

Secondary Procedure(s): _____

5

A 62-year-old female presents to her primary care physician's office complaining of an abrupt onset of a fiery-red swelling of her face. The physician's physical examination found that the swelling covered nearly all of the right side of the woman's face with well-demarcated raised borders. Her face was erythematous and edematous on the right side and the patient had a slightly elevated temperature. The patient stated her face felt hot but described feeling only mildly ill. An infectious disease physician's office was next door and he was asked to see this patient immediately, as her primary care physician had never seen this type of facial swelling and was concerned that her airway would eventually close. The infectious disease physician recognized the condition immediately as a superficial dermal and subcutaneous infection, usually caused by group A beta-hemolytic *Streptococcus*. He called the condition "acute erysipelas cellulitis" or "acute facial erysipelas" and advised immediate hospital admission for intravenous antibiotics. The patient was taken to the hospital by her family in a private vehicle because her primary care physician ordered a direct admission. After admission, it was determined that due to the severity of the acute facial erysipelas, the patient would require long-term IV antibiotic treatment and a centrally inserted venous catheter was inserted through the left subclavian vein. Imaging indicated that the catheter tip was located in the superior vena cava. After two days of initial antibiotic treatment, improvement was seen, and the patient was discharged home to continue IV antibiotic therapy as an outpatient.

Principal Diagnosis: _____

Secondary Diagnoses: _____

Principal Procedure: _____

Secondary Procedure(s): _____

6

An 18-year-old female, who attends a state university about 90 miles away from home, is brought to her family physician's office after her parents brought her home because of a mumps epidemic at the university. During the office visit, the patient complained of fever, malaise, myalgia, and anorexia. She also had an earache and, due to the swelling of her jaw, reported that it was difficult to chew and swallow. A physical examination found the classic findings of mumps. Both sides of the woman's face were swollen consistent with bilateral infectious parotitis. Given her recent exposure to other students diagnosed with mumps, the family physician concluded that the patient had mumps and diagnosed her with bilateral infectious parotitis, but could not find evidence of any complications in other body systems. The patient was sent home and was advised to avoid contact with people outside her family. The treatment included analgesics and warm compresses to the parotid area to relieve swelling and reduce symptoms. No medications are known to be effective in treating this viral infection.

First-Listed Diagnosis: _____

Secondary Diagnoses: _____

7

A 21-year-old male student came to the college health service center at this state university with complaints of urethral discharge, frequent urination, blood in the urine, and a stinging sensation during urination. The man, who admitted to several sexual partners, stated his symptoms had become obvious in the past week. A physical examination confirmed the presence of a urethral discharge and swollen glands in the groin region. A urinalysis and urine culture were ordered. The patient noted that his symptoms were similar to a previous episode when he was told he had an acute gonococcal infection. An oral antibiotic was prescribed, and the patient was advised to stop all sexual activity until the treatment was completed and inform his sexual partners of his diagnosis so that they could be tested and treated as necessary. The patient was given an appointment to return in 14 days. The college health service physician wrote acute gonococcal urethritis and acute gonococcal cystitis on the outpatient encounter form.

First-Listed Diagnosis: _____

Secondary Diagnoses: _____

8

A 65-year-old semi-retired nurse came to her primary care physician's office with the following complaints: coughing, chest pain, shortness of breath, fatigue, fever, sweating at night, and a poor appetite. She recently returned from volunteering at a clinic in Southeast Asia where there were many patients diagnosed with pulmonary tuberculosis. The patient previously had tuberculin skin tests that were negative. The physician ordered a chest x-ray, and a tuberculin skin test was administered. Sputum was obtained and submitted for culture. The physician made the diagnosis of pulmonary tuberculosis based on the patient's symptoms and recent exposure to the disease. The patient was given a prescription for an oral medication, isoniazid, which would probably be required for six months to one year. The patient is also known to have essential hypertension and is one-year status post percutaneous coronary angioplasty for coronary artery disease. Her cardiovascular status was also assessed and prescriptions were renewed. A follow-up visit in two weeks was scheduled.

First-Listed Diagnosis: _____

Secondary Diagnoses: _____

9

A 70-year-old female patient was referred to the neurologist's office by her primary care physician because of a new onset of weakness, fatigue, and pain in her left leg. This leg had been affected by acute poliomyelitis (polio), which she had 60 years ago. She had atrophy of the muscles of the left leg since having polio as a child. She walks with a limp because of the weakened, slightly shortened leg. On this occasion, following examination, the neurologist concluded that her symptoms reflect postpolio syndrome, which includes a progressive dysfunction and loss of motor neurons that had been compensating for the neurons lost during the original infection. The patient did not have a new onset of the polio infection. The consultant's diagnosis was progressive atrophy of the leg muscles due to postpolio syndrome.

First-Listed Diagnosis: _____

Secondary Diagnoses: _____

10

A 9-year-old boy was brought to the emergency department (ED) by his father, who stated that the child had an acute onset of fever, chills, headache, neck stiffness, photophobia, and pain in his eyes. He also had some nausea and vomiting. Upon physical examination, the ED physician found meningismus—a constellation of signs and symptoms—suggestive of meningitis. The child was admitted to an isolation room in the pediatric intensive care unit, and a spinal tap was performed by inserting a needle percutaneously into the spinal canal in order to obtain spinal fluid. The examination of the cerebral spinal fluid and results of other tests led the attending physician to conclude the patient had coxsackie-virus meningitis. Because this is a viral illness, medical treatments are limited and are directed at relieving symptoms. The patient had an uncomplicated recovery and was discharged home for continued rest.

Principal Diagnosis: _____

Secondary Diagnoses: _____

Principal Procedure: _____

Secondary Procedure(s): _____

11

The patient is a 67-year-old female admitted to the hospital from the emergency department. She reported that she had nausea and vomiting and a fever for the last two days. She had been eating poorly for at least three days and within the last 12 hours started having chills, racing heart, and shortness of breath. She noticed a strong odor and dark color in her urine. The complete blood count (CBC) on admission had a result of 24,000 white cells with a shift to the left. Other laboratory tests confirmed an electrolyte imbalance, with hyponatremia and hypokalemia. The urinalysis showed too many white blood cells to count and many bacteria present. She was admitted for intravenous antibiotics and rehydration fluids to correct the electrolyte imbalance. The patient had been undergoing chemotherapy for recently diagnosed metastatic carcinoma in her axillary lymph nodes. The patient had primary breast cancer diagnosed and treated five years ago with surgery and chemotherapy. Her diagnosis on admission was acute sepsis with a suspected urinary tract infection as the cause. A urine culture and two blood cultures were positive for Klebsiella pneumoniae, a Gram-negative organism. After the initiation of the IV fluids and antibiotics, the patient improved and was able to eat more and ambulate. She had no vomiting or diarrhea. The repeat urinalysis and blood counts showed values that were approaching a normal range. The oncologist examined the patient in the hospital and determined her next chemotherapy session would be delayed by two weeks to allow the patient to recover from this infection and regain her strength. Both the attending physician and the oncologist agreed that the patient's final diagnosis was sepsis due to underlying urinary tract infection, both due to Klebsiella pneumoniae Gram-negative organism infection, hyponatremia, hypokalemia, and history of primary breast cancer with metastatic disease in the axillary lymph nodes. The patient was discharged home with home care nurses to visit the next day.

Principal Diagnosis: _____

Secondary Diagnoses _____

Principal Procedure: _____

Secondary Procedure(s): _____

12

The mother of a 3-year-old female brought the child to the emergency department (ED) because of fast breathing, a fast heartbeat, and a generalized erythematous rash. The mother stated the child had been refusing food and drink and had not urinated much during the past 12 hours. The ED physician found the child, clinging to her mother, to be dehydrated, febrile, and lethargic. The child was started on IV fluid for rehydration and respiratory treatments of albuterol to improve her respiratory rate. Multiple chicken pox lesions were noted over the child's face, trunk, and legs, but the majority were crusted and nonvesiculating. The mother reported that her 6-year-old son had chicken pox recently. The physician also noted the child's abdomen to be distended. Examination of the ears showed a right otitis media with the left ear tympanic membrane normal. The chest exam demonstrated expiratory and inspiratory rhonchi with expiratory wheezes at the bases that were consistent with pneumonia. The child was placed into the pediatric observation unit. Over the next 12 hours the patient's symptoms improved after treatment. Amoxicillin medication was started for the ears. The child became more alert, smiling, and happy, but still clinging to her mother. The mother was allowed to take the child home the next day with pediatric home care follow-up ordered. Discharge instructions included bed rest and continuation of albuterol suspension and amoxicillin. Discharge diagnoses were chicken pox complicated by pneumonia, dehydration, and acute nonsuppurative right otitis media.

First-Listed Diagnosis: _____

Secondary Diagnoses: _____

13

A 21-year-old male made an appointment with his optometrist because he thought he had a problem with his new contact lenses. The patient complained of increasingly severe eye pain. When the optometrist questioned the patient on how he took care of his contacts, the patient described rinsing the lens in tap water at work (a sports and exercise facility) during the day and not always using the contact solution prescribed to store the lenses at night, again using tap water. The optometrist examined the patient and documented the patient had a mild to moderately severe case of acanthamoeba keratoconjunctivitis. The patient was told to throw out his current contacts, wear his eyeglasses until his next physician's appointment in one week, use only contact solution for rinsing and storage, and take nonsteroidal anti-inflammatory drugs to ease the eye pain.

First-Listed Diagnosis: _____

Secondary Diagnoses: _____

14

The patient is a 40-year-old female who is being seen today in the Transplant Clinic of the University Medical Center as part of her evaluation for a possible liver transplant. The patient is known to have chronic hepatitis C and autoimmune hepatitis. Her autoimmune hepatitis was diagnosed recently by antibody tests and a liver biopsy. The patient's symptoms from her disease have been significant, including fatigue, aching joints, jaundice, enlarged liver, and recurrent ascites. The patient's father and brother have died from "liver failure," and this patient's physician suspects there is a genetic factor in the family that leads to autoimmune hepatitis, in which the patient's liver is attacked by the patient's immune system. The patient is on the liver transplant list and waiting for an orthotopic transplant to occur. The patient or her husband carries her transplant beeper at all times. The patient's diagnosis listed on the encounter form for this visit is (1) chronic hepatitis C and (2) autoimmune hepatitis.

First-Listed Diagnosis: _____

Secondary Diagnoses: _____

15

On Monday evening, the parents of a 15-year-old female brought her to the emergency department (ED) complaining of abdominal cramps, headache, muscle aches, chills, diarrhea, nausea, and vomiting for the past 12 hours. The family had been at a family picnic on Sunday with food served throughout the day, and the weather was hot. The teenager ate mostly raw foods and salads at the event. Today, the mother learned that other members of her extended family had similar symptoms, but her daughter appeared to be the most acutely ill. The patient was very lethargic and continued to have diarrhea and vomiting in the ED after she arrived. Immediate laboratory testing found her to be dehydrated, and intravenous fluids were promptly started. Based on her symptoms and history, the physician concluded the patient had acute gastroenteritis caused by salmonella food poisoning, complicated by severe dehydration. The patient remained in the ED for 6 hours and then was discharged to her parents' care.

First-Listed Diagnosis: _____

Secondary Diagnoses: _____

16

The patient is seen in the office of an infectious disease specialist who treated her 1 year previously when she had Lyme disease. She complains of generalized joint pain and stiffness. Based on laboratory test results and physical examination, the physician concludes that the patient no longer has active Lyme disease. However, he concludes that her arthritis of multiple joints is the residual effect of the cured Lyme disease.

First-Listed Diagnosis: _____

Secondary Diagnoses: _____

17

A 2-year-old female was brought to the emergency department (ED) by her mother, who stated the child had a cold, runny nose, congestion, and a mild fever. The patient then developed a dry, hacking cough that progressed to prolonged coughing spasms. Overnight, the child became very ill. Upon physical examination, the ED physician noted a high fever and stiffness in the neck, and the child was very difficult to rouse. The mother reported the child had vomited at home. The child was admitted to the pediatric service. Infectious disease and pulmonary medicine specialists consulted with the attending pediatrician to make the diagnosis of whooping cough due to *Bordetella pertussis* with complicating pneumonia. The child was treated with intravenous antibiotics. The girl recovered from the bacterial illness and was discharged to the care of her mother with home health agency nursing follow-up.

Principal Diagnosis: _____

Secondary Diagnoses: _____

Principal Procedure: _____

Secondary Procedure(s): _____

18

The mother of a 3-year-old male brought him to the emergency department stating he developed vomiting followed by diarrhea and became very lethargic. Physical findings revealed a tired young child with a fever, increased bowel sounds, sunken eyes, dried lips, and dry mucous membranes. Laboratory findings included an abnormal electrolyte panel and an elevated white blood count with a left shift. He was admitted to the hospital and administered IV fluids with potassium added to correct the dehydration. It was determined the child had gastroenteritis caused by a rotavirus when another lab finding revealed a positive rotavirus antigen. After two days in the pediatric unit, the child was discharged having recovered from the gastroenteritis due to rotavirus and the resulting dehydration. The mother will bring the child to the pediatrician for a follow-up visit in one week.

Principal Diagnosis: _____

Secondary Diagnoses: _____

Principal Procedure: _____

Secondary Procedure(s): _____

19

A 45-year-old male presented to the emergency department (ED)complaining of fever and constant pain in his anal area. The ED physician examined the patient and immediately visualized a fluctuant, tender mass in the anal canal just past the anal orifice. The patient was also found to have a high fever with hypotension and tachycardia. The ED physician diagnosed the patient with sepsis and a perianal abscess. The patient was started on intravenous fluids and antibiotics and was taken to the operating room for incision and drainage of the abscess. In the operating room, the surgeon made an incision in the mucosa of the anal canal overlying the tender mass and purulent drainage immediately resulted from the incised abscess cavity. Cultures were obtained, which later came back positive for *B. fragilis*, an anaerobic Gram-negative bacterium. The abscess cavity was irrigated with sterile saline and left open to drain and heal. The patient was kept in the hospital for several days for continued administration of antibiotics and fluids and monitoring of his condition. At discharge, his diagnosis was *B. fragilis* sepsis due to perianal abscess.

Principal Diagnosis: _____

Secondary Diagnoses: _____

Principal Procedure: _____

Secondary Procedure(s): _____

Chapter 2

Neoplasms

Coding Scenarios for *Basic ICD-10-CM* *and ICD-10-PCS Coding Exercises*

The following case studies are organized following the sequence of the chapters in the ICD-10-CM Tabular List of Diseases and Injuries as published on the Centers for Disease Control and Prevention National Center for Health Statistics website (http://www.cdc .gov/nchs/icd/icd10cm.htm). The objective of this book is to provide the student with detailed clinical information to code, rather than one- or two-line diagnosis and procedure statements.

ICD-10-CM diagnosis codes are to be assigned to both the inpatient hospital admission and the outpatient visit case studies. In this book, the ICD-10-PCS procedure codes are to be assigned only to the inpatient hospital admission cases. In actual practice, outpatient cases are assigned CPT/HCPCS codes. The ICD-10-PCS codes are only required for inpatient procedures. In the answer key for the exercises, the Alphabetic Index entry is listed after the code to indicate the main terms and subterms used to locate the code that must be verified in the ICD-10-CM Tabular List or in the ICD-10-PCS Code Tables prior to assigning the code.

1

A 63-year-old male patient, known to have emphysema, was advised by this physician to be admitted to the hospital to evaluate and treat his worsening lung condition. The patient quit smoking cigars five years ago after he was told he had emphysema. The patient complained his coughing and wheezing had become worse, and his sputum was streaked with blood. A chest x-ray done on an outpatient basis the previous week showed a mass in the right main bronchus. After admission, a fiber optic bronchoscopy and excisional biopsy of the right main bronchial mass was performed. The pathologic diagnosis of the biopsy examination was small cell type bronchogenic carcinoma located in the right main bronchus. A nuclear medicine bone scan found areas of suspicious lesions that were determined to be bone metastasis. The diagnoses provided by the physician at discharge were bronchogenic, small cell carcinoma of the right main bronchus with metastatic disease in the bones, emphysema, and former nicotine dependence.

Principal Diagnosis: _____

Secondary Diagnoses: _____

Principal Procedure: _____

Secondary Procedure(s): _____

2

A 72-year-old male with a diagnosis of acute myeloid leukemia, M7, is admitted for the first scheduled chemotherapy infusion, which will last several days. The patient is administered chemotherapy intravenously the central venous catheter that had been placed during a previous hospital stay.

Principal Diagnosis: _____

Secondary Diagnoses: _____

Principal Procedure: _____

Secondary Procedure(s): _____

3

A patient with terminal carcinoma of the sigmoid colon with metastases to the liver was admitted to the hospital with hypotonic dehydration. The patient's dehydration was deemed by the attending physician to be due to the malignancy. The dehydration was the focus of the treatment with intravenous therapy, but the patient was also treated for hyponatremia and the patient felt relief from his symptoms. Chemotherapy had been recently discontinued after discussions with the patient about its ineffectiveness in curing his disease and how sick the treatment made the patient feel. During the hospital stay, the patient and his family agreed to palliative care only, which was ordered along with an order to "do not resuscitate" (DNR). The patient was discharged to home to consider electing hospice services.

Principal Diagnosis: _____

Secondary Diagnoses: _____

Principal Procedures: _____

Secondary Procedure(s): _____

4

A 98-year-old male was brought to his primary care physician by his family for his regular check-up. The man, who was very alert and oriented for his age, stated that he was feeling increasingly tired with each day, causing him to sleep 10 to 12 hours a day. He also stated he had a loss his appetite and felt slightly nauseated all the time. His physician, concerned by these symptoms present in a patient of advanced age, advised admission. The patient was admitted for probable dehydration, which was later confirmed by examination and laboratory findings. Intravenous hydration was started. Other laboratory tests showed evidence of chronic kidney disease (CKD) stage 4 and hypertension. Further workup revealed a mass at the head of the pancreas. The patient began to experience neoplasm-related pain and was administered low doses of morphine. The patient, having lived a long life, refused surgery, chemotherapy, and all other treatments, preferring to return home to die in peace. The patient and his family consented to hospice care at home and the patient was discharged. The physician's final diagnoses included the statement "probable carcinoma of the pancreatic head, hypertensive CKD stage 4, with neoplasm-related dehydration and pain."

Principal Diagnosis: _____

Secondary Diagnoses: _____

Principal Procedure: _____

Secondary Procedure(s): _____

5

A 39-year-old female with known cervical dysplasia had been seen in the outpatient surgery department the previous week for a colposcopy and biopsy. Pathologic exam of the biopsied tissue was inconclusive but suggested the possibility of a malignancy in the cervix. Before the patient could return to the outpatient surgery department for definitive treatment, she began bleeding heavily and was admitted to the hospital. A conization of the cervix was performed by loop electrosurgical excision (LEEP) using a colposcope for guidance in order to destroy the site of the possible malignancy. A portion of the cervix was submitted for histopathologic examination with the findings returned as carcinoma of the uterine cervix. The patient will follow up in the office.

Principal Diagnosis: _____

Secondary Diagnoses: _____

Principal Procedure: _____

Secondary Procedure(s): _____

6

This is a 56-year-old female who has biopsy-proven malignant melanoma of the left upper arm on the shoulder. The pathology diagnosis was superficial spreading malignant melanoma. The patient is brought to the hospital outpatient department for excision of the 2.5×1.5 cm lesion. She will be seen in the office in 14 days for suture removal and a discussion on what further treatment might be indicated.

First-Listed Diagnosis: _____

Secondary Diagnoses: _____

7.

This is a 46-year-old female who had biopsy-proven malignant melanoma and excision of the skin lesion on her forehead. Since the last visit, the patient learned that her brother and possibly her father (who is now deceased) had lesions and moles removed that were skin cancer and, in her father's case, probably a melanoma. All three people shared the same history of growing up in a southern state with year-round extensive sun-related radiation exposure. The patient, her brother, and her father enjoyed fishing at the beach and rarely applied sunscreen lotion. On this occasion, she is brought back to the hospital outpatient department for a "wide excision" of the same location on her forehead where the lesion had previously been removed, 4 × 3 cm in area, at the site of the original excision. Because the affected area was her forehead, the patient asked for a plastic repair of the site. The surgeon agreed and documented that the plastic repair, which required the insertion of synthetic substitute, was not done for cosmetic reasons but done to avoid future possible painful scarring. The reason for the second excision was stated as "further excision as margins of initial excision showed evidence of remaining malignancy." The physician said this procedure was to "finish" the original excision to make certain the "margins are clean" and no malignant tissue remains. The pathology report states: "Normal tissues, margin clean, no evidence of remaining malignant melanoma." The patient will be seen in the office for suture removal, and further treatment options are to be discussed.

First-Listed Diagnosis: _____

Secondary Diagnoses: _____

8

A 57-year-old male patient was admitted to the hospital with the known diagnosis of right ureteral obstruction caused by secondary neoplasm of the ureter. Known to have a primary malignancy of the stomach (body) that was surgically resected six months earlier, the patient was still receiving chemotherapy for the gastric malignancy. Outpatient testing showed evidence of minor ascites and right ureteral metastasis causing obstruction, resulting in right hydronephrosis. The patient was admitted for treatment of the hydronephrosis. The patient was taken to the radiation department where an interventional radiologist percutaneously inserted a nephrostomy tube directly into the right kidney for drainage. A percutaneous paracentesis was also performed for diagnostic purposes. Cytology examination of the peritoneal fluid showed evidence of peritoneal metastasis and malignant ascites. The patient did not want further aggressive therapy and was discharged home to consider using hospice services.

Principal Diagnosis: _____

Secondary Diagnoses: _____

Principal Procedure: _____

Secondary Procedure(s): _____

9

The patient is a 53-year-old female with left breast cancer, metastatic to the bone and brain, all diagnosed in the past six months with continued management. The patient is seen in the hospital's outpatient oncology clinic for her next cycle of intravenous infusion, through a peripheral vein, of Aredia (pamidronate disodium), a chemotherapy drug used as palliative treatment for bone metastases.

First-Listed Diagnosis: _____

Secondary Diagnoses: _____

10

A 73-year-old male was seen in his physician's office with a variety of gastrointestinal complaints, including vague abdominal pain, diarrhea, urinary frequency, and flushing across his face, neck, and chest. Laboratory and radiology tests were inconclusive, but based on his continuing symptoms the physician suspected the patient might have a chronic form of appendicitis. Because of the uncertainty of the etiology of patient's symptomatology and his advanced age, an inpatient laparoscopic appendectomy was scheduled and performed. The entire appendix was excised. The final pathology report confirmed the frozen section diagnosis of malignant carcinoid tumor of the appendix. The surgeon was informed of this diagnosis, agreed with the pathologist, and documented malignant carcinoid tumor of the appendix as the final diagnosis. Additional testing performed during the inpatient encounter determined that the patient was experiencing a "carcinoid syndrome" because of this tumor, which explained many of his vague symptoms, including the flushing. The appendectomy is considered curative treatment for the appendiceal tumor. Upon discharge, the patient will be seen in the oncologist's office for further recommendations, especially to treat the carcinoid syndrome.

Principal Diagnosis: _____

Secondary Diagnoses: _____

Principal Procedure: _____

Secondary Procedure(s): _____

11

The patient is a 59-year-old female who is admitted to the hospital after complaining of weakness and for her next cycle of chemotherapy. She has a primary malignancy of the transverse colon. On admission, blood work performed indicated severe anemia. The oncologist documented that the anemia was associated with malignancy. Chemotherapy was cancelled. The patient received a transfusion via a peripheral vein of (nonautologous) packed red blood cells and was discharged.

Principal Diagnosis: _____

Secondary Diagnoses: _____

Principal Procedure: _____

Secondary Procedure(s): _____

12

The patient is a 28-year-old male who was recently diagnosed with a seminoma and underwent an orchiectomy of his left testicle, which was normally descended. He has had several courses of retroperitoneal radiation therapy. Outpatient bloodwork scheduled before his next radiation therapy session indicated severe anemia. He was admitted for transfusion of nonautologous whole blood via a peripheral vein. Final diagnosis was stage I seminoma being treated with retroperitoneal radiation therapy, aplastic anemia due to adverse effect of radiotherapy.

Principal Diagnosis: _____

Secondary Diagnoses: _____

Principal Procedure: _____

Secondary Procedure(s): _____

13

The patient is a 49-year-old automotive mechanic who was working on his vehicle at his home over the weekend when he developed what he called the "mother of all headaches" or the worst headache of his life. He had nausea but no vomiting. He later noticed visual disturbances and dizziness. Thinking the headache would go away, he went to bed but was unable to sleep all night because of the intensity of the headache pain, which was not relieved by Tylenol. He also felt some vague discomfort in his chest. He called his physician the next morning and was advised to go to the emergency department and was subsequently admitted. CT of the thorax and MRI scans of the head were performed. The MRI found a three ring-enhancing lesion located in the parietal lobe of the brain associated with a large amount of edema extending into the occipital and temporal regions. The CT of the thorax found pulmonary lesions that seem to be cavitating in the right lung. The patient has been smoking cigarettes for the past 30 years. The patient consented to and underwent two procedures: (1) closed biopsy of the parietal lobe of the brain through a burr hole approach and (2) bronchoscopic right lung biopsy. Based on the pathologic findings, the physician concluded the patient had a giant cell glioblastoma multiform of the parietal region with metastases to the lung. In addition to these diagnoses, the physician gave other final diagnoses of pre-diabetes and nicotine dependence. Upon questioning the patient more, the patient admitted he had had headaches for several months but none as bad as the one this time that prompted him to go to the physician. The patient was discharged home as he wished to seek a second opinion at a major university medical center. Copies of his records and radiology films in CD format were given to the patient for this purpose.

Note: Many facilities, inpatient coders are not required to assign codes for CTs or MRIs. These procedures are "hard coded" during the charge entry process using the chargemaster.

Principal Diagnosis: _____

Secondary Diagnoses: _____

Principal Procedure: _____

Secondary Procedure(s): _____

14

The patient is a 69-year-old gravida 3, para 2, AB 1, female whose last menstrual period was 15 years ago. She originally came to the gynecologist's office complaining of postmenopausal bleeding. As an outpatient, she had an endometrial biopsy that revealed poorly differentiated adenocarcinoma with clear-cell features of the endometrium. Today the patient was admitted to the hospital for an open total abdominal hysterectomy and related surgery as deemed necessary by the surgeon during the hysterectomy. Her medical history includes ongoing treatment for hypertension, anxiety disorder, postsurgical hypothyroidism with a history of thyroid cancer, and type 2 diabetes mellitus. The surgery performed was a total abdominal hysterectomy, including the uterus and cervix. The patient failed to mention that her fallopian tubes and ovaries had been removed in the past as a fail-safe method of birth control. There was no evidence of metastasis into other pelvic organs. A consultation with an oncologist was performed prior to discharge. The patient had an uneventful recovery from the surgery and was discharged on day three to follow up with her gynecologist and oncologist in the next two weeks.

Principal Diagnosis: _____

Secondary Diagnoses: _____

Principal Procedure: _____

Secondary Procedure(s): _____

15

The patient is a 37-year-old female who was diagnosed with breast cancer two years ago and had a partial mastectomy of her left breast. Her estrogen receptor status is positive. Her chemotherapy and radiation therapy treatments ended six months ago. She has had follow-up CT imaging, and there is no evidence of residual disease. The patient is in the physician's office today to receive her third intravenous infusion of Herceptin (trastuzumab), which she will continue to receive on a weekly schedule for the next five years if she can tolerate it and there are no side effects. The physician reminds the patient that the drug is not an antineoplastic chemotherapy drug. It is an antineoplastic monoclonal antibody drug that attaches itself to cancer cells and signals the body's immune system to destroy them. It is antineoplastic in the sense that the drug decreases the risk of the cancer recurring in a patient like her with estrogen receptor positive status breast cancer. The drug is considered long-term therapy for consolidative treatment of her breast cancer.

First-Listed Diagnosis: _____

Secondary Diagnoses: _____

16

A 59-year-old female was admitted to the hospital for a scheduled open total abdominal hysterectomy (TAH) with a bilateral salpingo-oophorectomy (BSO). The patient also had type 2 diabetes that was well controlled by insulin. The patient first visited her gynecologist several months ago complaining of postmenopausal vaginal bleeding and abnormal vaginal discharge. An endometrial biopsy was taken in the office and was suggestive of uterine cancer. The TAH-BSO was performed, and the following postoperative diagnoses were recorded by the physician: Stage I endometrial adenocarcinoma (corpus uteri) and bilateral corpus luteum cysts of the ovaries, worse on the right side, fallopian tubes appeared normal. The patient continued to receive insulin while in the hospital.

Principal Diagnosis: _____

Secondary Diagnoses: _____

Principal Procedure: _____

Secondary Procedure(s): _____

17

HISTORY: A 55-year-old female presented to the office with a right breast mass, approximately 2.0 cm × 2.0 cm, in the upper inner quadrant. There was no lymphadenopathy. She has a significant family history of breast cancer being diagnosed in her mother, maternal aunt, and older sister. Three days ago, a fine needle aspiration procedure demonstrated cells suspicious for malignancy. She was admitted to the hospital for definitive surgical treatment with a right breast lumpectomy.

OPERATIVE FINDINGS: A hard 2.0 × 2.0 cm mass in the upper inner quadrant of the right breast with no lymphadenopathy was confirmed. Pathology reports the specimen to be confirmed as carcinoma. The surgical margins on the mass excised were found to be normal. It is felt the entire lesion was removed.

DESCRIPTION OF PROCEDURE: After preoperative counseling, the patient was taken to the operating room and placed in a supine position on the table. The chest, right breast, and shoulder were prepped with Betadine scrub and paint and draped in the usual sterile fashion. The skin around the mass was anesthetized with 1% lidocaine solution. An elliptical incision was made, leaving a 1.5-cm margin around the mass in a circumferential fashion. The mass was sharply excised down to the pectoralis fascia, which was excised and sent with the specimen of the breast. The deep medial aspect of the specimen was marked with a long suture and the deep inferior margin marked with a short suture. The wound was left open until the pathologist reported that the margins were negative under frozen section. The wound was copiously irrigated. Hemostasis was achieved with Bovie cauterization and 3-0 Vicryl suture ligatures. The skin was closed with a running subcuticular 4-0 Vicryl, Benzoin, and steri-strips. A sterile dressing was applied. The patient was subsequently transferred to the recovery room in stable condition. She tolerated the procedure well and will be advised of the procedural findings when she is returned to her room.

Principal Diagnosis: _____

Secondary Diagnoses: _____

Principal Procedure: _____

Secondary Procedure(s): _____

18

HISTORY: The patient is a 62-year-old female who was admitted to the hospital for scheduled surgery to treat her recently diagnosed carcinoma of the rectosigmoid colon. She had noticed a change in her bowel habits about six to seven months ago but did not seek medical care until two weeks ago when she went to her primary care physician. The patient was immediately scheduled for an outpatient colonoscopy, and a 10-cm tumor was found and biopsied, with carcinoma diagnosed. She has a long history of angina and had a percutaneous transluminal coronary angioplasty (PTCA) twice in the past 4 years, with two non-drug-eluting stents in the right coronary artery. She also has a history of tobacco use, but she is no longer smoking. She was cleared for surgery by her cardiologist with the diagnoses of coronary artery disease with stable angina and hypercholesterolemia that continued to be managed with her usual medications while she was in the hospital. The patient was discharged home with home health services following an uneventful postoperative recovery. She has an appointment with her oncologist in two weeks to discuss the next treatment options.

OPERATIVE FINDINGS: During an anterior resection of the rectosigmoid colon, the patient was found to have a tumor that extended into the muscular wall but not through the muscular wall of the rectosigmoid colon. No tumor was found outside the rectosigmoid intestine. The pathologist identified the tumor as a primary infiltrating papillary adenocarcinoma of the colon, rectosigmoid junction that extended focally into the outer muscular wall with no evidence of metastasis to pericolonic lymph nodes. The tumor staging was T2 N0 M0. The colon specimen was a sessile round lesion about 12 cm in length with the tumor measuring 3 cm × 2.5 cm. The tumor was elevated about 0.8 cm above the surrounding mucosal surface.

DESCRIPTION OF PROCEDURE: The patient consented to an anterior resection of the rectosigmoid colon. Under endotracheal anesthesia, the abdomen was prepped and draped in the usual surgical manner. It was opened through a lower abdominal midline incision extending to the left of the umbilicus using a hot knife. Exploration of the abdominal cavity revealed a normal-feeling-and-appearing stomach, liver, gallbladder, and large and small bowels. The aorta and iliac vessels had some atheromatous plaque. Both kidneys appeared and felt normal. The Bookwalter retractor was used. The rectosigmoid colon was freed from its attachment in the pelvis on the right and left side by sharp dissection. The ureters were both identified and avoided. The blood supply of the rectosigmoid area was serially clamped, divided, and tied with 2-3 Ethibond sutures. The tumor was palpated just below the peritoneal reflection. The colon was freed below the peritoneal reflection. Again, the blood supply was serially clamped, divided, and tied with 2-0 Ethibond sutures. Proximally, a portion of the rectosigmoid colon mesentery was serially clamped, divided, and tied as well. Satinsky clamps were placed proximally and distally, and the colon and specimen were removed. An end-to-end anastomosis was performed in a single layer with interrupted 3-0 silks. The wound was inspected for bleeding, and it was dry. A temporary post-operative Penrose drain was placed down near the anastomosis from the stab wound in the left lower quadrant. The first sponge and needle count was correct. The peritoneum was closed with continuous 2-0 Vicryl, fascia with interrupted 2-0 Ethibond, subcutaneous with Vicryl, and the skin with skin clips. The drain was sutured in place. All sponge and needle counts were correct. The patient tolerated the procedure well and left the operating room in satisfactory condition.

Principal Diagnosis: _____

Secondary Diagnoses: _____

Principal Procedure: _____

Secondary Procedure(s): _____

19

The patient is a 68-year-old male who was admitted to the hospital for a transurethral fulguration of a bladder tumor and a bladder biopsy. Two months ago the patient was diagnosed with papillary transitional cell carcinoma in situ of the anterior wall of the bladder. The patient was also taking medications for well-managed type 2 diabetes mellitus and hypertension that were continued in the hospital. On the day of admission, the patient was taken to the endoscopy suite and underwent a transurethral endoscopic fulguration of a bladder tumor on the anterior wall of the bladder and a transurethral endoscopic biopsy by excision of another small lesion on the lateral wall of the bladder. There were no postoperative complications. On the morning of the next day the patient was voiding clear urine and intravenous fluids were discontinued. The patient was discharged later that day with several prescriptions, including a postsurgical antibiotic as well as his regular medications for his diabetes and hypertension. The final pathology report of the resected tissue and the biopsy showed papillary transitional cell carcinoma in situ of the anterior and lateral walls of bladder that was acknowledged by the surgeon in the medical record. A follow-up visit was scheduled in the urologist's office one week after discharge.

Principal Diagnosis: _____

Secondary Diagnoses: _____

Principal Procedure: _____

Secondary Procedure(s): _____

20

The patient is a 78-year-old male who was diagnosed with carcinoma of the right upper lobe one year ago. He was recently hospitalized with massive pleural effusions that were attempted to be treated and found to be the result of metastatic carcinoma of the pleura. Further studies proved the existence of metastatic liver carcinoma as well. The patient is also known to have severe COPD that has been treated for 10 years. The patient is a former cigarette smoker who quit smoking at the time he was diagnosed with lung cancer. The reason for the visit in his oncologist's office today was to discuss advance care planning. The physician recently told the patient there were no options to cure him of his lung cancer and the metastatic disease. The patient, his wife, and son discussed his options for palliative care or hospice care with the physician. The patient and the physician completed the necessary advance directive documents to identify his wishes for care in the future.

Principal Diagnosis: _____

Secondary Diagnoses: _____

21

A 58-year-old patient with an established diagnosis of cancer of the left pelvic sidewall was admitted for excision of the left pelvic sidewall tumor and insertion of the CivaSheet® brachytherapy device. In the operating room the surgeon excised the tumor via a wide lower abdominal incision. After the tumor had been completely removed from the left pelvic sidewall, the surgeon placed the CivaSheet® brachytherapy device onto the tumor excision site. CivaSheet® is a low dose rate brachytherapy device containing embedded radioactive palladium-103 that is shielded on one side so that the radiation is emitted in only one direction (unidirectionally). Once the device is inserted, it begins delivering brachytherapy immediately. The patient tolerated the procedure well and proceeded to the recovery room in stable condition.

(Coding tip: According to Coding Clinic First Quarter 2019, page 27, pelvic sidewall should be coded using the Body Part *retroperitoneum*.)

Principal Diagnosis: _____

Secondary Diagnoses: _____

Principal Procedure: _____

Secondary Procedure(s):   _____

Chapter 3

Diseases of Blood and Blood-forming Organs and Certain Disorders Involving the Immune Mechanism

Coding Scenarios for *Basic ICD-10-CM and ICD-10-PCS Coding Exercises*

The following case studies are organized following the sequence of the chapters in the ICD-10-CM Tabular List of Diseases and Injuries as published on the Centers for Disease Control and Prevention National Center for Health Statistics website (http://www.cdc.gov/nchs/icd/icd10cm.htm). The objective of this book is to provide the student with detailed clinical information to code, rather than one- or two-line diagnosis and procedure statements.

ICD-10-CM diagnosis codes are to be assigned to both the inpatient hospital admission and the outpatient visit case studies. In this book, the ICD-10-PCS procedure codes are to be assigned only to the inpatient hospital admission cases. In actual practice, outpatient cases are assigned CPT/HCPCS codes. The ICD-10-PCS codes are only required for inpatient procedures. In the answer key for the exercises, the Alphabetic Index entry is listed after the code to indicate the main terms and subterms used to locate the code that must be verified in the ICD-10-CM Tabular List or in the ICD-10-PCS Code Tables prior to assigning the code.

1

A 20-year-old African-American male is admitted to the hospital from the emergency department with acute vaso-occlusive pain and pulmonary symptoms including shortness of breath, chills, and cough. He was known to have Hb-SE sickle-cell disease. A chest x-ray showed new pulmonary infiltrates. Treatment was focused on reducing the chest pain to improve breathing and treat the respiratory infection. The physician's discharge diagnosis was acute chest syndrome due to the sickle-cell crisis.

Principal Diagnosis: _____

Secondary Diagnoses: _____

Principal Procedure: _____

Secondary Procedure(s): _____

2

A severely anemic 75-year-old male patient with known inoperable carcinoma of the head of the pancreas is admitted to the hospital for nonautologous packed red blood cell transfusions, which were administered through a catheter inserted into a peripheral vein in the left arm. The discharge diagnosis was anemia of chronic disease due to inoperable carcinoma of the pancreas.

Principal Diagnosis: _____

Secondary Diagnoses: _____

Principal Procedure: _____

Secondary Procedure(s): _____

3

While an inpatient in an acute care hospital, a 60-year-old female was referred for consultation to a hematologist with a diagnosis of anemia. A bone marrow aspiration biopsy of the right iliac crest was performed. Pathologic analysis of the specimen concluded the patient had "hypercellular marrow with diminished iron consistent with iron deficiency anemia" with the iron deficiency anemia also documented by the consultant in a postprocedure note. The attending physician agreed with the pathologist's conclusion. Code only for the consultant's diagnosis and procedure performed.

Principal Diagnosis: _____

Secondary Diagnoses: _____

Principal Procedure: _____

Secondary Procedure(s): _____

4

An 80-year-old female was seen by her family practice physician in the office for symptoms of fatigue, palpitations, and weakness. She had recently moved from her home of 50 years to an assisted living center. Although she likes the new residence, she feels the move has caused her to become ill. She has no appetite and was distressed over all she had to do prior to the move. Laboratory tests were ordered, including a CBC, a comprehensive metabolic profile, and an EKG and chest x-ray. Her hemoglobin and hematocrit were abnormal and, given her history, especially the lack of adequate nutrition, the diagnosis of nutritional anemia was made. The patient was encouraged to take advantage of the assisted living center's on-site dietitian to review her nutritional needs. The patient was scheduled to return to the physician in two weeks. If the blood count does not improve by then, the option of administering packed cells via transfusion will be discussed. The only other finding of her diagnostic studies was known chronic obstructive pulmonary disease (COPD) that is under treatment and a healed myocardial infarction that occurred three years ago and is currently asymptomatic.

First-Listed Diagnosis: _____

Secondary Diagnoses: _____

5

The patient, a 40-year-old male, was diagnosed with acquired hemolytic anemia, auto-immune type with warm-reactive (IgG) antibodies (warm type), and had been treated with glucocorticoids (prednisone). The patient failed to respond to this medication, so it was stopped two months ago. The patient is also under treatment for systemic lupus erythematosus. Given the aggressive nature of his anemia, he was advised to be admitted to the hospital and have a total splenectomy to eliminate the body's further destruction of red blood cells. The open, total splenectomy was performed without complications, and the patient was discharged to be followed up in the physician's and surgeon's offices.

Principal Diagnosis: _____

Secondary Diagnoses: _____

Principal Procedure: _____

Secondary Procedure(s): _____

6

A 70-year-old male was admitted after seeing bright red blood in the toilet following a bowel movement. An esophagogastroduodenoscopy (EGD) revealed a chronic gastric ulcer with evidence of recent bleeding. The final diagnoses documented were chronic gastric ulcer with recent hemorrhage and resulting acute blood loss anemia.

Principal Diagnosis: _____

Secondary Diagnoses: _____

Principal Procedure: _____

Secondary Procedure(s): _____

7

A 60-year-old female was placed in the observation unit after complaining of chest pain. She was recently seen for a follow-up visit at the hematologist's office for recently diagnosed pernicious anemia. The patient is also known to have agammaglobulinemia that is frequently found in patients with pernicious anemia. The patient is also being treated for chronic atrophic gastritis that is a consequence of her pernicious anemia. The patient is treated with medications to replace the cobalamin deficiency of pernicious anemia. The chest pain was attributed to her chronic atrophic gastritis and she was discharged the same day.

First-Listed Diagnosis: _____

Secondary Diagnoses: _____

8

A 50-year-old female is admitted directly from her hematologist-oncologist's office after a follow-up visit concerning drastically reduced blood counts as reported on recent laboratory tests. After workup, the attending physician diagnosed acquired aplastic anemia. The physician also refers to her aplastic anemia as "pancytopenia with hypocellular bone marrow." The patient has been undergoing aggressive cytotoxic chemotherapy for left ovarian carcinoma. No chemotherapy was administered during this visit. The patient was discharged and scheduled to report to the hospital outpatient transfusion center tomorrow for two units of red blood cells to be infused for the aplastic anemia, documented as an adverse effect of her chemotherapy.

Principal Diagnosis: _____

Secondary Diagnoses: _____

Principal Procedure: _____

Secondary Procedure(s): _____

9

The patient is a 20-year-old male who was born with factor VIII deficiency and diagnosed with hemophilia, type A. He has been receiving factor VIII replacement therapy with some response to treatment. The patient is admitted to the hospital on this occasion for his first course of therapeutic plasmapheresis, specifically extracorporeal immunoadsorption. The procedure is performed by drawing blood from an antecubital vein through a needle and returning it to another vein in the other arm. The access vein is connected to a primed blood processor. Blood is drawn into a cell separator. The plasma is passed to a monitor that controls continuous plasma flow through one of two ECI protein A columns. One column absorbs antibodies and the other treats the remaining plasma. The treated plasma is returned to the blood processor, mixed with the patient's red blood cells, and reinfused back to the patient. This treatment took 4 hours and 10 minutes. The patient was kept in the hospital overnight to observe for any possible complications. The patient is known to have "hemophilic arthritis" of the knees as a result of bleeding into these joints. This arthropathy caused by his hemophilia was evaluated by an orthopedic physician during his hospital stay. No complications of his immunoadsorption treatment were detected, and the patient was discharged, accompanied by his parents, for a follow-up visit in 1 week in the physician's office.

Principal Diagnosis: _____

Secondary Diagnoses: _____

Principal Procedure: _____

Secondary Procedure(s): _____

10

The patient is a 55-year-old female with known chronic idiopathic thrombocytopenic purpura. The patient has been treated for this autoimmune disorder for approximately 1 year. The patient was previously seen in the office of her internal medicine specialist to discuss an elective splenectomy. The patient has failed to maintain a normal platelet count after a course of prednisone therapy. She also had major side-effect reactions to the prednisone medication. After hearing of the risks and benefits of the splenectomy versus another course of steroid therapy, the patient is admitted and consents to the surgery, a laparoscopic partial splenectomy.

Principal Diagnosis: _____

Secondary Diagnoses: _____

Principal Procedure: _____

Secondary Procedure(s): _____

11

A 68-year-old female was admitted to the hospital from a local nursing home because she has two large pressure ulcers on her sacrum and right hip with the sacral ulcer now bleeding. Lab results indicated severe anemia, and the patient received one nonautologous packed red blood cell transfusion percutaneously through a peripheral vein for her documented acute blood-loss anemia. The wound care physician and nurses treated her massive stage 3 sacral pressure ulcer and stage 2 right hip pressure ulcer. The patient was also treated for her well-controlled type 2 diabetes and hypertension. The patient also has chronic back pain (radiculopathy) from lumbar spinal osteoarthritis. Given the size of the pressure ulcers, the intensive care necessary to manage the ulcers, her chronic back pain, and subsequent immobility, a surgical consultation was obtained to consider creating a diverting colostomy to alleviate the fecal incontinence that she had for the past several months that failed to respond to medical management. The fecal incontinence had done damage to her skin and affected her skin ulcers. After completion of the red blood cell transfusion, she was stable enough for the permanent colostomy open procedure of the descending colon. There were no postoperative complications, and after two days the patient was transferred to the skilled nursing facility for recovery from surgery and continued wound care.

Principal Diagnosis: _____

Secondary Diagnoses: _____

Principal Procedure: _____

Secondary Procedure(s): _____

12

A 70-year-old female patient with metastatic bone carcinoma from carcinoma of the right breast, still under treatment by chemotherapy and radiation therapy, is admitted with vague complaints of weakness. After workup, she was diagnosed as having aplastic anemia caused by her radiation therapy.

First-Listed Diagnosis: _____

Secondary Diagnoses: _____

13

A 60-year-old male patient with end-stage renal disease (ESRD) requiring dialysis is seen in his nephrologist's office for an evaluation of his known anemia due to ESRD. Up until now, the anemia was not severe. However, based on the patient's hemoglobin, transferrin saturation, and serum ferritin laboratory values, the physician concludes the patient will need to receive Epogen to treat the anemia and avoid the need for blood transfusions. The medication will be administered intravenously three times a week at the dialysis center with the drug's dosage based on the patient's hemoglobin values and iron status. The patient will be monitored by the dialysis center physician and return to his nephrologist's office in one month.

First-Listed Diagnosis: _____

Secondary Diagnoses: _____

14

The patient, a 28-year-old female, is admitted with labor pains in her second trimester of pregnancy at 25 and 3/7 weeks. She is expecting a boy. While in the hospital, she has a discussion of recent testing to determine her sickle-cell genetic status. The patient is married to a 29-year-old male who is known to carry the sickle-cell anemia trait. The patient is informed she also is a carrier of the sickle-cell trait. The patient and her husband are anxious to begin a family. The physician informs the patient that the gene that causes sickle-cell anemia must be inherited from both parents to cause full-blown sickle cell anemia in a child. With both the father and mother carrying the sickle-cell trait, the couple has a 25 percent chance of having a child with the disease and a 50 percent chance of having a child who is a carrier. Otherwise, neither of the parents with the sickle-cell trait required treatment for the trait. She had a fetal ultrasound after the labor halted. The patient is discharged with the diagnoses false labor, sickle-cell trait.

Principal Diagnosis: _____

Secondary Diagnoses: _____

Principal Procedure: _____

Secondary Procedure(s): _____

15

A 40-year-old male of Mediterranean descent is admitted to the hospital after passing out. The patient has beta thalassemia major and requires blood transfusions every three to four weeks. On initial evaluation, the physician documents splenomegaly, which is unchanged. This sign, as well as the patient's reported fatigue and reduced appetite, are classic symptoms of this hereditary hemolytic anemia. Since his scheduled appointment for a blood transfusion of red blood cells coincides with the admission, he is transfused one unit of nonautologous packed red blood cells percutaneously through a peripheral vein. A neurologist is asked to see the patient. She does not believe that the patient passed out because of the beta thalassemia major but cannot determine another cause. The final diagnoses are syncope, etiology unknown, and beta thalassemia major.

Principal Diagnosis: _____

Secondary Diagnoses: _____

Principal Procedure: _____

Secondary Procedure(s): _____

16

The patient is a 61-year-old female who is being seen in the hematology-oncology clinic for a follow-up visit. Eighteen months ago, the patient was diagnosed with an aggressive form of breast cancer and was treated with a mastectomy and chemotherapy that was completed in the past six months. Recently, she was found to be anemic and underwent a bone marrow biopsy that revealed myelodysplastic syndrome. During this visit, the patient complained of generalized fatigue and shortness of breath for the past couple of days. Blood was drawn in the clinic for a hemoglobin/hematocrit and the results returned with hemoglobin of 3.4 and hematocrit of 8.4. On physical exam the patient was noted to be weak, orthostatic, and short of breath on exertion. She said she has not noticed any blood in her stools or blood in her urine. Arrangements were made for the patient to be taken to the hospital and placed in observation status. Blood transfusions will be administered over the next 24 hours, the number to be determined by her response to the first two units ordered. The physician documented the patient's reason for being in the clinic today as myelodysplastic syndrome in a patient with a past history of carcinoma of the breast. The physician also documented in the clinic notes that he was unable to determine during this visit whether the condition was the result of her previous chemotherapy. It was stated that while she is in the observation status at the hospital it would be investigated with more testing.

Principal Diagnosis: _____

Secondary Diagnoses: _____

Principal Procedure: _____

Secondary Procedure(s): _____

17

The patient is an 80-year-old male who was referred to the hematology clinic after being seen by his family practice physician, who had seen him for surgical clearance for scheduled right eye cataract surgery. During that exam, the patient was found to be weak and his hematocrit was 19. Prior to his visit in the hematology clinic, blood was drawn for iron studies.

The hematologist documented that the patient stated he was often dizzy when he changed positions from supine to erect. He said he only ate two small meals a day because he was never hungry. The physician noted the patient was a tall, thin man but the patient denied losing any weight recently. The physician documented the lab results of an iron of 2, TIBC of 384, and ferritin of 20. Blood was drawn in the office for type and crossmatch of two units of packed cells that the patient will receive later the same afternoon. The physician's documented impression at the end of the visit was nutritional anemia with poor iron absorption and right-sided senile cataract.

Principal Diagnosis: _____

Secondary Diagnoses: _____

Principal Procedure: _____

Secondary Procedure(s): _____

18

A 49-year old female was sent to the hospital from her gynecologist's office for treatment of acute blood loss anemia due to abnormal uterine bleeding. The patient was treated with a transfusion of nonautologous red blood cells through a peripheral vein, and was subsequently sent to the operating room, where she underwent endometrial ablation. The endometrial ablation was performed using a hysteroscope and the NovaSure device, which was inserted through the vagina into the cervix and uterus. Radiofrequency energy was delivered via the device for 90 seconds. The patient's final discharge diagnoses were menorrhagia and acute blood loss anemia.

Principal Diagnosis: _____

Secondary Diagnoses: _____

Principal Procedure: _____

Secondary Procedure(s): _____

Chapter 4

Endocrine, Nutritional, and Metabolic Diseases

Coding Scenarios for *Basic ICD-10-CM and ICD-10-PCS Coding Exercises*

The following case studies are organized following the sequence of the chapters in the ICD-10-CM Tabular List of Diseases and Injuries as published on the Centers for Disease Control and Prevention National Center for Health Statistics website (http://www .cdc.gov/nchs/icd/icd10cm.htm). The objective of this book is to provide the student with detailed clinical information to code, rather than one- or two-line diagnosis and procedure statements.

ICD-10-CM diagnosis codes are to be assigned to both the inpatient hospital admission and the outpatient visit case studies. In this book, the ICD-10-PCS procedure codes are to be assigned only to the inpatient hospital admission cases. In actual practice, outpatient cases are assigned CPT/HCPCS codes. The ICD-10-PCS codes are only required for inpatient procedures. In the answer key for the exercises, the Alphabetic Index entry is listed after the code to indicate the main terms and subterms used to locate the code that must be verified in the ICD-10-CM Tabular List or in the ICD-10-PCS Code Tables prior to assigning the code.

1

An older adult female who lives alone was brought to the hospital emergency department by fire department ambulance after being discovered on the front porch by neighbors. She was in a semiconscious state. She was known to have type 1 diabetes mellitus, maintained on insulin. The physicians described her diabetes as very brittle with hyperglycemia. There were many fluctuating blood sugar measurements during her hospital stay. A type and dosage of insulin was finally established. During her inpatient hospital stay the patient complained of vision problems. She was examined by an ophthalmologist and found to have mild nonproliferative diabetic retinopathy. The patient was able to be discharged home to be followed up in her physicians' offices, as well as by home health nurses. The discharge diagnosis was uncontrolled type 1 diabetes on insulin with mild nonproliferative retinopathy.

Principal Diagnosis: _____

Secondary Diagnoses: _____

Principal Procedure: _____

Secondary Procedure(s): _____

2

A 57-year-old female patient was sent to the hospital outpatient laboratory department by her physician with a written order for a blood glucose test. The patient has known type 2 diabetes mellitus with polyneuropathy and diabetic chronic kidney disease, stage 2; these diagnoses were documented on the order form as the reasons for the blood test.

First-Listed Diagnosis: _____

Secondary Diagnoses: _____

3

An 18-year-old female patient who has had type 1 diabetes for 10 years was admitted with ketoacidosis. She has an insulin pump. The pump was tested and found to have a breakdown; it was not pumping enough insulin, so there was an underdosing of the insulin, which is what caused the ketoacidosis. With intravenous hydration and insulin drip, the patient's ketones cleared quickly. The insulin pump was reset to the correct dosage.

Principal Diagnosis: _____

Secondary Diagnoses: _____

Principal Procedure: _____

Secondary Procedure(s): _____

4

A 36-year-old male is seen in his physician's office for ongoing management of diabetes mellitus. As of this time, no obvious manifestations of diabetes are affecting any other body system. The patient takes insulin daily and has received a renewed prescription for insulin and needles. The patient noted that he was very satisfied with the new glucose monitoring device he was advised to use during his last visit. A follow-up appointment was made for 60 days following this visit.

First-Listed Diagnosis: _____

Secondary Diagnoses: _____

5

A 47-year-old female was seen in her physician's office as a follow-up visit. Results for laboratory tests ordered during the previous visit revealed elevated calcium in the bloodstream. A second laboratory test found an excessive amount of parathyroid hormone in the bloodstream. Follow-up imaging studies confirmed the presence of a benign parathyroid adenoma. The patient is presently complaining of muscle weakness, fatigue, and some nausea and intermittent vomiting. Based on these findings, the physician concludes that the patient is demonstrating primary hyperparathyroidism. The physician explains to the patient that the hyperparathyroidism can only be cured by surgical excision of the parathyroid adenoma. The patient refuses surgery. The physician agrees the need for surgery is not urgent at this time and orders a bone density radiologic examination to be done next week. The patient will have a follow-up appointment in one month and measurement of calcium levels and renal functions in six months. Symptoms of the primary hyperparathyroidism were treated at this time.

First-Listed Diagnosis: _____

Secondary Diagnoses: _____

6

A 52-year-old female had been seen in her physician's office because of increasingly irritating symptomatology, including nervousness, irritability, increased perspiration, shakiness, and increased appetite with unexplained weight loss, increased heart rate, palpitations, sleeping difficulties, and other problems. The patient is returning to the office today to review her test results with her physician. The physician advised the patient of the following findings: the blood test for thyroid-stimulating hormone had an elevated measurement, and a nuclear medicine scan of the thyroid found hyperactivity in the entire gland. Based on these findings, the diagnosis of hyperthyroidism in the absence of a goiter (rule out Graves' disease) was made. The physician had eliminated a thyroid adenoma or a multinodular goiter as the cause of the hyperthyroidism. The patient was placed on an oral anti-thyroid medication to lower the level of thyroid hormones in the blood. Additional tests were ordered, and the patient was scheduled to return to the office in 10 days. Because the patient's heart palpitations were more pronounced than seen in other patients with hyperthyroidism, arrangements were made for her to have a consultation with a cardiologist tomorrow.

First-Listed Diagnosis: _____

Secondary Diagnoses: _____

7

The parents of a 16-year-old boy accompanied him to the hospital for admission for the insertion of a totally implantable insulin infusion pump and injection of insulin. The patient has had type 1 diabetes mellitus since the age of 11 years. The insertion of the pump into the subcutaneous tissue of his abdomen was successful. On numerous occasions during the admission, the patient has had hyperglycemia so his diabetes had been uncontrolled. The treatment has been administering various types and dosages of insulin through the pump. The patient was discharged and will return to the hospital's diabetic clinic in one week with his parents for insulin pump titration and training. For the next week, the pump will run with saline.

Principal Diagnosis: _____

Secondary Diagnoses: _____

Principal Procedure: _____

Secondary Procedure(s): _____

8

The patient is a 42-year-old female who is admitted for bariatric surgery for morbid obesity with alveolar hypoventilation. The patient, who has been obese since childhood, currently weighs 150 pounds more than her ideal body weight. The patient's BMI is 48.4. In the past 20 years, she has been treated for essential hypertension, hyperlipidemia, obstructive sleep apnea, insulin resistance, and primary osteoarthritis of the hips and knees. She has had repeated failures of other therapeutic approaches and various diets to lose weight and has been cleared by a psychiatrist who could find no psychopathology that would make her ineligible for this procedure. The patient underwent a laparoscopic Roux-en-Y gastric bypass (gastroenterostomy) procedure, consisting of the creation of a small gastric pouch connected to the jejunum. The procedure and postoperative course were uneventful, and the patient was discharged the following day. During this hospital stay, hypertension, hyperlipidemia, insulin resistance, and osteoarthritis of the multiple joints were also treated.

Principal Diagnosis: _____

Secondary Diagnoses: _____

Principal Procedure: _____

Secondary Procedure(s): _____

9

The patient is a 32-year-old male who is admitted for laparoscopic bariatric surgery for morbid obesity due to excess calories. The patient currently weighs 200 pounds more than his ideal body weight with a body mass index of 54. In the past 10 years he has lost and gained back more than 100 pounds, but now suffers from several major health conditions that require more aggressive management of his obesity. He has a strong family history of morbid obesity. It occurs in his parents, two sisters, and one brother. In the past 10 years, he has been treated for essential hypertension, dyslipidemia, obstructive sleep apnea, gallstone pancreatitis, type 2 diabetes with diabetic amyotrophy, and osteoarthritis localized to his knees, for which he has had bilateral knee replacements. He has had repeated failures of other therapeutic approaches to losing weight and has been cleared by a psychiatrist who could find no psychopathology that would make him ineligible for this procedure. The patient underwent a laparoscopic gastric restrictive procedure with an adjustable gastric band and port insertion. The patient had an uneventful postoperative recovery in the hospital and was discharged for follow-up in the office. During this hospital stay, the conditions of hypertension, dyslipidemia, and type 2 diabetes were also treated.

Principal Diagnosis: _____

Secondary Diagnoses: _____

Principal Procedure: _____

Secondary Procedure(s): _____

10

A 35-year-old male is seen in his physician's office for dietary counseling and ongoing surveillance of his familial hypercholesterolemia, low density lipoid type. He has been taking the HMG-CoA reductase inhibitor drug, lovastatin (Mevacor), as directed. He has no identifiable adverse effects from the medication. He recently quit smoking, having been nicotine dependent since his teenage years, and was counseled to maintain his smoke-free status. A follow-up appointment is made for a repeat visit in 3 months.

First-Listed Diagnosis: _____

Secondary Diagnoses: _____

11

The patient is a 57-year-old male who was seen in the office for a regular follow-up appointment for the management of secondary diabetes mellitus and his insulin dosage. The AccuChek performed in the office showed a result of 400. The patient stated his glucose is usually over 300 when he checks it at home. He reported feeling fairly well, with a little more fatigue than usual. The patient is a retired truck driver and is fairly active, including helping his neighbors with yard work and snow shoveling. He has a history of pancreatic cysts treated surgically by partial pancreatectomy that has produced his secondary diabetes and postoperative hypoinsulinemia. Since it was noted that his blood glucose was at a critically high level, he was advised admission. He was admitted and seen by an endocrinologist, who carefully monitored his glucose levels and adjusted his insulin dosage until his glucose levels remained at normal levels. No other complications of his diabetes were found. The patient was discharged with instructions to follow up with the endocrinologist in one week and to make an appointment for diabetic teaching in the diabetic clinic.

Principal Diagnosis: _____

Secondary Diagnoses: _____

Principal Procedure: _____

Secondary Procedure(s): _____

12

The patient was admitted to the hospital after outpatient laboratory testing revealed a potassium level of 6.3 with elevated creatinine. A nephrology consultation was obtained to evaluate his hyperkalemia. He was administered Kayexalate, and his potassium levels improved. The consultant's report suggested that two issues may be contributing to his high potassium. He was taking medications for high blood pressure and a prophylactic anticoagulant, and he did not avoid high potassium foods as previously instructed. The combination of medications and dietary indiscretion may have resulted in the inadvertent potassium intake excess. The attending physician and consultant took the opportunity of this hospital stay to evaluate the patient's many chronic conditions and encourage compliance with his medications and dietary restrictions. In addition to hyperkalemia, the physician included the following conditions in the discharge summary: acute renal insufficiency, hypertension with chronic kidney disease stage 1, coronary artery disease, status post cardiac pacemaker, chronic atrial fibrillation, and noncompliance with dietary instructions. He was seen by a dietician and provided with information about avoiding foods high in potassium. The patient was encouraged to return to the physician's office in two weeks.

Principal Diagnosis: _____

Secondary Diagnoses: _____

Principal Procedure: _____

Secondary Procedure(s): _____

13

The patient is a 70-year-old female who was a former office employee of her primary care physician. She had called the physician's office three days prior to admission complaining of general weakness and nausea, and, according to her niece who checked in on her every few days, was apparently not able to get around her house very well. The physician advised her to come to the office, and she agreed but did not show up. The patient had often been noncompliant with medications and treatments recommended. When the physician's office called her after she failed to show, she said she did not feel well enough to drive but her niece would drive her to the physician's office the next day. The patient did not show up the next day either. On the third day, the physician's office called her again. When she sounded less responsive on the telephone, one of the physician's office staff nurses was given permission to go to the house to check on the patient. When the nurse got to the home, she found the front door unlocked and the patient in bed very lethargic, feverish, and not responding clearly to questions. An ambulance was called, and the patient was brought to the emergency department and admitted as an inpatient. The patient was known to have type 2 diabetes with several body systems affected. She was also known to have alcohol dependence, consuming a pint of vodka on a daily basis. Initial laboratory work showed a glucose level of 245, urinalysis with 3+ bacteria and greater than 150 white cells with 10–20 RBCs, a positive blood alcohol level indicating acute intoxication, and ketoacidosis. A urine culture grew *E. coli* bacteria. She was started on IV antibiotics. She improved steadily and described herself as feeling the best she had felt in a long time. She was watched closely for signs of alcohol withdrawal, but nothing obvious was noted. During her hospital stay, the following conditions were treated: diabetes mellitus, type 2, with ketoacidosis with coma; diabetes mellitus with worsening nephropathy; diabetic severe nonproliferative retinopathy and macular edema; *E. coli* urinary tract infection; history of UTIs; alcohol dependence; and noncompliance with medical care. The attending physician was queried and documented that the diabetic ketoaci-dosis best met the definition of principal diagnosis. A social work consultation was requested, and the patient and her niece were given information about assisted living centers to help the patient live safely with some medical supervision. However, the patient flatly refused to consider the option and was discharged home with home health services requested for medical management.

Principal Diagnosis: _____

Secondary Diagnoses: _____

Principal Procedure: _____

Secondary Procedure(s): _____

14

The patient is a 10-month-old female infant who was discharged from the hospital 48 hours ago after treatment for a community-acquired pneumonia and gastroenteritis. The child received IV antibiotics in the hospital. The fever and the diarrhea abated, and the child was discharged to her parents' care. However, early this morning the child's father called the physician and said her fever and diarrhea had returned, she was increasingly lethargic, and was refusing to take fluids or food. The child was readmitted to the hospital for dehydration and hypokalemia. She was placed on IV fluids and medications to treat the dehydration and hypo-kalemia and continued on antibiotics for resolving pneumonia. Within 24 hours the child was afebrile with no diarrhea and a good appetite. Electrolyte laboratory values were back in the normal ranges. The infant also had a diaper rash that was treated in the hospital with medica-tion that was also given to the parents to take home. The patient was discharged to her parents' care with prescriptions given and a follow-up appointment made for 5 days later. The diagno-ses listed by the physician in the discharge summary were (1) dehydration, (2) hypokalemia, (3) gastroenteritis, (4) resolving pneumonia, community-acquired, and (5) diaper rash.

Principal Diagnosis: _____

Secondary Diagnoses: _____

Principal Procedure: _____

Secondary Procedure(s): _____

15

A 30-month-old male toddler was admitted to the university hospital for investigation of a complex group of symptoms. The child and parents live four hours away from the hospital. The child was admitted so that the majority of the testing could be done at one time without repeated long trips back and forth to the hospital. The mother reported she noticed changes in the child's facial appearance starting about six months ago. She also noted a loss of previously acquired skills, including language, and observed new aggressive behavior. Upon examination, the physician noted an enlarged liver and spleen with a distended abdomen and suspected there were cardiovascular complications as well. A series of laboratory tests were performed and an extensive medical history was taken from both parents. The physicians concluded the patient had a type of inherited metabolic disorder called mucopolysaccharidosis (MPS), specifically type MPS IIA, also known as Hunter Syndrome. The patient's problem is his body's inability to produce specific enzymes to carry out essential functions. The parents were told there is no cure for Hunter Syndrome at this time and treatment focuses on managing signs and symptoms of the disease to provide relief to the child as the disease progresses. Known life-threatening complications include cardiovascular, respiratory, brain, and nervous system, in addition to skeletal and connective tissue problems. Because this condition is known to be an X-linked recessive disease, the mother of the child was tested for the mutated gene known to cause Hunter's Syndrome. It was determined the mother was a carrier of this disease because she had the X-linked recessive disorder with the mutated gene located on one of her X chromosomes and the normal gene on the other. The mother is unaffected by the disease but can pass it on to children, most often to a son. The parents were told that enzyme replacement therapy and other emerging therapies may offer their son more help in the future. The family was given a follow-up appointment to return in three months for possible hematopoietic stem cell transplant planning. The family was also made aware of the National MPS Society that provides support for families and research support.

Principal Diagnosis: _____

Secondary Diagnoses: _____

Principal Procedure: _____

Secondary Procedure(s): _____

16

A 7-year-old girl was admitted for dehydration due to viral gastroenteritis. The patient had been seen in the pediatrician's office yesterday and was diagnosed with viral gastroenteritis based on the patient's symptoms and history, but the patient's family brought her to the emergency department today when she became increasingly lethargic and weak. Intravenous fluids were administered for rehydration, and the patient was admitted for treatment of the dehydration. During the two-day hospital stay, the patient's viral gastroenteritis was also treated, but the focus of her treatment was to correct her dehydrated status. The pediatrician noted that the patient would not have been admitted for treatment of the viral gastroenteritis alone.

Principal Diagnosis: _____

Secondary Diagnoses: _____

Principal Procedure: _____

Secondary Procedure(s): _____

17

The patient is a 60-year-old male who was seen in the Internal Medicine Clinic for follow up for his newly diagnosed type 2 diabetes mellitus with proliferative diabetic retinopathy. Based on recent laboratory testing, it appeared the current diabetic medications were beginning to bring the patient's diabetes under better control. Before the physician began the physical examination, the patient told the physician he had a "sore" on his left fourth and fifth toes. Upon examination, it was obvious to the physician that the patient had a small area of wet gangrene on both toes. The wounds were cleaned and dressings applied. The physician arranged for the patient to be seen in the Wound Clinic the next day to further treat the gangrene of the toes. The physician documented the following as the reasons for the visit in the Internal Medicine Clinic: Wet gangrene of the toes due to type 2 diabetes and proliferative diabetic retinopathy.

Principal Diagnosis: _____

Secondary Diagnoses: _____

Principal Procedure: _____

Secondary Procedure(s): _____

18

The patient is a 55-year-old male who is brought to the emergency department by his family. They tell the physician that over the past two weeks the patient has had difficulty walking to the point that, today, he cannot walk at all. The emergency physician identifies the problem as progressive ataxia and starts to investigate the cause. The patient states his legs do not hurt but he feels his legs are weak and cannot support him. The patient had a 40-year history of abusing alcohol and admits he is an alcoholic. He also admits to smoking a pack of cigarettes per day for the same amount of time. The physician concludes there are no other medical problems such as pancreatitis or cirrhosis of the liver as a result of the alcohol dependence. The patient was admitted to the hospital with the admitting diagnosis of ataxia. The attending physician and neurology consultant speculate the ataxia was cerebellar from alcoholic degeneration of the cerebellum or possibly Wernicke's encephalopathy. Over the next 24 hours, the patient became very confused and agitated with some violent outbursts and actions. After a couple days of confusion and disorientation, the patient's sensorium slowly cleared. The physicians considered whether the patient was experiencing delirium tremens, but his family said the patient had been sober for the two weeks prior to admission; his ataxia seriously concerned him, so he stopped drinking. The patient had several abnormalities in his laboratory tests, including a severe thiamine deficiency that could be causing the encephalopathy. The pulmonary medicine physician examined the patient and concluded his chronic cough was due to chronic bronchitis/COPD. Because the neurologist was looking for evidence of Wernicke's encephalopathy, an MRI of the brain was performed and showed the cerebellum as normal in size and shape, but a CT of the brain showed an area of calcification in the right occipital region. Over the next 5 days, the patient's ataxia lessened and the patient was able to ambulate slowly with a walker and physical therapy. It was also determined the patient had essential hypertension and was started on antihypertensive medications. The patient was discharged with medications prescribed including antihypertensive oral medicine, folic acid, and multivitamins as well as an inhaler to treat the chronic bronchitis. The patient was encouraged to maintain his sobriety by joining the local Alcoholics Anonymous organization and to discontinue smoking. The discharge diagnoses documented were possible Wernicke's encephalopathy, chronic alcohol dependence, nicotine dependence, COPD/chronic bronchitis, and hypertension.

Principal Diagnosis: _____

Secondary Diagnoses: _____

Principal Procedure: _____

Secondary Procedure(s): _____

19

The patient is a 37-year-old obese male who underwent a laparoscopic gastric banding surgery one year ago. The patient presented to the emergency department complaining of persistent nausea, vomiting, weakness, and epigastric abdominal pain. Imaging studies were performed, which revealed probable malposition of the gastric band. The patient consented to removal of the band. He was taken to the operating room where he underwent a laparoscopic evaluation of his gastric band. This examination confirmed that the band had indeed slipped from its proper position. It was this displacement that was causing the patient's symptoms and abdominal pain. The surgeon removed the band and its attached port laparoscopically. The patient was kept in the hospital for several days to monitor his condition and intake and treat his dehydration. His discharge diagnoses were: complication of gastric band, obesity with BMI of 40, and dehydration.

Principal Diagnosis: _____

Secondary Diagnoses: _____

Principal Procedure: _____

Secondary Procedure(s): _____

Chapter 5

Mental, Behavioral, and Neurodevelopmental Disorders

Coding Scenarios for *Basic ICD-10-CM* *and ICD-10-PCS Coding Exercises*

The following case studies are organized following the sequence of the chapters in the ICD-10-CM Tabular List of Diseases and Injuries as published on the Centers for Disease Control and Prevention National Center for Health Statistics website (http://www.cdc.gov/nchs /icd/icd10cm.htm). The objective of this book is to provide the student with detailed clinical information to code, rather than one- or two-line diagnosis and procedure statements.

ICD-10-CM diagnosis codes are to be assigned to both the inpatient hospital admission and the outpatient visit case studies. In this book, the ICD-10-PCS procedure codes are to be assigned only to the inpatient hospital admission cases. In actual practice, outpatient cases are assigned CPT/HCPCS codes. The ICD-10-PCS codes are only required for inpatient procedures. In the answer key for the exercises, the Alphabetic Index entry is listed after the code to indicate the main terms and subterms used to locate the code that must be verified in the ICD-10-CM Tabular List or in the ICD-10-PCS Code Tables prior to assigning the code.

1

A 30-year-old male was brought to the emergency department by police who found him walking down the middle of a highway. The patient was obviously intoxicated and initially unco-operative, experiencing visual hallucinations. Based on the physical examination and laboratory work, and with information later provided by the patient, the physician concluded the patient had impending delirium tremens that required admission. He was also monitored for nicotine withdrawal, as he smoked two packs of cigarettes daily. He was administered a nicotine patch and did not experience nicotine withdrawal. The patient's discharge diagnosis was delirium tremens and psychotic disorder/hallucinations due to alcohol dependence and nicotine dependence.

Principal Diagnosis: _____

Secondary Diagnoses: _____

Principal Procedure: _____

Secondary Procedure(s): _____

2

A 35-year-old female was admitted to the hospital by the psychiatrist after being seen in the community mental health center for group therapy to deal with her escalating anxiety and depression. The patient also has agoraphobia with panic disorder symptoms, so going to the group meetings is often difficult for her. During her admission she participated in group therapy with good results. The psychiatrist also conducted supportive individual therapy sessions with her during the hospital stay. Upon discharge, she felt able to return to the community mental health center for outpatient group therapy sessions.

Principal Diagnosis: _____

Secondary Diagnoses: _____

Principal Procedure: _____

Secondary Procedure(s): _____

3

After numerous drug possession arrests, a 40-year-old male was mandated to the substance abuse treatment facility for admission to undergo detoxification for his cocaine use disorder, moderate. He was suspected of criminal activity to support his cocaine dependence, but repeatedly denied breaking the law even though he had difficulties with his memory. He agreed to an administration of intravenous barbiturate (narcosynthesis) in order to release any possible suppressed or repressed thoughts. Upon conclusion of the test, it was determined he was telling the truth. The procedure of detoxification occurred over the first three days of stay at the residential center. The patient was transferred to a residential center for rehabilitation services to be continued for the next 25 days.

Principal Diagnosis: _____

Secondary Diagnoses: _____

Principal Procedure: _____

Secondary Procedure(s): _____

4

A patient with type I bipolar disorder without psychosis, most recently in a mild depressed state, was admitted to the hospital with side effects due to the prescription lithium carbonate she had been taking. According to her caregivers, the drug had been administered correctly, and there was no possibility of a drug overdose. The patient had been sleeping 20 hours a day and was diagnosed with a drug-induced hypersomnia as a result of lithium toxicity. A therapeutic drug level for the lithium carbonate was found to be increased. The dosage was adjusted, and the patient received individual supportive verbal psychotherapy for the bipolar disorder while in the hospital. The patient was able to be discharged to the residential living center where she resided.

Principal Diagnosis: _____

Secondary Diagnoses: _____

Principal Procedure: _____

Secondary Procedure(s): _____

5

A 48-year-old male was brought to the emergency department after suffering an episode of syncope at a family picnic. The patient had been involved in a heated argument with several family members when he suddenly grabbed his chest and neck and collapsed to the ground. He awoke prior to the arrival of emergency medical personnel but was weak, diaphoretic, and confused. He was brought to the hospital emergency department. Once in the emergency department, cardiovascular studies were performed, but no cardiovascular disease was immediately evident. There was no history of alcohol or substance abuse, and the patient had not consumed a large amount of alcohol at the party. After admission, the patient's private physician performed a comprehensive history and a physical examination. The patient admitted to a similar episode during a past business meeting, but this episode of syncope was more profound and disturbing to the patient. Upon questioning, it was learned that his mother had suffered similar attacks when the patient was a child, but he knew nothing of their causes and did not think she was ever treated by a physician for the attacks. Other diagnostic tests failed to reveal any cardiovascular or pulmonary pathology to account for the syncope or feelings of panic. A psychiatric consultation was obtained, and the patient was started on antidepressant medication and recommended to begin psychotherapeutic interventions with the psychiatrist in his office. The patient agreed and was discharged in improved condition on day 3. The patient was much relieved that his problem was taken seriously and committed to ongoing treatment and management. The family physician agreed with the psychiatrist's conclusion of panic disorder without agoraphobia and added the secondary diagnosis of non-cardiac chest pain, resolved.

Principal Diagnosis: _____

Secondary Diagnoses: _____

Principal Procedure: _____

Secondary Procedure(s): _____

6

A 30-year-old female is referred to the psychiatrist for an office visit for continued management of her somatization disorder. The patient has a history of many physical complaints over the past 10 to 12 years and has suffered significant impairment in social, occupational, and other areas of normal functioning. The patient is receiving an antidepressant medication, and this seems to be helping her. The medication is also helping with her obsessive ruminations that were identified through psychotherapeutic interventions. After each investigation of her complaints, there has been no known medical condition to explain them. Her treatment of choice by this psychiatrist is behavior modification therapy as an attempt to control her access to other physicians for repeated physical investigations and to give her support that her psychological condition is treatable. The patient will return for follow-up visits three times per week.

First-Listed Diagnosis: _____

Secondary Diagnoses: _____

7

A 38-year-old male was admitted to the drug treatment unit of the local hospital for detoxification from heroin, an opioid drug he has been dependent on for several years. The addiction medicine physician describes his dependence as severe opioid use disorder. In anticipation of expected withdrawal symptoms, the patient is managed medically, pharmacologically, and psychologically over the next five days with individual and group motivational substance abuse counseling. The patient suffers multiple symptoms of withdrawal but copes with the process appropriately. By day six, the patient is actively engaged in individual and group therapy to reach his goal of an "opioid-free lifestyle" within his drug rehabilitation therapy. He has undergone drug detoxification in the past but appears much more committed during this hospital stay. The patient is discharged from the hospital on day eight to immediately enter a 21-day residential program at a local residential treatment facility. Long-term plans include a future stay at a drug-free recovery center and job training to enable the patient to improve his chances of recovery.

Principal Diagnosis: _____

Secondary Diagnoses: _____

Principal Procedure: _____

Secondary Procedure(s): _____

8

The patient is seen in his psychologist's office for individual psychotherapy as part of his long-term treatment for borderline personality disorder. The psychologist describes his condition as a "cluster B borderline personality disorder." The patient has been faithfully taking his monoamine oxidase inhibitor (MAOI) medication and reports he feels it has helped him manage his impulsive, overly emotional, and erratic behavior. The patient is also a recovering cocaine addict whom the therapist describes as being "in remission." The patient attends Narcotic Anonymous (NA) meetings twice a week and enjoys the interactions with other recovering individuals. The patient will return next week for his scheduled appointment.

First-Listed Diagnosis: _____

Secondary Diagnoses: _____

9

The patient was brought to the emergency department (ED) by city police after exhibiting extremely erratic behavior in jail. He was arrested for a fight with the owner of a local restaurant in which he frequently dines. The business owner reports the man can be very nice and reasonable one day and completely "crazy" the next time he is in the restaurant. Today the patient got into a fight with another person in the restaurant, and the police were called. His family members arrived at the emergency department and informed the emergency department physician on duty that the patient is known to have paranoid-type schizophrenia and is under treatment by a physician at the VA Medical Center. He is treated with Perphenazine. The family also suspected the patient had not been taking his medications regularly because he claims that he cannot afford them and had exhibited more paranoia recently. The ED physician contacted the VA physician and arranged for an immediate transfer to the psychiatric unit at the VA Medical Center. Ambulance transfer was also approved. The ED physician used the diagnosis provided to him by the VA psychiatrist as chronic paranoid schizophrenia in acute exacerbation with medication noncompliance.

First-Listed Diagnosis: _____

Secondary Diagnoses: _____

10

A 17-year-old female is admitted to the eating disorders/psychiatric unit of the University Hospital for anorexia nervosa. The patient's current weight is less than 80 percent of her expected weight for height and age, and her body mass index (BMI) is 18.2 or the 80th percentile for her pediatric age group. A thorough history, physical, and psychological examination is performed. It is determined the patient has a "restricting" subtype of anorexia nervosa because she loses weight by use of caloric restriction accompanied by excessive exercise. The patient is also known to "fast" two days a week to "cleanse her system of food toxins." The patient is extremely reluctant to gain even a small amount of weight. Intensive medical and psychological support was given to the patient. Weight restoration to 90 percent of her predicted weight was her primary treatment goal. After admission, laboratory tests revealed a serious electrolyte imbalance, which was treated. Along with medical and psychological support, the patient established a positive relationship with a young female dietitian who gained the patient's trust and respect, and this was extremely positive in helping the patient regain control of her disease. The patient was discharged on day eight with a small weight gain recorded. The patient was transferred to a residential treatment facility with a successful eating disorders management program for further care.

Principal Diagnosis: _____

Secondary Diagnoses: _____

Principal Procedure: _____

Secondary Procedure(s): _____

11

A 25-year-old male was brought to the hospital emergency department by fire department ambulance after being found by his father hanging from a rope in an attached garage at their house. The father cut the rope, and the patient fell to the ground. When paramedics arrived on the scene, the patient was unconscious but became responsive after being administered oxygen. The patient complained of a sore neck and a "cold." The patient's past medical history includes methadone for heroin dependence, continuous basis, and chronic pain syndrome as the result of an old back strain. The patient was taking the following medications: Xanax, Lithium, Methadone, Seroquel, and Norco. The patient was first admitted to the medical floor for "depression" and then consented to be transferred to the inpatient psychiatric unit for treatment. His psychiatric diagnosis was recurrent severe depressive disorder. He admitted to the suicide attempt and said it was impulsive after an argument with his parents and not planned ahead of time. He admits to depressive symptoms for the past one to two months, if not longer. While on both units in the hospital he was diagnosed with a mild form of pneumonia and treated with antibiotics. The orthopedic surgeon evaluated his neck and diagnosed an acute cervical sprain. The pain management physician, who knew the patient, evaluated the patient and agreed with the present medical management. The patient was discharged from inpatient status on day 10 and was scheduled to begin outpatient therapy through the partial psychiatric hospitalization program the next day.

Principal Diagnosis: _____

Secondary Diagnoses: _____

Principal Procedure: _____

Secondary Procedure(s): _____

12

The male patient was brought to the emergency department by fire department ambulance after being found unresponsive lying under a bench at a bus stop. People in the area told the paramedics they saw the man sitting on the bench then have a "seizure" and fall under the bench. When they checked on him, they thought he had stopped breathing and died, and they called 911. When paramedics arrived, they found the patient breathing very shallowly and placed him on oxygen. The patient was not able to be aroused but reacted to painful stimuli. Blood and urine were obtained for laboratory testing, and the patient was placed on a cardiac monitor, which showed a slow but regular heart rhythm. The lab result documented by the physician was a very high blood alcohol level, 225 mg/100mL. Based on the information in his wallet, his identity was determined, and his brother was called. The brother stated the patient had long suffered from chronic alcoholism but had been living independently and working part-time as a custodian, cleaning office buildings at night. The brother promised to come to the hospital and pick up the patient when he got off work in about 8 hours. The patient slept in the ER for several hours and then awoke. He was pleasant, cooperative, appreciative of the attention, and hungry. He was fed dinner and, later, a snack. His brother arrived to drive him home. The patient was given information about alcohol treatment programs and encouraged to consider. The patient knew all about such programs and told the staff he would call his "sponsor" when he got home and return to Alcoholics Anonymous meetings to resume his recovery. His final diagnosis was acute alcoholic intoxication in a patient with chronic alcoholism.

First-Listed Diagnosis: _____

Secondary Diagnoses: _____

13

The patient is a 15-year-old male who was recently released from a long stay in an adolescent psychiatric therapeutic hospital and has entered a five-days-per-week day program to continue the management of his challenging behavioral health conditions. The young man has been followed by his psychiatrist and psychiatric social worker for two years prior to the recent hospital stay. For many years he has had difficulties in school, having been dismissed from two traditional schools and more recently threatened to be discharged from an alternative school, which, along with major family conflicts and an encounter with the police, led to his recent hospitalization. He has been arrested on multiple occasions for battery but never convicted of the charges. He was first thought to be suffering from a conduct disorder and attention deficit hyperactivity disorder, and these have been confirmed. As time passed it became evident that the patient's main disability was chronic schizophrenia of a schizophreniform type. Also, since the age of four, the patient has been attracted to matches, lighters, and fires, and a diagnosis of pyromania was also established. The patient was raised in a chaotic household. His father has a long history of psychiatric disorders, and an older brother left home four years ago and had no contact with the family until recently, when the family learned he was incarcerated in another state's psychiatric prison. During the patient's recent hospital stay, his physicians were able to determine which medications were most beneficial to him. Since joining the day program, the patient has reported that his home life is more peaceful, he has not had a fight with anyone, has not set anything on fire, has enjoyed cooking meals with his mother, and has written several letters to his brother in prison. He has been able to comply with his behavioral contract and reports that he has not had any flare-up of his auditory hallucinations and feels more in control of his hyperactivity disorder. The patient attributes his "success" to the medications, which he initially resisted because he didn't want to become an "addict" but realizes he must take them the rest of his life. He also recognizes the importance of continuing his outpatient behavioral therapy, family therapy, and other group therapy, along with his psychiatric drug therapy. His current Axis I diagnoses are (1) schizophreniform disorder, (2) conduct disorder, socialized type, (3) attention deficit hyperactivity disorder, hyperactive type. Axis II diagnosis is (1) learning disabilities. There are no Axis III disorders. His Axis IV is moderate to severe. Axis V is a GAF score of 40 upon discharge from the hospital.

First-Listed Diagnosis: _____

Secondary Diagnoses: _____

14

The patient is a 32-year-old male admitted to the hospital for medical detoxification for his cocaine and cannabis dependency. The patient has been free-basing and snorting cocaine sporadically with increasing frequency over the past 10 years. He is now considered to have a moderate cocaine use disorder or dependence. He has also been using marijuana on an almost daily basis for 14 years, which is also considered a severe cannabis use disorder or dependence. He has been totally unable to quit using either drug on his own and now agrees to enter a residential treatment program for his drug addictions with the full support of his family and employer in order to save his marriage and his job. Prior to entering the residential program, the patient must complete at least a 48-hour detoxification program, and this is the reason he is admitted at this time. The patient was treated with Chlorazepate for cocaine withdrawal and agitation. He received Phenobarbital for cocaine-related insomnia. He was also treated with Thiamine hydrochloride and Allbee with vitamin C capsules. His admission drug screen was positive for cocaine and marijuana. For his persistent cocaine-related insomnia, he received L-tryptophan. His very controlling personality in detoxification gradually subsided over the next 72 hours, and he became very cooperative and interested in becoming fully invested in the chemical dependency rehabilitation program he was about to enter. He was discharged on day 4 after a difficult detoxification experience to enter the predicted month or longer residential program. If successful, this stay is to be followed with transition to a very strong outpatient day hospital rehabilitation program and later phase into a full 2-year aftercare program and lifelong Narcotics Anonymous meetings.

Principal Diagnosis: _____

Secondary Diagnoses: _____

Principal Procedure: _____

Secondary Procedure(s): _____

15

The patient is a 28-year-old male veteran of the Iraq war who served two tours of duty. He was referred to a Veterans Affairs Medical Center for evaluation. He experienced combat and survived two improvised-explosive-device (IED) explosions while riding in military vehicles. Four fellow soldier friends were killed in the two vehicle explosions. After returning from Iraq two years ago, the patient began experiencing anxiety-like symptoms, including a pounding heart, sweating, and trouble breathing on occasions. He also reported bad dreams of his war experiences. He had difficulty falling and staying asleep. He also reported trouble getting along with his family members and coworkers in his civilian job because of his angry outbursts over relatively minor things. He describes himself as "emotionally numb" and admits to having thoughts of and plans for suicide. The patient is diagnosed with chronic posttraumatic stress disorder with suicide ideation. To fully evaluate the patient and begin therapy, the patient is admitted to an inpatient unit. Over the next five days, the patient is treated with supportive psychotherapy and cognitive-behavioral therapy. At the time of discharge, the patient reported feeling better and is scheduled to continue receiving outpatient cognitive-behavior therapy.

Principal Diagnosis: _____

Secondary Diagnoses: _____

Principal Procedures: _____

Secondary Procedure(s): _____

16

The patient is a 22-year-old male brought to the emergency department (ED) by his probation officer, who said the patient told him the patient wanted to kill himself. The psychiatrist came to the ER and interviewed the patient. He documented the patient had recurring ego-dystonic thoughts, ambivalent feelings about his parents, was hearing voices, seeing visions, was depressed, and expressed a sense of hopelessness and a strong desire to end his life. The patient was hospitalized two years earlier for similar psychiatric complaints and had been shuffling back and forth between his parents' homes since that discharge. The patient said he had not gone back to his psychiatrist in the past six months since he was arrested for robbery but did like talking to his probation officer, which he thought "helped" him. The patient consented to be admitted to the psychiatric unit at the hospital. During his hospital stay, the patient started out as withdrawn and suspicious and continued to express his suicide ideation. His laboratory examinations were all reported as normal results. The patient authorized the release of his records from the hospital where he was hospitalized two years ago. The diagnoses documented by the previous physicians were consistent with what the current psychiatrist considered the young man's conditions, with the primary reason for being admitted on this occasion as the schizophrenia. Different medications were started and discontinued during the hospital stay until a particular combination of medications seemed to control the patient's thoughts and symptoms and allowed him to better participate in therapy and build a more trusting relationship with his father and therapist. The patient and the father agreed to continue outpatient counseling upon discharge. The final diagnoses provided by the psychiatrist in the patient's discharge summary were (1) undifferentiated type schizophrenia, (2) suicide ideation, and (3) anxious personality disorder. The therapies performed included individual cognitive-behavioral psychotherapy, group psychotherapy, and family mental health psychotherapy.

Principal Diagnosis: _____

Secondary Diagnoses: _____

Principal Procedure: _____

Secondary Procedure(s): _____

17

This is the second psychiatric admission for the 59-year-old white female who was admitted to the hospital because she had not been responding to outpatient treatment for her major depression that had been part of her life for over 20 years. The patient had become more withdrawn, isolated herself from friends and family, and lost interest in everything that had been important to her. She had trouble sleeping, was tired all the time, had a loss of appetite, felt weak, and had many somatic gastrointestinal complaints. She reported she had a difficult time getting started each morning and tended to feel better later in the afternoon and evening. An internal medicine consultation was performed that included many laboratory tests, cardiology exams, and gastrointestinal investigations. No abnormal findings were identified, so it was concluded there was no medical explanation for her symptoms. Her psychiatric treatment was primarily medication management with antidepressant and antianxiety medications started and discontinued in various combinations. Finally, on the day before discharge, the patient declared "you finally got it right" and the particular present medications relieved her symptoms and helped her feel optimistic about the future. The psychiatrist concluded the patient had a typical depressive diurnal pattern that meant her problems were more depressive in nature, but her response to certain medications indicated that an anxiety disorder was also present. The physician documented recurrent major depressive disorder, anxiety disorder, and somatization disorder. He described the procedures performed as mental health "medication management."

Principal Diagnosis: _____

Secondary Diagnoses: _____

Principal Procedures: _____

Secondary Procedure(s): _____

18

The patient is a 27-year-old female admitted to the hospital for treatment of her recurrent major depressive disorder with psychotic features. Her family has become concerned over her persistent suicidal ideation. The patient and her family are convinced that the current medications that the patient is taking are not adequately treating her condition. The patient consents to undergo electroconvulsive therapy. The patient is placed under general anesthesia and bilateral electrodes are placed on the patient's scalp. The stimulus is delivered, causing a single seizure lasting 30 seconds. The patient is monitored after the procedure to ensure her safe recovery. The patient's diagnoses are specified as major depressive disorder with psychotic features and suicidal ideation.

Principal Diagnosis: _____

Secondary Diagnoses: _____

Principal Procedures: _____

Secondary Procedure(s): _____

Chapter 6

Diseases of the Nervous System

Coding Scenarios for *Basic ICD-10-CM* and *ICD-10-PCS Coding Exercises*

The following case studies are organized following the sequence of the chapters in the ICD-10-CM Tabular List of Diseases and Injuries as published on the Centers for Disease Control and Prevention National Center for Health Statistics website (http://www.cdc.gov/nchs/icd/icd10cm.htm). The objective of this book is to provide the student with more detailed clinical information to code, rather than one- or two-line diagnosis and procedure statements.

ICD-10-CM diagnosis codes are to be assigned to both the inpatient hospital admission and the outpatient visit case studies. In this book, the ICD-10-PCS procedure codes are to be assigned only to the inpatient hospital admission cases. In actual practice, outpatient cases are assigned CPT/HCPCS codes. The ICD-10-PCS codes are only required for inpatient procedures. In the answer key for the exercises, the Alphabetic Index entry is listed after the code to indicate the main terms and subterms used to locate the code that must be verified in the ICD-10-CM Tabular List or in the ICD-10-PCS Code Tables prior to assigning the code.

1

An 85-year-old female was brought to the family physician's office by her family to better treat the symptoms of her severe dementia due to Alzheimer's disease. She is becoming increasingly difficult to manage at home. At times, she becomes aggressive and attempts to strike family members with household objects. She also has repeatedly wandered away from the home's backyard and has had to be located by calling police to assist in the search. The family members have refused to admit the patient to a long-term care facility. The family members will continue to care for the woman in their home. The physician's diagnosis is late onset Alzheimer's dementia with behavioral disturbances such as aggression and wandering.

First-Listed Diagnosis: _____

Secondary Diagnoses: _____

2

The patient is an 18-year-old male with spastic cerebral palsy with quadriplegia. He is brought to the Neurology Clinic for ongoing management. The patient also has recurrent seizures and asthma treated sporadically with an aerosol. He had a gastrostomy tube placed five years ago and an intrathecal pump for baclofen inserted last year. The patient also had intermittent fecal impactions. During this examination the patient was found to be alert but could not answer questions, which is his normal state. He was not in any acute distress. The sites of the intrathecal pump and G-tube were clean and clear of infection. The patient has contracture deformities of his upper extremities with flexion of his elbows as well as clenching of his fingers. His skin was examined, especially on his back, buttocks, and legs, and was found to be free of any pressure sores. The patient was continued on his present medications: baclofen, Keppra, albuterol, and milk of magnesia and will return to clinic in six months or sooner if medically necessary.

First-Listed Diagnosis: _____

Secondary Diagnoses: _____

3

The patient is a 65-year-old male with a past medical history of progressive Parkinson's disease for the past several months with a history of Parkinson's disease for the past 23 years. He was brought to the emergency department by his wife because of his increasing rigidity, loss of speech, and a new development—his inability to walk and stand. The patient was admitted to inpatient status by his primary care physician. The patient was seen by his neurologist, who adjusted the patient's antiparkinson agent, carbidopa-levodopa, to 25 mg/200 mg. On physical examination, a small abscess was noted over the left lower back area. The patient's wife stated it had been present for several months and was likely irritated by the transfer belt that had been used on the patient for gait stability, but the area was not as red at home as it appeared in the hospital. Over the next three days, the cutaneous abscess bloomed in size and began draining. The patient was recommended incision and drainage of the abscess while the patient was in the hospital because of the difficulty of bringing the patient back to the hospital as an outpatient for day surgery. A surgeon examined the patient and agreed with the plan. Because the patient was almost completely stiff and contracted, the surgeon recommended performing the surgery under general anesthesia for the patient's comfort. After general anesthesia induction in surgery, the patient was placed in the right lateral decubitus position, and the area was infiltrated with 0.5% plain Marcaine. An elliptical incision was made, and the cutaneous abscess was unroofed and drained. Aerobic culture was taken. The wound was irrigated and hemostasis obtained. The subcutaneous wound was packed with saline-soaked 2 × 2 gauze, and a pressure dressing was applied. The patient tolerated the procedure well and was taken to the recovery room in good condition. Postoperatively, the patient was placed on intravenous antibiotics for 48 hours and then discharged in good condition with prescriptions for his new antiparkinson agent and an oral antibiotic. He will be followed by home health nursing for postoperative wound care.

Principal Diagnosis: _____

Secondary Diagnoses: _____

Principal Procedure: _____

Secondary Procedure(s): _____

4

An 8-year-old male was seen in the pediatric neurologist's office for his absence attack or petit mal childhood epilepsy. The mother reports two episodes of motor seizures over the past month that consisted of localized twitching of his right arm and leg. The patient has an older brother (age 18 years) who had the same type of epilepsy during childhood but has been seizure-free for four years. The young patient is treated with mild anti-seizure medications and is scheduled for a repeat EEG in two weeks.

First-Listed Diagnosis: _____

Secondary Diagnoses: _____

5

The patient, a 75-year-old male, was brought to the emergency department with progressive deterioration of his overall mental and physical status, lethargy, and difficulty swallowing. The patient's family continued to try to feed the patient. The patient was found to be hypothermic with a temperature of 33.7 °C and hypotensive with an initial pressure of 58/34 mm Hg that did not improve much with treatment. The patient was admitted to the intensive care unit, but his blood pressure and overall status did not improve with two liters of fluids, and he was started on Levophed and antibiotics. A chest x-ray showed a right lower lobe infiltrate consistent with aspiration pneumonia, probably due to food. The attending physician concluded that aspiration pneumonia was present. The patient was known to have Lewy body dementia, bed-bound status, and a stage III pressure ulcer of the sacrum. Upon discharge the patient's diagnoses were severe sepsis with septic shock, acute renal failure, acute hepatic failure, and aspiration pneumonia. Given the patient's overall very poor prognosis, the patient was made DNR status by his physician after discussing the situation with the patient's family. On hospital day 2, the family decided to elect hospice care with no further aggressive care to be ordered. The patient was transferred to the inpatient hospice unit at the hospital.

Principal Diagnosis: _____

Secondary Diagnoses: _____

Principal Procedure: _____

Secondary Procedure(s): _____

6

A 42-year-old female patient was admitted to the hospital for surgery to correct her long-standing trigeminal neuralgia. She also had essential hypertension treated with atenolol medication. The patient has suffered from unremitting facial pain for the past eight months and has failed to respond to medical therapy. The patient was given the option of continued medical management with the drug carbamazepine, gamma knife radiosurgery, or open microvascular decompression to release the trigeminal nerve. She selected the open surgery to release the nerve. She was taken to surgery, and a right side suboccipital craniotomy was performed. Microvascular decompressive release of the trigeminal nerve was performed after clearly visualizing the trigeminal nerve. The patient was transferred to the intensive care unit for overnight monitoring. In the ICU she had serial neurologic monitoring, blood pressure control to minimize hypertensive-related bleeding, aggressive pulmonary toilet, as well as stress gastritis prevention and mechanical DVT prophylaxis treatment. No complications were experienced. The patient was transferred to a surgical unit and was discharged in two days to be followed up at home by home health intermittent nursing services.

Principal Diagnosis: _____

Secondary Diagnoses: _____

Principal Procedure: _____

Secondary Procedure(s): _____

7

The patient is a 60-year-old female who comes to her primary physician's office complaining of right-sided facial droop. She had decreased eye blinking on the right side and could not completely close her right eye. She was drooling out of the right side of her mouth. She also complained of a headache with throbbing. Based on these complaints and the physical exam, the physician diagnosed the patient with Bell's Palsy, facial palsy or seventh cranial nerve palsy. The patient was placed on oral prednisone but must be watched carefully as the patient has type 2 diabetes and the prednisone could elevate the blood sugar. The patient takes glipizide orally for the diabetes. The patient was advised to wear gauze over the right eye at night to avoid drying out the eye and getting a corneal ulcer. She was also told to use artificial tears to moisten the eye. The patient is also a two-pack-a-day smoker and was, once again, strongly encouraged to quit smoking cigarettes. The patient was given a prescription for Zyban to take as the patient was trying to cut down on her smoking. The patient was sent to the outpatient laboratory after the office visit to have blood drawn for the Lyme titer and sedimentation rate that were ordered by the physician. An appointment was made for the patient to return to the office in two weeks.

First-Listed Diagnosis: _____

Secondary Diagnoses: _____

Principal Procedure: _____

Secondary Procedure(s): _____

8

A 4-year-old male was brought to the emergency department by his mother, who stated the child had become ill very rapidly over the course of one day. He had been treated for a right ear infection at the pediatric clinic last week. Upon physical examination, the emergency department physician noted a high fever, drowsiness, and stiffness in the neck. The mother reported the child had said his head hurt and also reported that he had vomited at home. The physician noted slight rash on the child's upper trunk and axilla bilaterally. Suspicious for meningitis, a pediatric consult was requested and obtained. The emergency department physician and pediatrician obtained consent for a spinal tap and the child was admitted to the pediatric unit.

Over the next couple of days, the pediatrician made the diagnosis of bacterial meningitis with the causative organism of *Haemophilus influenzae (H. influenzae)* based on the physical findings and the examination of the cerebrospinal fluid obtained by the spinal tap. The child is treated with intravenous antibiotics and other medications as well as supportive care. The pediatrician found the acute suppurative otitis media still needed treatment. The child made a full recovery but will be followed closely as an outpatient to determine whether any effects of the meningitis, such as hearing loss, occur later. The child was discharged to the care of his mother.

Principal Diagnosis: _____

Secondary Diagnoses: _____

Principal Procedure: _____

Secondary Procedure(s): _____

9

A 75-year-old patient is admitted to the hospital with the acute onset of neurologic symptoms including double vision, speech difficulty, and loss of balance. Because the patient had a cerebral infarction five years previously, with residual hemiparesis on her left non-dominant side, the physician is concerned the patient is having another stroke. Physical and neurologic examination along with CT scanning and blood tests prove the patient has not had another stroke. The physician describes this episode of illness as a "TIA" or transient ischemic attack. The patient's symptoms completely resolve, but she is seen by a physical therapist for the residual hemiparesis on her left side that was the result of her previous cerebral infarction. The patient's essential hypertension is also treated. The stage II chronic kidney disease due to her type 2 diabetes mellitus was monitored and treated. The patient is discharged from the hospital on day 3 for follow up in her physician's office in one week.

Principal Diagnosis: _____

Secondary Diagnoses: _____

Principal Procedure: _____

Secondary Procedure(s): _____

10

The patient is a 35-year-old female who was in a motor vehicle crash four months ago. She was treated in the emergency department of a local hospital and in this physician's office following the crash and had been diagnosed with concussion. The patient reported to her physician during this visit that she has had headaches almost every day since the crash. She stated that over-the-counter pain medication helps relieve the pain but she is concerned that the headaches are still present. The physician examines the patient and makes the diagnosis of "post-concussion syndrome with chronic headaches due to old intracranial injury from a previous vehicle crash." The patient is referred to a neurologist for a consultation and will return to this physician's office in two weeks to determine the next course of treatment.

First-Listed Diagnosis: _____

Secondary Diagnoses: _____

11

The patient is a 78-year-old male who was admitted to the hospital today for the implantation of a dual-chamber permanent pacemaker device. The patient had a several-month history of syncope that was investigated on a couple of encounters. Finally, it was determined that the patient's neurocardiogenic syncope was caused by carotid sinus syndrome, which another physician referred to as carotid sinus hypersensitivity. The dual-chamber cardiac pacemaker was implanted into the subcutaneous tissue of the patient's chest, followed by insertion of leads into the right atrium and right ventricle via a percutaneous approach to treat the carotid sinus syndrome. The patient had no complications from the procedure and was discharged home with an appointment with his cardiologist in 10 days.

Principal Diagnosis: _____

Secondary Diagnoses: _____

Principal Procedure: _____

Secondary Procedure(s): _____

12

A 45-year-old male was admitted to the hospital for a decompressive laminectomy to treat his long-standing lumbar spinal stenosis. The back pain from the spinal stenosis has not been relieved by pain management treatment or physical therapy. The man has been off work for three months due to the chronic back pain and agreed to the spinal surgery as his last option to relieve the pain and support his family. The patient is healthy and has no other medical problems, including any neurogenic claudication associated with the spinal stenosis. The surgery was performed on the day of admission and involved removal of a small portion of a lumbar disc, open approach. During the surgery, a dural tear was noted as the result of an unintended durotomy. The tear was immediately repaired during the same procedure. The patient was informed of the unintended durotomy and the necessary repair. Otherwise the patient had no complications from the procedure and recovered well enough to go home in three days. The patient will be seen in his surgeon's office in one week.

Principal Diagnosis: _____

Secondary Diagnoses: _____

Principal Procedure: _____

Secondary Procedure(s): _____

13

The patient is a 60-year-old male farmer who was treated a month ago for the apparent toxic effects of herbicide chemicals that he was applying to his crops. Since that time the patient has had severe vertigo, headaches, nausea, and loss of sensation in his hands and feet. The patient was admitted to evaluate the relationship between his past toxic exposure and his current symptoms. The most recent toxicology studies indicated a moderate level of herbicides in the blood—less than one month ago when it was initially tested. The physician documented the final diagnosis as toxic polyneuropathy due to herbicide toxicity. Medications were prescribed to manage the symptoms the patient continued to experience, and the patient will return to the physician's office for additional blood tests in one month. In the interim, the patient is advised not to operate machinery or drive a vehicle.

Principal Diagnosis: _____

Secondary Diagnoses: _____

Principal Procedure: _____

Secondary Procedure(s): _____

14

A 35-year-old male was admitted to the hospital. The admitting diagnosis documented on the history and physical examination report was "chronic pain syndrome and chronic lower back pain with exacerbation of lower back pain and lower extremity pain." Also included in the patient's history is the fact that the patient was injured in a serious motor vehicle crash three years ago and has had back pain ever since that injury. However, the patient's pain has increased over the past three months and has become excruciating over the past week. The patient was admitted to the hospital specifically for pain management. The patient received intravenous and intramuscular pain medications as well as a peripheral nerve block to manage his pain, which he reported as much improved at the time of discharge. The peripheral nerve block involved percutaneous injection of a regional anesthetic. The final diagnosis written by the physician was acute exacerbation of chronic pain syndrome, chronic lower back pain, and lower extremity pain, both right and left legs. The physician also wrote that the pain was likely the consequence of sympathetic lumbar spinal nerve root damage from the injuries sustained in the motor vehicle crash.

Principal Diagnosis: _____

Secondary Diagnoses: _____

Principal Procedure: _____

Secondary Procedure(s): _____

15

A 20-year-old male college student was brought to the emergency department complaining of a sudden onset headache, fever, and stiffness with pain in the neck. He had been treated in the college health service center for an ear infection in the past week. After admission, the patient also complained of chest pain, fatigue, cough, and nausea. A diagnostic lumbar puncture was performed and the findings were positive for meningitis. A chest x-ray revealed pneumonia. Sputum and spinal fluid cultures grew the pneumococcus organism (*Streptococcus pneumoniae*). The physical examination also confirmed the presence of acute otitis media of both ears. The patient was treated with intravenous antibiotics for the infections. The discharge diagnoses written by the physician were pneumococcal meningitis with pneumococcal pneumonia and acute bilateral suppurative otitis media.

Principal Diagnosis: _____

Secondary Diagnoses: _____

Principal Procedure: _____

Secondary Procedure(s): _____

16

The patient is admitted to the hospital and diagnosed with chronic postviral fatigue syndrome. The patient is known to have had infectious mononucleosis several months previously and has never felt well since that time. Laboratory tests and neurologic studies are used to evaluate the patient's condition and possible underlying cause. The physician concludes that the current condition is a late effect of chronic Epstein-Barr infection. The patient was discharged home for rest and recovery.

Principal Diagnosis: _____

Secondary Diagnoses: _____

Principal Procedure: _____

Secondary Procedure(s): _____

17

The patient is a 56-year-old male who was seen in his internist's office complaining of weakness and tingling sensations in both of his legs. Five days later the patient called his internist to say the weakness had spread to both his arms and his upper body and that is when the internist admitted the patient to the hospital. Ten days ago the patient had a viral respiratory infection. Given that fact and the sudden unexpected onset of the symmetrical weakness and abnormal sensations that spread from both legs to his upper body and both arms, the internist suspected the onset of Guillain-Barre Syndrome (GBS). A neurology consultant examined the patient and concluded the patient was having an initial attack of GBS. A diagnostic spinal tap was performed which revealed more protein in the spinal fluid than usual. The internist and neurologist recommended a treatment with plasmapheresis, where the patient's blood is drawn and then the plasma is removed and the blood cells are infused back into the patient. The patient was discharged with the final diagnosis of GBS to be followed up within the offices of the internist and the neurologist. The patient was scheduled for a nerve conduction study and physical therapy as an outpatient.

Principal Diagnosis: _____

Secondary Diagnoses: _____

Principal Procedure: _____

Secondary Procedure(s): _____

18

The patient, a 52-year-old female, is referred by her family practice physician to the neurologist for a consultation in her office with the reason for the referral as "possible spasmodic torticollis." Upon examination, the neurologist found the patient's neck muscles were contracted involuntarily, causing her head to turn to one side with her chin pointing toward her shoulder. The neurologist learned by taking the patient's history that the patient's mother had the same condition for the past 10 years of her life. The neurologist concluded the patient had spasmodic torticollis. The patient was very upset and frightened that she would have the same fate as her mother. The neurologist reassured the patient there are more treatments available to her than were available to her mother 30 years ago. The patient was given a prescription for a mild muscle relaxant, prescription for physical therapy, and an order for the fitting of a special neck brace. The neurologist recommended injections of botulinum toxin into the affected muscles but the patient wanted to think it over and was asked to make a follow-up appointment in one month or sooner if she decided to have the Botox injections. The patient was also given information about the National Spasmodic Torticollis Association that offers patient education and support to people with spasmodic torticollis.

First-Listed Diagnosis: _____

Secondary Diagnoses: _____

19

The patient is a 65-year-old male who was brought to the emergency department by his wife after he complained of acute worsening of his chronic lower back pain and a sudden difficulty in urinating. The patient is also experiencing numbness and weakness in his legs. The patient states that he has been diagnosed with lumbar spinal stenosis with neurogenic claudication in the past. Imaging studies are performed and severe spinal stenosis at the level of L5 is confirmed. The patient is diagnosed with cauda equina syndrome and is taken to the operating room for an emergent decompression of the spinal cord. An L5 laminectomy is performed to relieve the pressure on the spinal cord. The patient is kept in the hospital for further monitoring of his neurological condition after the surgery. The patient's final diagnoses are cauda equina syndrome and lumbar spinal stenosis with neurogenic claudication.

Principal Diagnosis: _____

Secondary Diagnoses: _____

Principal Procedure: _____

Secondary Procedures: _____

Chapter 7

Diseases of the Eye and Adnexa

Coding Scenarios for *Basic ICD-10-CM* *and ICD-10-PCS Coding Exercises*

The following case studies are organized following the sequence of the chapters in the ICD-10-CM Tabular List of Diseases and Injuries as published on the Centers for Disease Control and Prevention National Center for Health Statistics website (http://www.cdc.gov /nchs/icd/icd10cm.htm). The objective of this book is to provide the student with more detailed clinical information to code, rather than one- or two-line diagnosis and procedure statements.

ICD-10-CM diagnosis codes are to be assigned to both the inpatient hospital admission and the outpatient visit case studies. In this book, the ICD-10-PCS procedure codes are to be assigned only to the inpatient hospital admission cases. In actual practice, outpatient cases are assigned CPT/HCPCS codes. The ICD-10-PCS codes are only required for inpatient procedures. In the answer key for the exercises, the Alphabetic Index entry is listed after the code to indicate the main terms and sub-terms used to locate the code that must be verified in the ICD-10-CM Tabular List or in the ICD-10-PCS Code Tables prior to assigning the code.

1

A patient is seen in the eye clinic at the University Medical Center. After taking a thorough history and conducting an extensive physical eye examination, the physician orders several tests to be done over the next week. At the conclusion of the visit, the physician writes the diagnosis of mild bilateral open angle glaucoma.

First-Listed Diagnosis: _____

Secondary Diagnoses: _____

2

The patient is an 88-year-old female who was remarkably alert and cogent for her age. She was living with her grandson, an Army captain, until he was deployed overseas. She now lives alone in her own home and has no relatives in the area. The type of procedure planned for the patient could usually be performed on an outpatient basis but, because of her lack of support, the patient's procedure is scheduled as an inpatient procedure. The patient was diagnosed with retinal detachment, single break in the right eye. The patient has vision of 20/400 in the right eye. She is status post cataract extraction in the left eye. The procedure performed was a pars plana vitrectomy, gas/fluid exchange with autologous serum injection, C#3/F#8 gas injection, which are components of the procedure of cryoretinopexy of the right eye. The procedure was performed percutaneously to repair the detached retina using intravenous moderate sedation. At the conclusion of the procedure, injections of dexamethasone and gentamicin were administered subconjunctivally. The patient was kept in the hospital two days, until Friday when a neighbor was able to pick up the patient and care for her over the weekend.

Principal Diagnosis: _____

Secondary Diagnoses: _____

Principal Procedure: _____

Secondary Procedure(s): _____

3

A 40-year-old female came to the ophthalmologist's office last week complaining of a fleshy fold of tissue that appeared in the corner of her left eye near her nose and started growing toward the center of her eye. She reported that it had begun to obstruct her vision. Upon examination, the physician found a progressive peripheral pterygium that starts in the conjunctiva and attaches to the cornea as it grows. The patient was scheduled for an excision of the pterygium of the left eye with corneal graft. This will be performed next week at the outpatient surgery center.

First-Listed Diagnosis: _____

Secondary Diagnoses: _____

4

A 3-year-old female was admitted to the hospital for strabismus surgery. The physician states her condition is concomitant convergent strabismus or early-acquired esotropia, monocular. The physician described the deviation as 25 prism diopters and stable. The child was otherwise healthy and able to receive general anesthesia. Surgery was recommended to reestablish binocular vision. The extraocular muscle surgery performed was an open unilateral resection of a 6-mm portion of the lateral rectus muscle on the left eye. The child was discharged in the care of her parents on the day after surgery.

Principal Diagnosis: _____

Secondary Diagnoses: _____

Principal Procedure: _____

Secondary Procedure(s): _____

5

A 50-year-old male who has had type 2 diabetes for more than 10 years complains of vision problems that are worse on the left side. He is seen in the ophthalmologist's office upon the recommendation of his family physician. The patient's diabetes is treated with oral medications and diet. After examining the patient, the physician concludes that the patient has moderate nonproliferative diabetic retinopathy as a result of his type 2 diabetes.

First-Listed Diagnosis: _____

Secondary Diagnoses: _____

6

The patient is a 30-year-old male who has chronic allergic conjunctivitis, which causes him to rub his eyes continually. He had bilateral entropion repair four years ago and did well for at least three years. Over the last few months, he has had problems with rubbing of his right eye and with discharge from it. On examination by the ophthalmologist in her office, he was noted to have significant right upper eyelid laxity. He also has inversion of his right lower lashes. Surgical correction of his eyelid problems, his right upper and right lower lid entropion was discussed. The patient agreed to the proposed procedure. The physician's nurse will schedule the procedure and call the patient with the date and time of the procedure to be performed in the ambulatory surgery center in the next week. The physician provided recommendations on how to relieve the irritation from the chronic allergic conjunctivitis.

First-Listed Diagnosis: _____

Secondary Diagnoses: _____

7

The patient is a 40-year-old female with Down syndrome who was admitted to the hospital for a repeat penetrating keratoplasty (corneal transplant). The patient lives 120 miles away from the hospital with elderly parents and, because of the distance to be traveled, was being admitted instead of having an outpatient procedure. The patient had a penetrating keratoplasty on the left eye in the past. She developed a corneal ulcer and perforation, requiring a repeat penetrating keratoplasty via percutaneous approach in the left eye. The patient did understand the procedure and agreed to it, but the consent form was signed by her father. At the time of the corneal transplant it was noted again that her eye was soft and appeared to be perforated, with a flat anterior chamber. The donor cornea was prepared. The previous donor cornea was removed from the patient's eye. Four interrupted 10-0 nylon cardinal sutures were placed to secure the new donor tissue to the host, and a symmetrical rhomboid crease on the donor was noted. A total of 12 more interrupted 10-0 nylon sutures were placed equally distant from each other to secure the donor to the host, and the chamber was intermittently formed. The wound was checked for leaks, and none were seen. Subtenon injections of 80 mg Depo-Medrol and 40 mg gentamicin were administered as part of the procedure. Vigamox eye drops were placed in the eye. A bandage contact lens was placed in the eye with a shield on top. The patient was awakened and transferred to the recovery room. She stayed in the hospital overnight for pain control and management. She was examined the next morning by the ophthalmic surgeon and discharged to the care of her adult brother and parents to be driven home.

Principal Diagnosis: _____

Secondary Diagnoses: _____

Principal Procedure: _____

Secondary Procedure(s): _____

8

The patient is a 35-year-old male construction worker who suffered a traumatic intraocular foreign body and secondary cataract formation about one year ago. The eye condition was successfully surgically repaired after the injury. However, he is intolerant of contact lens wear and spectacle correction of his aphakia primarily because of his occupation and the safety equipment he must wear. His visual acuity with a contact lens in place is about 20/40. Without his eyeglasses or contact lens his visual acuity is 20/400. During this office visit, the physician recommended another surgical procedure—a capsulectomy and sector iridectomy and secondary sulcus intraocular lens placement. The patient was undecided about more surgery but agreed to think it over and will call the office if he decides to proceed with surgery. The physician listed traumatic aphakia with pupillary membranes, left eye with status post cataract extraction as the diagnoses on the encounter form.

First-Listed Diagnosis: _____

Secondary Diagnoses: _____

9

The patient is a 68-year-old male with a visually significant nuclear sclerotic cataract in addition to chronic angle closure glaucoma (severe stage) in his right eye that requires multiple glaucoma medications, including pills and drops. After discussion with his ophthalmologist in her office, the patient agreed to have surgery, specifically the cataract extraction with a trabeculectomy with mitomycin-C. The procedure was scheduled for the following week at the free-standing ambulatory surgery center near the patient's home.

First-Listed Diagnosis: _____

Secondary Diagnoses: _____

10

A 50-year-old female had a malignant skin tumor removed from her left upper eyelid about one year ago, followed by lid reconstruction surgery. Due to scarring of the left upper eyelid, the patient was examined in the ophthalmologist's office. The ophthalmologist found the patient to have several conditions, specifically the cicatricial entropion, cicatricial ectropion, exposure keratoconjunctivitis, and scarring from the previous surgery all on the left upper eyelid. The physician proposed an excision and repair of the eyelid with adjacent tissue transfer, correction of the lid retraction, and possibly a full-thickness graft to repair the eyelid completely. The ophthalmologist explained that further reconstruction may also be necessary. The patient agrees to read the educational material provided by the ophthalmologist and call the physician assistant to schedule the procedure if she decides to proceed.

First-Listed Diagnosis: _____

Secondary Diagnoses: _____

11

The patient, a 45-year-old male, was seen in the intensive care unit by the ophthalmologist in consultation. The patient was acutely ill with sepsis and infected joints. The patient was noted to have a very red swollen eye. The consultant concluded the patient had acute panophthalmitis and received consent from the patient's wife to perform an anterior sclerotomy and drainage of the right eye vitreous as well as an intra-vitreal injection of anti-infective agents into the eye. The patient was taken to surgery and the eye was examined again. There was significant pus in the anterior chamber with layered hypopyon inferiorly. No view of the posterior segment was possible. An ultrasound of the eye showed the retina to be flat. A lid speculum was placed in the right eye and Betadine dripped on the conjunctival surface. A needle was placed through the temporal pars plana into the mid vitreous cavity and 0.5 cc of liquid vitreous was aspirated without difficulty. Vancomycin 1 mg in 0.1 cc and ceftazidime 2 mg in 0.1 cc were each injected into the mid-vitreous by way of the temporal pars plana without difficulty. The vitreous sample was sent for culture. The eye was protected with a dressing for surgical recovery.

Code only for the eye condition and procedure.

Ophthalmic Diagnosis Code: _____

Principal Procedure: _____

Secondary Procedure(s): _____

12

The patient is a 75-year-old female who has experienced increasingly hooded lateral vision due to dermatochalasis. This was interfering with her driving her car. She also had left eyebrow and upper eyelid ptosis due to Bell's palsy. The patient was seen in the ophthalmologist's office upon recommendation of her primary care physician. The physician explained the proposed blepharoplasty to treat the bilateral upper eyelid dermatochalasis, which was worse on the left, and the procedure to repair the paralytic ptosis of the left upper eyelid. The patient signed the consent for surgery and agreed to a surgery date two weeks later at a local hospital for the outpatient procedure.

First-Listed Diagnosis: _____

Secondary Diagnoses: _____

13

The patient is a 26-year-old male seen in the ophthalmologist's office upon request of his primary care physician. The patient sustained an accidental chemical burn to the right eye several months ago. The burn has healed, but the patient has increased intraocular pressure in the right eye. This moderate stage glaucoma is the sequela of the chemical burn trauma. The intraocular pressure is not controlled with conventional medications. Therefore, the recommendation was made by the ophthalmologist to place an Ahmed valve in the eye to reduce the pressure. The patient consented to the procedure and agreed to meet the physician the next morning at the outpatient surgery center for the procedure.

First-Listed Diagnosis: _____

Secondary Diagnoses: _____

14

The patient is a 75-year-old male who had a right penetrating keratoplasty (corneal transplant) recently for a previous infectious keratitis. He was seen today in the Corneal Disease Clinic and found to have a ruptured descemetocele in the right eye. This problem is a mechanical complication due to the corneal graft. The patient had a prior temporary tarsorrhaphy with sutures pulling through. The patient agreed to the recommended surgery of a more permanent tarsorrhaphy to prevent potential exposure keratopathy. The patient will meet the physician later the same day at the outpatient surgery center to have the procedure performed.

First-Listed Diagnosis: _____

Secondary Diagnoses: _____

15

The patient is an 80-year-old female who has been treated at the University Medical Center Glaucoma Clinic for many years. She has been seen several times in the past few months with increasing right eye pain. The patient's chronic eye pain exists in a visually useless eye. The severe eye pain is the result of long-standing glaucoma, which is now considered absolute glaucoma. The patient is requiring increasing amounts of pain medications and is very tired of the constant eye pain. Surgical options were discussed with the patient and her daughter. Today, the patient was admitted to the hospital and underwent an open evisceration of the ocular contents with placement of an ocular implant. Admission was warranted since the physician was concerned about post-operative bleeding due to the patient's long-standing hemophilia A history.

Principal Diagnosis: _____

Secondary Diagnoses: _____

Principal Procedure: _____

Secondary Procedure(s): _____

16

The patient is a 50-year-old female who made an appointment with an ophthalmologist because she thought she was having vision changes and wondered if she had cataracts. The ophthalmologist did a complete bilateral eye exam including dilation of the lens and concluded the patient had tiny flakes built up in the front of both eyes, leaving deposits on both lenses. The condition was worse on the right eye, but present in both eyes. The ophthalmologist explained this condition was known as "pseudoexfoliation syndrome." She described it as a condition when flaky material comes off the outer layer of the lens capsule of the eye. This material usually clogs the angle between the cornea and the iris. This in turn blocks the drainage system of the eye and leads to increased intraocular pressure and can cause glaucoma. The ophthalmologist explained the patient was six more times likely to develop glaucoma because of the exfoliations. The good news was, while the patient did have mildly elevated intraocular pressures in both eyes, she did not have high enough pressures to make the diagnosis of glaucoma at this time. The ophthalmologist prescribed a medication for the patient and requested that she return for another exam in six months or sooner if she noticed more changes in her vision. The patient asked if this condition was the same as having a cataract, and the ophthalmologist explained that some physicians may call it a specific type of cataract, but the concern was more about the potential for glaucoma and the need for laser therapy and filtering surgery in the future.

First-Listed Diagnosis: _____

Secondary Diagnoses: _____

17

The patient is an 82-year-old female who was known to have a vitreous hemorrhage of her left eye. She was seen in her ophthalmologist's office to check on the status of her left eye. She said her left eye vision was worse than at the time of the last office visit. During this examination, the patient was found to have a traction detachment of the retina in her left eye too. The patient was counseled on her options to treat her left eye and she agreed to surgery. She was tentatively scheduled in four days for the endolaser photocoagulation of the left retina. First the patient had an appointment made with her primary care physician to get medical clearance for surgery because she had hypertension and rheumatic heart disease with abnormal EKGs in the past. The ophthalmologist documented the diagnoses for this office visit as (1) left vitreous hemorrhage, (2) traction retinal detachment left eye, (3) hypertension, (4) abnormal EKG and, (5) rheumatic heart disease.

First-Listed Diagnosis: _____

Secondary Diagnoses: _____

18

The patient is a 75-year-old female who is currently in the hospital undergoing treatment for dehydration due to food poisoning. The patient was found to have a large, painful hordeolum on her external right lower eyelid. Due to the size of the pustule and the pain it was causing the patient, the decision was made to incise and drain the hordeolum.

Code only the eye diagnosis and procedure.

Ophthalmic Diagnosis: _____

Ophthalmic Procedure: _____

Chapter 8

Diseases of the Ear and Mastoid Process

Coding Scenarios for *Basic ICD-10-CM and ICD-10-PCS Coding Exercises*

The following case studies are organized following the sequence of the chapters in the ICD-10-CM Tabular List of Diseases and Injuries as published on the Centers for Disease Control and Prevention National Center for Health Statistics website (http://www.cdc.gov /nchs/icd/icd10cm.htm). The objective of this book is to provide the student with more detailed clinical information to code, rather than one- or two-line diagnosis and procedure statements.

ICD-10-CM diagnosis codes are to be assigned to both the inpatient hospital admission and the outpatient visit case studies. In this book, the ICD-10-PCS procedure codes are to be assigned only to the inpatient hospital admission cases. In actual practice, outpatient cases are assigned CPT/HCPCS codes. The ICD-10-PCS codes are only required for inpatient procedures. In the answer key for the exercises, the Alphabetic Index entry is listed after the code to indicate the main terms and subterms used to locate the code that must be verified in the ICD-10-CM Tabular List or in the ICD-10-PCS Code Tables prior to assigning the code.

1

A 30-year-old male who is a member of a well-known musical band is seen in the "Performing Arts Clinic" at the University Medical Center. The musician complained of ringing, buzzing, and clicking in his ears and hearing loss on the right side. The musician said he was told by other musicians that he had "rock and roll deafness." Upon examination and audiometric testing consisting of auditory processing using a computer, the physician diagnosed the patient as having sensorineural hearing loss of the right ear as a result of acoustic trauma from performing loud music over the past 12 years. His left ear was fine. The patient was advised to return for further evaluation and possible hearing aid fitting because this type of sensorineural deafness is likely to be permanent.

First-Listed Diagnosis: _____

Secondary Diagnoses: _____

2

The patient is a 60-year-old male who is seen in his primary care physician's office complaining of a buzzing and hissing sound in his right ear. The sounds make hearing difficult out of the same ear. The patient thinks sometimes the sounds are in both ears but definitely worse in the right ear. An extensive history is taken from the patient and it was determined the patient has not had any ear infections, wax in the ears, or foreign body in the ear. Medically the patient did not have a history of cardiovascular disease, anemia, or hypothyroidism that can have a relationship to tinnitus. Other risk factors discovered were that the patient is a farmer who is around noisy equipment, and he had a head injury five years ago when he fell down a long flight of stairs. The patient agreed to go to the local hospital for a comprehensive audiologic assessment and a CT scan of the temporal bone. Depending on the findings, an MRI scan of the head may be ordered later. The physician advised the patient that treatment for tinnitus is usually directed to the underlying disease. If an underlying disease is not found, the patient may find that a hearing aid suppresses the tinnitus. The patient agrees to a follow-up appointment in one week after completion of the outpatient tests ordered. The physician's diagnosis for the encounter is right ear tinnitus.

First-Listed Diagnosis: _____

Secondary Diagnoses: _____

3

An 82-year-old female is seen in the ENT physician's office at the request of her primary care physician. The patient is complaining of short episodes of dizziness that occur when the patient turns over in bed or attempts to get out of bed or out of her recliner chair. She feels lightheaded and nauseous, but all except the dizziness passes if she sits still for a few minutes before attempting to ambulate. The patient had the same symptoms a year ago but they disappeared as suddenly as they occurred. Prior to coming to the ENT physician's office, the patient had outpatient testing completed, specifically, hearing tests and tests of the vestibular system and an MRI scan of the brain. Upon considering all the facts of the case and the test results, the physician concluded the patient had benign paroxysmal positional vertigo of both ears. Various physical maneuvers and exercises were prescribed by the physician to relieve symptoms. The patient has a follow-up appointment with her primary care physician in two weeks.

First-Listed Diagnosis: _____

Secondary Diagnoses: _____

4

A 70-year-old male was seen in his primary care physician's office with complaints of not being able to hear out of both ears, but the right ear seemed to be worse. He said his ears felt "plugged." Several years ago, a different physician cleaned wax out of the patient's ears. Upon physical examination, the physician found the patient had bilateral hard impacted ear wax in both ears. The physician's nurse gently worked to soften and remove the ear wax out of both ears. Afterward, the patient commented on how much better his ears felt and how his hearing had improved. The patient and his wife were counseled on how to use over-the-counter ear drops to soften ear wax. The patient was encouraged to come back to the office if he felt that his ears were plugged in the future. The diagnosis for this encounter was documented as cerumen, both ears.

First-Listed Diagnosis: _____

Secondary Diagnoses: _____

5

The patient is a 25-year-old male who came to the emergency department (ED) on his own complaining that he was deaf in his left ear. When he was questioned, the patient was vague about his recent activities or illnesses or whether he suffered any trauma to his head. He claimed he did not have any trauma to his ear or any other medical problems. Upon examination, the physician found a small central perforation of the tympanic membrane of the left ear with some discharge in the ear canal. The right ear appeared normal. The patient did not have a primary care physician or health insurance. The patient was advised that the perforation was small and would probably heal on its own but he was strongly encouraged to keep the appointment made for him at the local public health clinic. He was also advised to avoid getting water in his ear and to avoid any potential for trauma to his head because if the perforation did not heal he could have permanent hearing loss. The discharge diagnosis documented on the ED record was small central perforation of the left tympanic membrane.

First-Listed Diagnosis: _____

Secondary Diagnoses: _____

6

The patient is a 28-year-old female who has a complicated otologic history. She had recent surgery by another otorhinolaryngologist where a myringotomy tube was placed with difficulty. The patient noticed significant hearing loss in her left ear after the procedure and presented to this ENT physician in his office for evaluation. Upon examination it was noted that the patient had a retained myringotomy tube and possible perforation of the tympanic membrane. There was also marked crusting of the tympanic membrane. The patient's hearing was tested, and she was found to have significant mixed hearing loss as well as a drop in sensorineural hearing in the higher frequencies. The diagnoses written by the physician in the patient's record were (1) left side only sensorineural hearing loss, (2) chronic serous otitis media, left and (3) possible perforation of tympanic membrane, left. The patient consented to a left exploratory tympanotomy with removal of the myringotomy tube and possible placement of a paper patch on the tympanic membrane. The procedure will be performed in two days at the ambulatory surgery center.

First-Listed Diagnosis: _____

Secondary Diagnoses: _____

7

The patient is a 20-year-old male who has a long history of left chronic otitis media. The patient has failed numerous medical treatments. During the examination in the ENT physician's office, he was found to have a large cholesteatoma filling up the left auditory canal. The left external canal was also filled with pus. This physician has treated the patient for several years and suspects there may be destruction of the incus, malleus, stapes, and stapes footplate as a result of the long-term ear infections. In the office record, the physician wrote the diagnoses cholesteatoma left external ear and left chronic otitis media. The patient was admitted for an open left mastoidectomy and total ossicular replacement procedure (with synthetic device) (TORP) so that his comorbid condition of Marfan's syndrome with associated cardiovascular conditions, namely aortic dilation, could be monitored with the associated risks managed.

First-Listed Diagnosis: _____

Secondary Diagnoses: _____

Principal Procedure: _____

Secondary Procedure(s): _____

8

The patient is a 28-year-old female, who had just returned from her honeymoon, was brought to the emergency department (ED) by her husband, complaining of severe bilateral ear pain and difficulty hearing. The couple came directly to the hospital from the airport after a long flight home. The couple had gone deep-sea diving several times during the past week. The husband had no ear pain or other symptoms. The patient, however, had an acute upper respiratory tract infection when she left on the trip but had fewer symptoms of it today. Upon examination, the physician saw possible bleeding in the ear with swelling and possibly a ruptured ear drum on the right side. The ED staff arranged for the patient to see an otolaryngologist tomorrow morning in his office. The final diagnoses entered in the ED record by the physician were (1) bilateral ear pain, (2) acute upper respiratory infection, (3) possible otitic barotrauma, and (4) possible perforated ear drum.

First-Listed Diagnosis: _____

Secondary Diagnoses: _____

9

A mother brought her 18-month-old male to the pediatric emergency department (ED) at 2200 hours. The mother stated the child has been very irritable this evening, pulling on his left ear, crying, and unable to go to sleep. The child has been diagnosed with acute suppurative otitis media on another occasion in the past six months. When the physician examined the child, she saw an erythematous bulging tympanic membrane in the left ear but did not see a perforation. The right ear did not appear to have an infection. There is no smoking in the household or at day care. The child's pediatrician was phoned to discuss the child's care and the pediatrician asked the ED physician to prescribe the same antibiotics the child received during the last ear infection that resolved the condition. The final diagnosis on the ED record was recorded as recurrent acute suppurative otitis media, left.

First-Listed Diagnosis: _____

Secondary Diagnoses: _____

10

A 22-year-old female came to the neighborhood health center complaining of tenderness, redness, and swelling over the mastoid area. The patient said she started having ear pain about two weeks ago and thinks she has a fever and some drainage out of her right ear. Since neither the patient nor her parents had health insurance, she did not go to a physician's office or to the emergency department of the local hospital. The physician was certain the patient had acute right mastoiditis as a result of her untreated acute otitis media on the right side that was still present. An initial antibiotic was prescribed and a sample of the otorrhea fluid was taken for culture. The patient was referred to the university medical center's ENT clinic for follow-up in one week. The diagnosis written by the health center physician on the referral form was "acute right-sided mastoiditis and acute purulent right otitis media."

First-Listed Diagnosis: _____

Secondary Diagnoses: _____

11

An 80-year-old male returned to his physician's office to review the findings of the tests that were performed in the past week. The patient had been in his physician's office a week ago complaining of severe unrelenting ear pain, a temporal headache, purulent discharge from his ears, dysphagia, and hoarseness. These conditions were still present. The physical exam again demonstrated marked tenderness in the soft tissue between the mandible ramus and the mastoid tip. The tympanic membrane was intact in both ears. The physician reviewed the results of the chemistry tests, cultures, and bone scan that showed possible osteomyelitis of the mandible. The patient had type 2 diabetes, and it was always poorly controlled. The patient was informed that he had malignant externa otitis of the right ear and uncontrolled type 2 diabetes with hyperglycemia. The management of his condition was proposed to be meticulous glucose control and aural toilet with systemic and ototopic antimicrobial medications. The patient was given a follow-up appointment in three weeks with a repeat bone scan to be performed prior to that visit.

First-Listed Diagnosis: _____

Secondary Diagnoses: _____

12

The mother of a 14-year-old male brought him to the emergency department. When interviewed, the young man said he had severe pain, itchiness, and a feeling of fullness in both ears. On physical examination and gentle otoscopic inspection, the physician found otorrhea, diffuse external ear canal edema and erythema, and tenderness of both ears, particularly the pinna and tragus. He was unable to visualize the tympanic membranes due to the swelling. The young man was a competitive swimmer and spent hours practicing in his school's pool. The physician informed the patient and his parent and documented in the record that the patient had "swimmer's ear" bilaterally. A prescription was given to the patient for medicated ear drops and he was advised to discontinue swimming practice and avoid getting water in his ears. The mother agreed to make an appointment with the primary care physician in two days to recheck the patient, especially to visualize the ear drums to ensure there was no perforation.

First-Listed Diagnosis: _____

Secondary Diagnoses: _____

13

The patient was a 60-year-old female known to have bilateral Meniere's disease. On this visit to her primary care physician's office, the patient reported she was having a familiar "attack" of this condition. She was experiencing fluctuating hearing loss, whirling vertigo, and a low, roaring tinnitus. The patient had been examined numerous times in the past to find an underlying reason for this disorder of the inner ear, and none had been found. The patient again was treated for her symptoms. A repeat audiometry test was ordered to compare her perceived hearing loss to her baseline test of two years ago. The patient was given prescriptions again for Antivert for the vertigo and a diuretic to reduce the fluid in the inner ears and was advised to continue her salt-restricted diet and to avoid caffeine and alcohol, which were suspected to be triggers of her symptoms. The patient's condition, bilateral Meniere's disease, was again documented in her health record for this visit.

First-Listed Diagnosis: _____

Secondary Diagnoses: _____

14

The father of a 6-year-old male child brought him to the pediatrician's office for a follow-up visit to reexamine him for the acute otitis media with effusion in his left ear that was diagnosed three days before this visit. Once again, the physician noted fluid present in the middle ear but this time found the infection to be resolving in the left ear. The tympanic membrane was intact. No evidence of fluid was obvious in the right ear. The physician advised the parent that an appointment will be made for the child with an otolaryngologist to determine if a myringotomy with insertion of a ventilating tube will be necessary.

In addition, the physician examined the patient's surgical sites for healing after his operation three weeks ago for his juvenile scoliosis where magnetic rods that could be remotely lengthened (reducing the need for multiple surgical procedures) had been percutaneously inserted for his early-onset thoracic scoliosis. The MAGEC rods would be lengthened periodically to correct the scoliosis.

Although the surgical procedure took place prior to this office visit, assign codes for the idiopathic scoliosis and growth rod insertion for practice. In addition, code the reason(s) for the office visit today.

Surgery

Principal Diagnosis: _____

Secondary Diagnoses: _____

Principal Procedure: _____

Secondary Procedure(s): _____

Office Visit

First-Listed Diagnosis: _____

Secondary Diagnoses: _____

15

A 19-year-old female was seen in the otolaryngology consultant's office one week after an emergency department visit because of severe vertigo with repeated nausea and vomiting. There was persistent nystagmus as well. The condition is minimally better as the nausea and vomiting have stopped. The patient had also seen her primary care physician in the prior week and completed outpatient testing including an audiologic assessment and an MRI of the head. Based on the test results and the physician's examination of the patient, including a detailed history interview, the physician concluded the patient had bilateral vestibular neuronitis and documented the diagnosis in the health record and in the report returned to the primary care physician. The physician explained to the patient that the disease is considered to be a neuronitis affecting the 8th cranial nerve and suspected to be viral in origin. The patient was advised that some patients only have one attack such as the one she suffered, while other individuals have repeated episodes over a period of one year or more.

First-Listed Diagnosis: _____

Secondary Diagnoses: _____

16

The patient is a 50-year-old male who comes to the Family Practice Clinic at the University Medical Center complaining that he felt dizzy, like his head was "spinning," and this makes him very nauseous. He said he has hearing loss in his right ear. He also said he has trouble with his vision, especially focusing because his eyes were moving erratically on their own. Upon questioning, the patient said he had what the physician interpreted as a viral upper respiratory infection last month and his symptoms started after the "cold." The patient also admits to consuming large amounts of alcohol on an almost daily basis and is a smoker. Based on the patient's history and the physical examination performed, the physician concluded the patient had labyrinthitis because the patient's history makes him at high risk for developing this condition. The physician prescribed antihistamine and anti-nausea medications to reduce his symptoms. He advised the patient to avoid alcohol, not to drive, and to avoid bright lights and video games. The patient was given a return appointment in two weeks. The final diagnoses documented by the physician for the visit were viral labyrinthitis, chronic alcoholism, and cigarettes/nicotine dependence.

First-Listed Diagnosis: _____

Secondary Diagnoses: _____

17

The mother of a 16-year-old female brought the patient to the ENT physician's office based on a recommendation from their primary care physician. The patient had redness, pain, swelling, and pus-fluid discharge from the cartilage of her left upper ear and a fever. The primary care physician had examined the patient three days ago and ordered a culture and sensitivity from the pus discharge from the ear. The ENT physician reviewed the culture results on the hospital electronic health record and found the bacteria identified was pseudomonas aeruginosa. The patient's girlfriend had pierced the upper part of her left ear, probably without sterile precautions. Based on the trauma of the piercing and the appearance of the infected area, the ENT physician concluded the patient had acute bacterial perichondritis of the left ear cartilage or pinna. The patient was a prescription for an antibiotic and an appointment for a return visit in 14 days.

First-Listed Diagnosis: _____

Secondary Diagnoses: _____

18

The patient is a 70-year-old male with intractable Meniere's disease of the left ear. He has continued to suffer from vertigo, nausea, and sensorineural hearing loss with tinnitus in the left ear despite trying various treatments. Dietary modification, vestibular suppresant and antiemetic medications, and vestibular rehabilitation therapy have all failed to alleviate the patient's symptoms. Since the patient's intractable Meniere's disease is severely impacting his quality of life, and since he already has very poor hearing in his left ear, he presents to the hospital for labyrinthectomy surgery. In the operating room, the patient is placed under general anesthesia and the surgeon exposes the site of the procedure by making a postauricular incision. The surgeon then performs the labyrinthectomy, completely removing the structures of the inner ear. The patient is kept in the hospital for several days to monitor the vertigo, nausea, vomiting, balance disturbance, and hearing loss that are expected consequences of the surgery.

Principal Diagnosis: _____

Secondary Diagnoses: _____

Principal Procedure: _____

Secondary Procedure(s): _____

Chapter 9

Diseases of the Circulatory System

Coding Scenarios for *Basic ICD-10-CM and ICD-10-PCS Coding Exercises*

The following case studies are organized following the sequence of the chapters in the ICD-10-CM Tabular List of Diseases and Injuries as published on the Centers for Disease Control and Prevention National Center for Health Statistics website (http://www.cdc.gov /nchs/icd/icd10cm.htm). The objective of this book is to provide the student with more detailed clinical information to code, rather than one- or two-line diagnosis and procedure statements.

ICD-10-CM diagnosis codes are to be assigned to both the inpatient hospital admission and the outpatient visit case studies. In this book, the ICD-10-PCS procedure codes are to be assigned only to the inpatient hospital admission cases. In actual practice, outpatient cases are assigned CPT/HCPCS codes. The ICD-10-PCS codes are only required for inpatient procedures. In the answer key for the exercises, the Alphabetic Index entry is listed after the code to indicate the main terms and subterms used to locate the code that must be verified in the ICD-10-CM Tabular List or in the ICD-10-PCS Code Tables prior to assigning the code.

1

A 50-year-old male was admitted to the hospital complaining of chest pain that was determined to be a result of an acute inferior wall (type 1) myocardial infarction (MI). The patient was treated for the acute MI. In addition, a right and left heart catheterization was performed with a Judkin's fluoroscopic coronary angiography of multiple coronary arteries, and a right and left fluoroscopic angiocardiography was performed using a low osmolar contrast dye. The patient has no history of CABG surgery in the past. He was found to have coronary arteriosclerosis due to lipid-rich plaque. The patient was also treated for persistent preexisting atrial fibrillation and discharged on day five in stable condition.

Principal Diagnosis: _____

Secondary Diagnoses: _____

Principal Procedure: _____

Secondary Procedure(s): _____

2

A 59-year-old male patient with aortocoronary artery disease of the native arteries was admitted to the hospital for scheduled coronary artery bypass grafts using left greater saphenous vein grafts (harvested by open technique) of four vessels performed under cardio-pulmonary bypass. Postoperatively, the patient developed pulmonary artery emboli attributed to the procedure that were treated successfully with no catastrophic consequences. After three days in the surgical ICU, the patient was transferred to a surgical floor and monitored closely. Phase I of cardiac rehabilitation was started on day 4, and the patient was able to be discharged on day 6. The patient will be seen in the surgeon's office seven days later and is scheduled to begin Phase II cardiac rehabilitation within the next month.

Principal Diagnosis: _____

Secondary Diagnoses: _____

Principal Procedure: _____

Secondary Procedure(s): _____

3

An 80-year-old female was seen in her physician's office for a follow-up visit. Six months previously she had a cerebral infarction for which she was admitted to the hospital at that time. As a consequence of her cerebral infarction, she has right-side (dominant) hemiparesis and dysphasia. She has been receiving outpatient physical therapy and has made good progress. She also is being treated for essential benign hypertension and atrial fibrillation. The patient's prescription medications were renewed, and she will be seen in the office in six months. She was advised to call her physician if she does not feel well or if new problems develop.

First-Listed Diagnosis: _____

Secondary Diagnoses: _____

4

The patient, a 75-year-old male, collapsed at home and was brought to the emergency department by fire department ambulance and admitted to the hospital. A CT scan of the brain using low osmolar contrast showed an acute cerebral embolus of the right middle cerebral artery with cerebral infarction. NIHSS scored at 17. Dysphagia and left hemiparesis were present on admission. The patient is right-handed. The patient is also under treatment for hypertension. At the time of discharge, the dysphagia had cleared, but the hemiparesis was still present. The patient was transferred to a rehabilitation facility.

Principal Diagnosis: _____

Secondary Diagnoses: _____

Principal Procedure: _____

Secondary Procedure(s): _____

5

A 65-year-old male collapsed in his garage after shoveling heavy, wet snow from the driveway of his single-family home. Fire department ambulance brought the man to the nearest hospital in full cardiac arrest. Family members stated the patient had an enlarged heart and had been on prescription medication for hypertensive heart disease in the past but had not seen a physician for over one year. Cardioversion and external chest compression cardiopulmonary resuscitation was initiated but was unsuccessful, and the man was pronounced dead 50 minutes after arriving at the hospital. The patient was never admitted to the hospital, with all of his medical care received in the emergency department (ED). The ED physician's conclusion in the ED record was "Cardiac arrest, probably due to acute myocardial infarction triggered by strenuous exertion, unknown as to exact cause with hypertensive heart disease."

First-Listed Diagnosis: _____

Secondary Diagnoses: _____

First-Listed Procedure: _____

Secondary Procedure(s): _____

6

A 70-year-old female was seen in her physician's office for ongoing management of several medical conditions. The patient has congestive heart failure, as a result of hypertension and chronic kidney disease, stage 2, and longstanding type 2 diabetes with polyneuropathy. Her main reason for being at the physician's office today is to renew medication for her heart failure.

First-Listed Diagnosis: _____

Secondary Diagnoses: _____

7

The patient is a 70-year-old male who was admitted by his cardiologist with the diagnosis of acute coronary syndrome. The patient had not had coronary angioplasty or coronary bypass surgery in the past. The patient consented to and underwent a diagnostic left heart cardiac catheterization and fluoroscopic coronary arteriography of multiple arteries with low osmolar contrast by Judkin technique, which showed extensive arteriosclerotic coronary occlusion of the left anterior descending (LAD). Other vessels also had minor coronary artery disease. Prior to the procedure, the patient understood there was the possibility that he would require a coronary stent placement, to which he also consented. Following completion of the diagnostic catheterization, the physician performed a coronary angioplasty of the LAD with the insertion of one nondrug-eluting coronary stent into the LAD. A platelet inhibitor drug (Integrilin) was also infused through the peripheral IV. The physician's final diagnosis was "acute coronary syndrome due to arteriosclerotic coronary artery disease." The patient was discharged for follow-up evaluation and possible cardiac rehabilitation therapy.

Principal Diagnosis: _____

Secondary Diagnoses: _____

Principal Procedure: _____

Secondary Procedure(s): _____

8

A 72-year-old retired family practice physician called an ambulance from his home to take him to the hospital in which he had practiced medicine for 40 years. En route to the hospital, he asked the paramedics to call the interventional radiologist at the hospital to meet him in the emergency department (ED). The radiologist was waiting for the physician-patient when the ambulance arrived in the driveway. The physician-patient described his symptoms to the ED physician and radiologist and said "I'm certain I have an abdominal aortic aneurysm." The symptoms he experienced—abdominal pulsatile mass, abdominal pain and tenderness, rigidity, lower back pain, rapid pulse, paleness, nausea, clammy skin, sweating— were classic symptoms of what physicians call a "triple A." The patient was admitted and taken immediately to the interventional radiology suite. Based on a quick physical examination and intravascular ultrasound of the abdominal aorta, an aneurysm was found. The patient consented to a repair by the interventional radiologist, and within 1 hour of arrival the following procedure was started. A synthetic graft was implanted endovascularly in the abdominal aorta to reinforce the vessel and prevent a ruptured aneurysm. After the procedure, the patient was taken to the ICU for postoperative monitoring. The patient was also treated for long-standing essential hypertension, as well as for chronic gouty arthritis of the right hip that was current. The patient had an uneventful recovery and was able to leave the hospital within five days for further recovery at home.

Principal Diagnosis: _____

Secondary Diagnoses: _____

Principal Procedure: _____

Secondary Procedure(s): _____

9

The patient, a 68-year-old female known to have congestive heart failure currently controlled by medication, is admitted to the hospital by her physician because of posterior calf pain with warmth and swelling of the proximal right lower leg. A duplex venous ultrasonography with pulse-wave Doppler detected a thrombus of the right popliteal vein intravascularly. Anticoagulant therapy was started to prevent pulmonary embolism or further venous embolization. The patient was stabilized and was able to be discharged home. Home health nurse services were arranged to take blood samples for ongoing prothrombin time (PT) laboratory tests to ensure the therapeutic level of the anticoagulant therapy in the blood. The patient was also treated for her compensated congestive heart failure while in the hospital.

Principal Diagnosis: _____

Secondary Diagnoses: _____

Principal Procedure: _____

Secondary Procedure(s): _____

10

The same patient described in question 9, a 68-year-old female known to have congestive heart failure, was readmitted to the hospital three months later with fatigue, shortness of breath, and swelling of the legs, especially the right leg. Upon questioning, the patient admitted to eating food that was not on her low-fat, low-salt diet over the past week, and her symptoms returned. Intravenous medications, including diuretic and cardiotonic drugs, were started, and the patient's heart function improved. The patient was still receiving maintenance warfarin sodium (Coumadin) to prevent recurrence of the right leg deep vein thrombosis she experienced three months previously. The physician described this condition in the progress notes as DVT and history of DVT. A duplex intravascular venous ultrasonography with pulse-wave Doppler did not detect a recurrent thrombus in the right leg. The patient was stabilized and was able to be discharged home. Home health nurses were arranged to take blood samples for ongoing prothrombin time (PT) laboratory tests to ensure the therapeutic level of the anticoagulant therapy in the blood. The patient was admitted to the hospital for the acute on chronic left sided systolic congestive heart failure she was experiencing.

Principal Diagnosis: _____

Secondary Diagnoses: _____

Principal Procedure: _____

Secondary Procedure(s): _____

11

The patient is a 102-year-old female (a retired teacher) who was admitted to the hospital for further management of her congestive heart failure. The patient, who lives with her 80-year-old son in a single-family home, has been remarkably well in spite of her advanced age. Six months ago, she was admitted to the hospital, was found to be in congestive heart failure with chronic respiratory failure, and became oxygen dependent. The heart failure was described as chronic combined systolic and diastolic congestive type. These conditions continue to be present with her hypertension. Her son states the patient has been sleeping more and has less energy. A couple of days ago she fell while getting up from the bedside commode in her bedroom but insisted she was fine. Her son noticed her left wrist was slightly swollen and bruised. The patient has been treated for hypertension for many years and has a history of urinary tract infections. During this admission, she was found to have another urinary tract infection and was treated for it. She was continued on oxygen, and her hypertension and congestive heart failure medications were adjusted. An x-ray of the wrist showed a minimally angulated fracture involving the left distal radius. The wrist was placed in a splint for support. On day two of the hospital stay, the patient was noticeably weaker, in mild respiratory distress, and sleeping almost continually. Whenever she was attended to by the nurses, physicians, or her son, she asked them to "just let me be." The patient and her son were offered the services of palliative care and accepted. Within 48 hours of receiving palliative, supportive, and comfort care, the patient died peacefully in her sleep.

Principal Diagnosis: _____

Secondary Diagnoses: _____

Principal Procedure: _____

Secondary Procedure: _____

12

The patient is a 35-year-old male who drove himself to the emergency department (ED) early in the morning because he had chest pain. The patient had been gambling in a casino overnight, drinking alcohol and snorting cocaine as well as smoking cigarettes. As the night progressed, the patient became aware of chest discomfort that advanced to chest pain. He had had chest pain on previous occasions, but this time it lasted longer and was more severe. He became scared and came to the ED. The patient does not have a family physician but does see a psychiatrist intermittently for his bipolar I disorder and is taking Lamictal 100 mg daily for this condition. The patient was admitted after the EKG was found to be abnormal and the patient's troponin lab values were found to be elevated. The admitting diagnosis was rule out myocardial infarction. Cardiology consultation was obtained. During his hospital stay the patient was monitored on cardiac telemetry, and the myocardial infarction was ruled out. A chest x-ray showed evidence of bilateral basilar pneumonia. He did have subsequent episodes of chest pain but refused further cardiac workup and insisted on being discharged on day three. The attending (family practice) physician assigned to the patient provided the following final diagnoses: Angina, cocaine addiction, alcohol abuse, tobacco dependence, pneumonia, and bipolar I disorder. The patient was given instructions to call the physician's office for an appointment within one week.

Principal Diagnosis: _____

Secondary Diagnoses: _____

Principal Procedure: _____

Secondary Procedure(s): _____

13

The physician went to the nursing home to see his 83-year-old male patient who was complaining of difficulty breathing and fatigue. The patient was known to have congestive heart failure. After examination, the physician diagnosed the patient as having chronic congestive diastolic heart failure and ordered new medications. In addition, the patient continued to receive treatment for his hypertension and type 2 diabetes mellitus with peripheral neuropathy. He instructed the nurses at the nursing home to closely monitor the patient and notify him if the patient's symptoms worsened because the patient may have to be admitted to the hospital for treatment if that occurred.

Principal Diagnosis: _____

Secondary Diagnoses: _____

Principal Procedure: _____

Secondary Procedure(s): _____

14

The same patient described in question 13, an 83-year-old male resident of a nursing home, developed more significant shortness of breath, increased edema in his legs, and chest pain during the two days after the physician had evaluated the patient in the nursing home. The patient was admitted to the hospital and treated for congestive heart failure with acute exacerbation of his chronic diastolic heart failure. In addition, the patient continued to receive treatment for his hypertension and type 2 diabetes with peripheral neuropathy. The patient improved with treatments and was transferred to a skilled nursing facility for further recovery.

Principal Diagnosis: _____

Secondary Diagnoses: _____

Principal Procedure: _____

Secondary Procedure(s): _____

15

The patient is a 62-year-old male who was initially admitted to Hospital A and diagnosed with an acute type 1 ST elevation anterolateral wall myocardial infarction (STEMI). He had a cardiac catheterization done at Hospital A with the findings of native vessel coronary artery disease in four vessels. The patient's condition was stabilized, and the patient elected to be transferred to a larger hospital for recommended angioplasty and coronary artery stenting. Records and films were transferred with the patient directly to Hospital B for admission. At Hospital B, the patient had percutaneous transluminal angioplasty of three vessels with coronary artery disease. In addition, two non-drug-eluting stents were inserted into two coronary arteries. The patient had an uncomplicated recovery and was scheduled to begin the cardiac rehabilitation program in four weeks. Code for Hospital B.

Principal Diagnosis: _____

Secondary Diagnoses: _____

Principal Procedures: _____

Secondary Procedure(s): _____

16

A 65-year-old male with a history of hypertension was admitted to the hospital through the emergency department with progressive episodes of angina while watching political talk shows on the television. His admission diagnoses were severe angina pectoris, rule out both myocardial infarction and coronary artery disease. His history and physical report noted that he had experienced episodes of angina pectoris in the past but always refused any diagnostic cardiology workup or procedure, consenting only to an EKG that was performed last year in his physician's office. The EKG showed no abnormalities. He was compliant with taking medication for essential hypertension. The patient has not had any bypass surgery in the past. The workup in this hospital for this encounter did not reveal a myocardial infarction, but because of the severity of his unstable angina symptoms the patient was advised to have a cardiac catheterization and possible angioplasty, to which he consented. The patient was taken to the cardiac catheterization laboratory, where he had a left heart catheterization, left ventriculogram, and arteriography of multiple coronary arteries performed using the double catheter technique (Judkins) under fluoroscopy using low osmolar contrast. He was found to have severe three-vessel coronary artery disease as the etiology of his unstable angina pectoris. Because of the extent of the patient's coronary artery disease, angioplasty was not performed, and the patient was transferred to another hospital for expected coronary artery bypass graft surgery.

Principal Diagnosis: _____

Secondary Diagnoses: _____

Principal Procedure: _____

Secondary Procedure(s): _____

17

HISTORY: The patient is a 50-year-old female who was transferred for admission to this academic medical center from a community hospital. She was admitted to the community hospital for a coronary angiogram. The angiogram findings noted an ejection fraction of 30–35 percent with global dyskinesia. The physician documented that the echocardiogram revealed severe aortic valve stenosis, moderate mitral valve regurgitation, and a calcified tricuspid value. The patient is also known to have hypertensive kidney disease with end-stage renal disease (ESRD) requiring dialysis. She also has anemia of chronic disease (ESRD) and dyslipidemia. The patient also has a history of hepatitis C. Because the three valve disease (described as old rheumatic disease by the physician) has caused significant chronic diastolic and congestive heart failure, the patient agreed to open heart surgery. The procedures performed at the academic medical center are aortic valve replacement with 19-mm tissue valve, mitral valve annuloplasty with 3-mm annuloplasty ring, left radial artery cutdown for arterial line insertion, Swan-Ganz catheter insertion, and cardiopulmonary bypass.

DESCRIPTION OF PROCEDURE: After detailed and informed consent was signed, the patient was brought to the operating room and placed supine on the operating table. General anesthesia was initiated and endotracheal intubation performed. Left radial artery cutdown was performed. She was prepped and draped in the usual sterile fashion. A Swan-Ganz catheter was placed via the left subclavian vein. A sternotomy was performed. The patient was heparinized. A standard cannulation was performed with arterial cannula in the ascending aorta and a single dual-stage venous cannula via the right atrial appendage. Antegrade cardioplegia catheter was inserted. Aortic cross clamp was applied, she was placed on the bypass pump, and the heart arrested. The aorta was opened. The patient had a calcified tricuspid valve. The aortic valve leaflets were excised and passed off the field. We then opened the left atrium. The echo had shown a central jet. The mitral valve sized to a 30-mm ring, and a 30-mm CG annuloplasty ring was sewn in place. The area was closed with running 4-0 Prolene. We then sized the aorta (valve) annulus to 19 mm and a Magna porcine bioprosthesis tissue graft valve was sewn in with interrupted simple sutures. Once the valve was in, the aortotomy was closed with running two layers of 4-0 Prolene. De-airing was performed through this aortotomy. The aortic cross clamp was removed. Once the patient was warmed, ventricular pacing wires were placed. Ventilation was begun, and the patient was weaned from bypass. Protamine was administered. All cannulae were removed and hemostasis ensured. Two 32-French chest tubes were placed. The sternum was closed with four figure-of-8 sternal wires, and the soft tissue was closed in three layers. The patient was taken to the adult cardiovascular intensive care unit in stable condition.

Principal Diagnosis: _____

Secondary Diagnoses: _____

Principal Procedure: _____

Secondary Procedure(s): _____

18

An 82-year-old male was admitted to inpatient care through the emergency department with severe heart failure after complaining of fatigue and increasing difficulty in breathing. He also had type 2 diabetes mellitus that had been controlled by oral medications. During his stay, he was administered insulin to control his blood sugar during this severe illness. He also had hypertension that was monitored and treated with oral medications. The physician described the type of heart failure this patient has as "acute on chronic systolic congestive heart failure."

Principal Diagnosis: _____

Secondary Diagnoses: _____

Principal Procedure: _____

Secondary Procedure(s): _____

19

A 55-year-old female patient was admitted to her local community hospital with pre-infarction angina. She underwent a combined right and left heart cardiac catheterization with coronary angiography, Judkins technique, and was determined to have significant atherosclerotic heart disease. She has no history of bypass surgery. Triple coronary artery bypass graft (CABG) surgery was recommended for the 80 percent to 90 percent occlusion found in three native coronary vessels. The patient was an active cigarette smoker, documented as nicotine dependent. With counseling and upon consent, the patient was transferred to a medical center licensed to perform open heart surgery and scheduled for the CABG. Once the patient was safely placed under anesthesia, the left greater saphenous vein was harvested through an open approach. Once the saphenous vein that was to be used as the bypass vascular graft was harvested, it was immediately flushed with DuraGraft Endothelial Damage Inhibitor and then placed into the DuraGraft solution until the anastomoses were performed. This new intraoperative technology was performed to prevent vein graft disease or vein graft failure. Next, the triple coronary artery bypass grafting was performed on the left anterior descending, the circumflex, and the diagonal arteries. The origin of the bypass was the aorta. This procedure was performed using extracorporeal circulation while the patient was placed on cardiopulmonary bypass for the duration of the procedure. The final diagnosis documented by the provider at the medical center was triple vessel coronary artery disease, unstable angina, no myocardial infarction. Smoking cessation was strongly advised. Code the medical center procedure(s) only.

Principal Diagnosis: _____

Secondary Diagnoses: _____

Principal Procedure: _____

Secondary Procedure(s): _____

20

This 85-year-old male was brought to the emergency department by his family because of right-sided temporary blindness that lasted only a few minutes on one day but then occurred two more times on different days. The patient was admitted with a diagnosis of transient monocular blindness. The physician described his condition as a unilateral temporary blindness, also known as amaurosis fugax. After study, the physician documented that the underlying cause of the amaurosis fugax was carotid artery stenosis. As documented in the record, the physician explained to the patient that transient ischemia resulting from carotid artery disease affects the optic nerve and the retina and causes blindness. This may be seen as a warning of internal carotid disease. Carotid arteriography (plain radiography, no contrast) confirmed the presence of carotid artery stenosis and occlusion of both carotid arteries. The left carotid stenosis and occlusion was minor. The right carotid stenosis and occlusion was significant and thought to be the cause of the patient's symptoms. The patient consented to a percutaneous endoscopic right internal carotid endarterectomy with a Dacron patch graft and was discharged the next day in good condition.

Principal Diagnosis: _____

Secondary Diagnoses: _____

Principal Procedure: _____

Secondary Procedure(s): _____

21

The 80-year-old female patient is seen in the neurology clinic at the request of her family physician for assessment of her aphasia due to her past stroke. The patient has facial weakness due to her past cerebrovascular accident that is also evaluated during the visit.

First-Listed Diagnosis: _____

Secondary Diagnoses: _____

22

The 57-year-old male patient is a resident of a long-term care facility after suffering a stroke two months previously, with bilateral quadriplegia as a result. The patient is being discharged from this facility to be readmitted to another long-term care facility that specializes in the type of care the patient requires for his paralytic syndrome.

Principal (Nursing Home) Diagnosis: _____

Secondary Diagnoses: _____

23

The patient is a 77-year-old female who is a resident of a nursing home. She had a stroke 10 months ago and since that time has had several seizures that have been determined to be a consequence of her stroke. None of the seizures has been very significant, but the patient has been placed on anticonvulsant medication. In the last progress note documenting his visit, her physician wrote the diagnosis of "Patient stable, seizure disorder over the past nine months due to her previous stroke."

Principal (Nursing Home) Diagnosis: _____

Secondary Diagnoses: _____

24

A patient who had a stroke seven months ago was admitted to the hospital for a surgical tendon transfer on his left hand. The patient acquired a contracture of the left hand as a result of the stroke. Otherwise the patient had recovered well from the stroke. During the hospital stay the orthopedic surgeon performed an open hand tendon transfer with no complications, and the patient was discharged from the hospital on the day after surgery. The patient also had two chronic conditions managed while in the hospital: essential hypertension and simple chronic bronchitis. The patient was discharged with instructions for postoperative care including a follow-up appointment in the orthopedic surgeon's office in five days.

Principal Diagnosis: _____

Secondary Diagnoses: _____

Principal Procedure: _____

Secondary Procedure(s): _____

25

The 80-year-old male patient was admitted to the hospital and diagnosed with symptomatic sick sinus syndrome. The cardiologist explained to the patient that sick sinus syndrome refers to a combination of symptoms the patient experienced as well as marked sinus bradycardia diagnosed by the cardiac workup. On admission, the patient's symptoms were dizziness, confusion, fatigue, and syncope that were attributed to the sick sinus syndrome. The patient was known to have congestive heart failure, though under reasonable control with treatment continued during the hospital stay. The cardiologist recommended to the patient that he needed a dual-chamber pacemaker, and the patient consented to the procedure.

PROCEDURE DESCRIPTION: The patient was brought to the pacemaker procedure suite and placed under conscious sedation. Fluoroscopic guidance was used during the procedure. One percent lidocaine was used to anesthetize the area under the left clavicle and an incision was used to create a pacemaker pocket was created in the subcutaneous tissue for the generator and leads. The left subclavian vein was cannulated percutaneously using two micro puncture sets with a regular 035 wire under fluoroscopic guidance. A 7-French sheath and a 7-French right ventricular lead was placed in the right ventricular upper septum and sutured down. The right atrial lead was placed with a 7-French sheath under fluoroscopy and sutured down. The leads were attached to the generator, which was sutured down into the pocket. The wound was irrigated with antibiotic solution and inspected for hemostasis. The wound was closed in layers. The patient was taken to the cardiology procedure recovery area and awoke from the conscious sedation. No obvious complications were noted following the procedure.

Principal Diagnosis: _____

Secondary Diagnoses: _____

Principal Procedure: _____

Secondary Procedure(s): _____

26

A 65-year-old female who recently underwent a partial colectomy for treatment of a bowel obstruction presents to the emergency department complaining of worsening swelling and acute pain in her right leg. The patient states that due to her recent surgery she has been spending more time lying down in bed. The patient is diagnosed with acute deep vein thromboses of her right popliteal and right peroneal veins. Since she recently had major gastrointestinal surgery, her risk of bleeding is high and anticoagulation is contraindicated. Therefore, she is taken to the operating room for insertion of an inferior vena cava filter. The patient's right femoral vein is accessed and a guidewire is inserted into the inferior vena cava. A catheter is inserted over the guidewire and the filter is deployed into the inferior vena cava through the catheter. The patient tolerates the procedure with no complications. The patient's discharge diagnoses are: acute DVT of the right popliteal vein, acute DVT of the right peroneal vein, status post partial colectomy. The procedure performed was insertion of an inferior vena cava filter due to the acute proximal DVT in the right popliteal vein.

Principal Diagnosis: _____

Secondary Diagnoses: _____

Principal Procedure: _____

Secondary Procedure(s): _____

Chapter 10

Diseases of the Respiratory System

Coding Scenarios for *Basic ICD-10-CM and ICD-10-PCS Coding Exercises*

The following case studies are organized following the sequence of the chapters in the ICD-10-CM Tabular List of Diseases and Injuries as published on the Centers for Disease Control and Prevention National Center for Health Statistics website (http://www.cdc.gov /nchs/icd/icd10cm.htm). The objective of this book is to provide the student with more detailed clinical information to code, rather than one- or two-line diagnosis and procedure statements.

ICD-10-CM diagnosis codes are to be assigned to both the inpatient hospital admission and the outpatient visit case studies. In this book, the ICD-10-PCS procedure codes are to be assigned only to the inpatient hospital admission cases. In actual practice, outpatient cases are assigned CPT/HCPCS codes. The ICD-10-PCS codes are only required for inpatient procedures. In the answer key for the exercises, the Alphabetic Index entry is listed after the code to indicate the main terms and subterms used to locate the code that must be verified in the ICD-10-CM Tabular List or in the ICD-10-PCS Code Tables prior to assigning the code.

1

A 70-year-old male patient with long-standing chronic obstructive pulmonary disease (COPD) was admitted through the emergency department with increasing shortness of breath, weakness, and fatigue. His admitting diagnosis was acute respiratory insufficiency. Treatment included respiratory therapy and medications. It was confirmed with the patient that he has not resumed his 50-year history of smoking, and he was encouraged to remain smoke-free. The final diagnoses written by the physician was acute respiratory insufficiency due to acute exacerbation of COPD. History of smoking.

Principal Diagnosis: _____

Secondary Diagnoses: _____

Principal Procedure: _____

Secondary Procedure(s): _____

2

An 80-year-old female patient from a nursing home was admitted to the hospital with symptoms of weakness, coughing, shortness of breath, and mental status changes. Swallowing studies revealed she had difficulty swallowing and easily aspirated particles into her respiratory tract. It was determined that she suffered from aspiration pneumonia. She also was found to have a superimposed bacterial pneumonia. Both conditions were treated with intravenous antibiotics, and the patient's condition improved. She was transferred back to the long-term care facility for care.

Principal Diagnosis: _____

Secondary Diagnoses: _____

Principal Procedure: _____

Secondary Procedure(s): _____

3

A 10-year-old male was treated in the allergist's office for childhood asthma. He was treated for his allergic rhinitis due to pollen and animal dander with his asthma. The patient's conditions were well controlled with his current medications.

First-Listed Diagnosis: _____

Secondary Diagnoses: _____

4

A bilateral tonsillectomy and adenoidectomy was performed on a 9-year-old patient to resolve his recurring infections due to adenotonsillar hyperplasia. No infection was present at the time of the surgery. The patient was admitted as an inpatient for an overnight stay.

Principal Diagnosis: _____

Secondary Diagnoses: _____

Principal Procedure: _____

Secondary Procedure(s): _____

5

The patient is a 65-year-old male who is receiving chemotherapy for multiple myeloma from an oncologist on staff at this hospital. The patient came to the emergency department stating he had a cough, fever, chills, and felt extremely weak. The patient was admitted. The chest x-ray at the time of admission showed evidence of pneumonia in the left lower lobe. During the hospitalization, the patient received respiratory therapy treatments, intravenous antibiotics, and supportive care. His chemistry profiles showed an abnormal BUN and glucose. Cultures of the sputum showed no pathologic organism. Blood cultures were negative. The patient's hemogram was abnormal with a hemoglobin of 9.3, hematocrit of 27, white blood cell count of 3,200 and platelets 126,000. A repeat CBC showed the hemogram had dropped to 7.5 with the hematocrit at 22. There was no evidence of GI or other source of bleeding. His oncologist also followed his care during the hospital stay and determined the pancytopenia shown on the CBC was a result of the chemotherapy the patient was receiving. For this reason, the patient was administered two units of nonautologous packed red blood cells via the patient's existing IV line in his peripheral vein. Follow-up CBC test showed hemoglobin at 9.6 and hematocrit at 28.

Follow-up chest x-ray showed significant clearing of the pneumonic process. The patient was switched to oral antibiotics at the time of discharge and administered a prescription to continue taking both antibiotics for another week. The patient appeared significantly anxious, and this was discussed with him. A psychiatric consultation and possible medications were recommended, which the patient refused. The patient has a follow-up appointment with his oncologist and with the private physician within the next 10 days.

Principal Diagnosis: _____

Secondary Diagnoses: _____

Principal Procedure: _____

Secondary Procedure(s): _____

6

The patient is a 45-year-old male who comes to the physician's office for his three-month follow-up visit for asthma. He is using a bronchodilator and steroid for control of his asthma. He is having no problems with the asthma at this time. He denies a change in cough and reports no increase in shortness of breath, no fluid retention, and no increase in wheezing. He is taking his medication regularly and not missing any doses. Upon physical examination, the lungs are clear with decreased breath sounds in both lung fields, heart is regular rhythm with no murmurs, and extremities are free of edema. Oximetry and pulmonary function tests have not changed since the last visit. The patient's diagnosis is stable asthma, on long-term systemic steroid therapy. The patient was advised to continue his present medications and return for a follow-up visit in three months.

First-Listed Diagnosis: _____

Secondary Diagnoses: _____

7

The patient is a 19-year-old male who comes to the physician's office complaining of a sore throat with fever for the past four days with pain in his right ear. He has difficulty swallowing and has been taking Tylenol for fever and throat lozenges for the sore throat. He feels weaker today. He has no known allergies. Physical examination showed the tonsillar arch reddened with tonsillar exudates. There are enlarged anterior cervical lymph nodes. The examination of the ears showed acute suppurative otitis media in both ears, but worse in the right ear.

A rapid strep screening test was positive. The diagnoses given were (1) possible early tonsillar abscess, (2) strep pharyngitis, and (3) acute suppurative otitis media. The patient was administered an injection of antibiotics and a prescription for an antibiotic to be taken for the next 10 days.

First-Listed Diagnosis: _____

Secondary Diagnoses: _____

8

A physician in private practice admitted this patient to the hospital. The patient is a 78-year-old female who has coronary artery disease and is status post coronary artery bypass graft 8 years ago. She is also under treatment for hypertension and mild congestive heart failure. The patient was admitted at this time for shortness of breath starting two days prior to admission and worse on the day of admission. She complained of wheezing and cough productive of white sputum. She thought she had a mild fever this morning but was afebrile on admission. She had no chills, nausea, or vomiting. Her paroxysmal nocturnal dyspnea and orthopnea remain unchanged. Physical examination showed the patient to be in mild distress but alert and oriented. Her blood pressure was 150/70 mm Hg, heart rate 70, and respiratory rate 16. Cardiovascular system examination revealed regular rate and rhythm. Lungs had poor air entry and patient was wheezing. Abdomen was soft, nontender. The extremities were 2+ edema bilaterally. Neurologically, her left upper extremity and left lower extremity have weakness as the result of a CVA 2 years ago. The patient was admitted with COPD, acute exacerbation. She responded well to respiratory therapy treatments and intravenous medications. She was discharged home with the following prescriptions: Prednisone, aspirin enteric-coated tablet, Albuterol inhaler, Persantine, Captopril, Theophylline, Diltiazem, Nitro paste, Lasix, and Digoxin. She will be seen in the office in five days. Discharge diagnoses are acute and chronic bronchitis/COPD, hypertension, CAD, status post CABG, CHF, old stroke with weakness/hemiparesis, left side in a right-handed woman.

Principal Diagnosis: _____

Secondary Diagnoses: _____

Principal Procedure: _____

Secondary Procedure(s): _____

9

The patient is a 9-year-old male who is brought to the pediatrician's office by his mother because of the following: runny nose, fever, yellow discharge from the nose, swelling around the eyes, and tenderness in the cheeks. The child is snoring during sleep. The mother had given the child Children's Tylenol. Physical examination confirmed most of the subjective complaints and detected fluid in the sinuses. A prescription was administered for 14-day oral antibiotic treatment and the physician recommended continued use of Children's Tylenol for fever. The physician documented the child had acute sinusitis in the frontal and maxillary sinuses.

First-Listed Diagnosis: _____

Secondary Diagnoses: _____

10

A 62-year-old female, on disability because of emphysema, is brought to the emergency department (ED) from home by fire department ambulance. The patient complained of sudden sharp chest pain, shortness of breath, and a nonproductive hacking cough. The patient has been under treatment for COPD and emphysema for more than 5 years and is dependent on oxygen. The patient described the pain as being on the left side with referred pain up to the shoulder. The patient was cautious when moving to protect her chest and shoulder. In the ED a chest x-ray and continuous pulse oximetry was ordered. Pulse oximetry showed low oxygen saturation. Physical examination revealed diminished breath sounds bilaterally, but significantly worse on the left side. The chest x-ray revealed a collapsed lung on the left side and fluid in the pleural space. The patient was admitted. A chest tube was inserted for pleural drainage and to aspirate air and re-expand the lung. Follow-up chest x-ray showed the lung had re-expanded to its normal size, and the pleural effusion's fluid appeared to be reabsorbed and resolved. The physician's discharge diagnoses were COPD and emphysema with left side secondary spontaneous pneumothorax and pleural effusion.

Principal Diagnosis: _____

Secondary Diagnoses: _____

Principal Procedure: _____

Secondary Procedure(s): _____

11

The patient is a 50-year-old female with known systemic lupus erythematosus with nephritis. Her renal function has been worsening over the past several months. Today the patient came to the emergency department complaining of pain in her chest that was worse when she coughed or took a deep breath. The ER physician heard a "friction rub," but a chest x-ray was inconclusive that any pleural effusion was present. The patient was admitted to the hospital. It was determined that the patient had pleurisy, but it was uncertain if it was related to her lupus. The patient also had diarrhea, dehydration with hyponatremia, hypokalemia, and azotemia. Intravenous fluids and medications were administered to correct her metabolic disorders, diarrhea, relieve the pain of the pleurisy, and treat her worsening renal function from her lupus.

Principal Diagnosis: _____

Secondary Diagnoses: _____

Principal Procedure: _____

Secondary Procedure(s): _____

12

The patient is an 89-year-old male with advanced COPD who was admitted to the hospital complaining of cough, shortness of breath, and fever. It was determined that he was suffering from COPD with acute bronchitis. He is supplemental oxygen dependent and also has cor pulmonale. He was treated with bronchodilators and antibiotics. The patient was on "do not resuscitate" (DNR) status. The patient was becoming progressively weaker with more respiratory distress. During this hospital stay, the family members decided to initiate comfort care measures after speaking with the physician about the patient's prognosis. The family elected to receive hospice care and took the patient home to receive home end-of-life and comfort care.

Principal Diagnosis: _____

Secondary Diagnoses: _____

Principal Procedure: _____

Secondary Procedure Code(s): _____

13

A 5-year-old male was brought to the emergency department by his mother, who gave the patient's two-day history of increasing lethargy, decreased appetite, and vomiting. The mother stated the child's sister had similar symptoms and was seen in the physician's office and diagnosed with viral syndrome during the past week. A physical examination and laboratory tests were performed on the 5-year-old male that showed evidence of dehydration and decreased breath sounds. A chest x-ray showed some diffuse areas in the right lower lobe, possibly involving pneumonia. The patient was admitted with an admitting diagnosis of dehydration and possible pneumonia of a viral or bacterial type. During the hospital stay, the child received IV antibiotics and fluids to treat the infection and dehydration. Within 12 hours, the child became alert, active, and back to normal per his mother. He was given a clear liquid diet and later wanted more to eat, with no vomiting reported. Repeat chemistry, hematology, and urinalysis lab tests were repeated the following morning and showed results back to normal. The child was discharged to his mother's care on day 2 with a follow-up appointment made in the primary care physician's office for day 5. The physician's conclusion on the discharge summary written the day of discharge was "pneumonia, possibly viral origin, complicated by dehydration."

Principal Diagnosis: _____

Secondary Diagnoses: _____

Principal Procedure: _____

Secondary Procedure(s): _____

14

The patient was a 59-year-old male brought to the emergency department (ED) by ambulance with increasing shortness of breath and worsening color. The patient's skin was mottled below the knees. Due to shortness of breath, the patient was not able to give any history in the ED before his family arrived. When they arrived, his family reported that he had become more lethargic at home over the past 24 hours. The patient had been a smoker for 45 years and had continued to smoke until one week ago. He had chronic obstructive asthma that was steroid dependent for many years and developed steroid-induced diabetes in the past 5 years. He was diagnosed with status asthmaticus upon admission. He was able to work up until the age of 55, when he received disability retirement benefits from his company and Social Security because of his poor health. Since his retirement he was also diagnosed with congestive heart failure. A month ago he was found to have a large left chest mass when a chest CT exam was performed because of an increasing cough. After this finding was described to him, he refused any further workup and signed an advance directive that specified no heroic efforts in his final days. After admission, an order was written for "no code" or do not resuscitate status per his advance directive, but the patient did allow respiratory therapy and intravenous medications for his heart and lung disease. Over the next 24 hours he seemed to improve with the breathing treatments of Solu-Medrol and Lasix, but his pulse oximetry was rarely above 80% without an oxygen mask. A portable chest x-ray showed his left lower lobe obstructing mass, larger than imaged one month ago, and pneumonia. Testing proved it to be pneumonia due to pseudomonas aeruginosa. His blood sugars improved, and he appeared to be stabilizing much to the surprise of his family and physicians. He had brief periods of alertness and was able to converse with his family and eat small meals. However, the evening before his passing, palliative care orders were written to make him as comfortable as possible, as his lung function was worsening again. Early in the morning of the third day he became unresponsive and then was noted to be without respirations or pulse at 0130. His wife and son were at his bedside when he was pronounced dead by the hospitalist on duty. His final diagnoses included pneumonia due to pseudomonas, systemic therapy steroid-dependent chronic obstructive asthma/COPD with exacerbation, steroid-induced diabetes, large left lung mass, congestive heart failure, and acute respiratory failure—all probably related to his tobacco dependence. No autopsy was performed.

Principal Diagnosis: _____

Secondary Diagnoses: _____

Principal Procedure: _____

Secondary Procedure(s): _____

15

The patient, a 60-year-old male, was taken to the emergency department of a local hospital from a wedding reception after he developed symptoms of shortness of breath and chest pain. He also reported that he felt very tired after traveling to this city for the wedding and has learned he cannot tolerate as much walking as he had even one month ago. The patient knew he had lung cancer. The ER physician contacted his family physician, who told him the patient had small cell carcinoma of the left upper lobe of the lung, diagnosed 14 months ago, and he had been followed for possible malignant pleural effusion that resolved without treatment three months ago. The patient was admitted to the hospital and examined by an oncologist and cardiologist. After several tests were performed, it was determined the patient had exudative pleural effusion, which the oncologist referred to as "malignant pleural effusion of the left lung."

The cardiologist performed a therapeutic thoracentesis on the left side that provided immediate relief. However, the relief was short lived and the fluid re-accumulated. A second procedure was then performed.

The patient came to the OR and was placed in a supine position on the table. General anesthesia was administered and video-assistance was used for the procedure. The right lateral decubitus position was utilized as the sterile prepping and draping of the left chest was done. Local anesthetic of the skin overlying the sixth rib was injected, and an incision was made. Subcutaneous dissection was performed. Dissection over the left pleural space continued with a curved hemostat until I entered the pleural space. Thoracostomy dilation was achieved and 1000 mL of pleural effusion drained by suction. Once most of the fluid had been drained, I inserted a 0 degree thoroscope and was able to drain a little pocket of effusion from the costophrenic recess. The thoroscope was then used to instill talc, 4 grams which had been aerosolized, covering both the pleura and the lung. Instruments were removed. Anesthesia was reversed, the patient extubated, and sent to the PACU in stable condition. All counts were correct at the end of the procedure with very minimal blood loss during the procedure.

The patient rested in the hospital for one more day and was discharged to the care of his family. The physicians advised the patient to rest at least two more days in this city before driving 250 miles with his family back to his hometown. Records were given to the patient to take to his oncologist at home.

Principal Diagnosis: _____

Secondary Diagnoses: _____

Principal Procedure: _____

Secondary Procedure(s): _____

16

HISTORY: The patient is a 75-year-old male with stage IV gastroesophageal junction carcinoma. He developed severe respiratory distress and was brought to the hospital emergency department and admitted. A large left pleural effusion was noted on CT scan and chest x-ray. His condition progressed to acute hypoxic respiratory failure, and he required intubation and mechanical ventilation for 25 hours. A chest tube insertion was recommended to relieve the patient's hypoxic respiratory failure caused by the left pleural effusion, and the patient consented to the procedure.

DESCRIPTION OF PROCEDURE: The patient was placed in the supine position in the medical intensive care unit on propofol drip. His left anterior chest was prepped and draped. One percent plain Xylocaine was administered, and a small incision was made. Using the hemostat, the chest cavity was entered and fluid was returned. Then, using the trocar, the chest tube was placed in the superior portion of the left pleural cavity. There was approximately 1,000 mL of fluid returned. The patient tolerated the procedure well, and the chest tube was sewn in place. A follow-up chest x-ray confirmed good positioning of the tube, and a decrease in the amount of pleural effusion was noted. Cytology examination of the pleural fluid did not show malignant cells.

Principal Diagnosis: _____

Secondary Diagnoses: _____

Principal Procedure: _____

Secondary Procedure: _____

17

An 80-year-old male who has been a long-term nursing home resident with chronic obstructive pulmonary disease (COPD) was admitted to the hospital by his primary care physician with shortness of breath, elevated white blood count, and bibasilar infiltrates. A pulmonary disease consultant agreed with the attending physician that the patient had aspiration pneumonia and acute respiratory failure, both present on admission. In addition, the pulmonologist describes the man's COPD as obstructive chronic bronchitis. The patient had an Advance Directive that indicated he did not want to be placed on a ventilator. Intravenous antibiotics were administered, and the patient agreed to be placed on intermittent positive airway pressure breathing for 48 hours. Fortunately, appropriate treatment was able to control the conditions quickly, and the patient was taken to a skilled nursing facility for extended recovery from the aspiration pneumonia and respiratory failure.

Given the patient had symptoms of three conditions (chronic lung disease, aspiration pneumonia, and respiratory failure) all present on admission, and any could have been the reason after study for the admission to the hospital, the coder asked the attending physician's assistance in identifying the principal diagnosis as determined by the circumstances of admission, the diagnostic workup, and therapy provided. The physician chose the aspiration pneumonia as patient's principal diagnosis, as it was one of the main reasons for the admission and required the greatest intensity of care and use of resources. According to the physician, the respiratory failure was suspected to have resulted from either the aspiration pneumonia or the worsening chronic lung disease affected by the aspiration pneumonia.

Principal Diagnosis: _____

Secondary Diagnoses: _____

Principal Procedure: _____

Secondary Procedure(s): _____

18

This was the first admission to a long-term acute-care hospital (LTACH) for the 45-year-old male patient who was unconscious and respiratory dependent because of his chronic respiratory failure. He acquired the respiratory failure after suffering a multi-drug overdose two weeks ago and this hospital stay was to manage the consequences of the drug overdose during this subsequent encounter. According to his family, it was believed the patient was addicted to multiple illegal drugs, but exactly which drugs was unknown. The patient had a tracheostomy in place for connection to the mechanical ventilator. The patient is admitted to the LTACH for managing his respiratory failure and possibly weaning from mechanical ventilation. All attempts to wean the patient from the ventilator were unsuccessful. After 30 days in the LTACH, the patient was transferred to a long-term care ventilator unit at a skilled nursing facility for further care. His final diagnoses were noted to be chronic respiratory failure from multiple drug overdose, polysubstance dependence, ventilator dependency, and tracheostomy status. He remained on the ventilator the entire time he was in the LTACH.

Principal Diagnosis: _____

Secondary Diagnoses: _____

Principal Procedure: _____

Secondary Procedure(s): _____

19

OPERATIVE REPORT

PRE-OPERATIVE DIAGNOSIS: Acute on Chronic Respiratory Failure with Hypoxia

POST-OPERATIVE DIAGNOSIS: Same

PROCEDURE: Permanent tracheostomy

INDICATIONS: The patient is a 64-year-old male who had long suffered from pan-lobular emphysema and became respirator dependent after being admitted to the hospital because of an onset of a gram-negative pneumonia. Because the patient was unable to be weaned from mechanical ventilation and will need long-term respiratory support, a tracheostomy was recommended to the patient's wife, the patient's agent according to his advance directive for healthcare, who consented to the procedure because her husband was unconscious and unable to consent.

PROCEDURE: The patient was brought to the operating room. After being placed under general anesthesia, the neck was prepped and draped for the procedure. A 2.5 cm incision was made approximately two fingerbreadths above the sternal notch. The strap muscles were identified and divided exposing the thyroid thymus. Dissection was taken down to the cricoid. The thyroid isthmus was divided, exposing the trachea. An incision was made between the second and third tracheal rings, and an inferior based tracheal flap was created. The flap was sewn to the skin edge creating a skin flap in order to mature the tracheal stoma with 3-0 vicryl. The endotracheal tube was withdrawn to just above the tracheostomy site. An appropriate sized Shiley trach was inserted with no difficulties. The balloon was inflated and connected to the anesthesia circuit and CO2 was confirmed. The tracheostomy was secured to the skin with 2-0 silk sutures. Straight ties and a drain sponge were applied. The patient was returned to the ICU in stable condition with no obvious adverse reactions to the procedure.

Assign the diagnosis identified as the reason for the procedure as the first diagnosis for this exercise as well as the underlying conditions.

Diagnosis for the operative procedure: _____

Other Diagnoses: _____

Principal Procedure: _____

Secondary Procedure(s): _____

20

OPERATIVE REPORT

PRE-OPERATIVE DIAGNOSIS:	Cystic fibrosis with pulmonary manifestations including atelectasis
POST-OPERATIVE DIAGNOSIS:	Cystic fibrosis with pulmonary manifestation including atelectasis
PROCEDURE:	Bronchoscopy with removal of mucus plug

INDICATIONS: The patient is a 15-year-old female who is known to have cystic fibrosis and recently developed pulmonary manifestations and was admitted for treatment of atelectasis that was caused by a mucus plug in the right main bronchus. A bronchoscopy was recommended to remove the plug that was not able to be dissolved by other techniques. The patient's parents consented to the procedure after being informed of the steps to the procedure, the risks and benefits.

PROCEDURE: The patient was brought to the endoscopy suite and placed under conscious sedation using Versed and fentanyl. The fiberoptic bronchoscope was passed through the oral cavity. The vocal cords were visualized. A large mucus plug was identified in the right main bronchus, and it was removed completely by lavage suction. Otherwise, a normal trachea was found with some secretions collecting in the bronchi that were suctioned into a canister for cytology evaluation. No other lesions or abnormalities were found. The patient's conscious sedation was reversed and the patient was awake when removed from the endoscopy suite and taken to the recovery area. No obvious complications or adverse reactions to the procedure were observed immediately after the procedure.

Code the diagnosis as described as the postoperative diagnosis.

Postoperative Diagnosis: _____

Other Diagnoses: _____

Principal Procedure: _____

Secondary Procedure(s): _____

21

The patient is a 45-year-old female who recently completed treatment for empyema. Although the infection has resolved, the patient continues to suffer from a loculated pleural effusion complicated by numerous septations within the pleural cavity. She is admitted to the hospital to have tissue plasminogen activator (tPA) administered into her pleural cavity in order to break up the septations and help drain the persistent pleural effusion. Through a percutaneously placed catheter, tPA is infused into the patient's pleural cavity. The patient tolerates the procedure without any complications.

Principal Diagnosis: _____

Secondary Diagnoses: _____

Principal Procedure: _____

Secondary Procedure(s): _____

Chapter 11

Diseases of the Digestive System

Coding Scenarios for *Basic ICD-10-CM and ICD-10-PCS Coding Exercises*

The following case studies are organized following the sequence of the chapters in the ICD-10-CM Tabular List of Diseases and Injuries as published on the Centers for Disease Control and Prevention National Center for Health Statistics website (http://www.cdc.gov /nchs/icd/icd10cm.htm). The objective of this book is to provide the student with more detailed clinical information to code, rather than one- or two-line diagnosis and procedure statements.

ICD-10-CM diagnosis codes are to be assigned to both the inpatient hospital admission and the outpatient visit case studies. In this book, the ICD-10-PCS procedure codes are to be assigned only to the inpatient hospital admission cases. In actual practice, outpatient cases are assigned CPT/HCPCS codes. The ICD-10-PCS codes are only required for inpatient procedures. In the answer key for the exercises, the Alphabetic Index entry is listed after the code to indicate the main terms and subterms used to locate the code that must be verified in the ICD-10-CM Tabular List or in the ICD-10-PCS Code Tables prior to assigning the code.

1

A 40-year-old female has been treated for symptoms of gallstones without improvement. The patient also was known to have chronic cholecystitis. She was admitted for a laparoscopic cholecystectomy. After the laparoscopy procedure was started, the physician stated the gallbladder could be visualized but could not be removed. The procedure was converted to an open procedure and the gallbladder was removed. The pathology report confirmed the preoperative diagnosis of chronic cholecystitis with cholelithiasis.

Principal Diagnosis: _____

Secondary Diagnoses: _____

Principal Procedure: _____

Secondary Procedure(s): _____

2

A 30-year-old female has been treated for Crohn's disease of the small intestine since 18 years of age. She has had several exacerbations of the disease over the past years. At this time, the patient comes to the emergency department in extreme pain. A small bowel x-ray shows a small bowel obstruction. The patient was admitted to the hospital. Later the obstruction was found to be a result of mural thickening. The patient is taken to surgery and a partial resection of the terminal ileum is performed to release the obstruction. An end-to-end anastomosis is performed to close the small intestine. The patient was also noted to have flat, firm, hot, and red painful small lumps on the shins of both legs. Consultation with the wound-care physician determined the ulcers to be erythema nodosum, a known complication of Crohn's disease. The wound care physician prescribed oral and topical medications.

Principal Diagnosis: _____

Secondary Diagnoses: _____

Principal Procedure: _____

Secondary Procedure: _____

3

A 68-year-old male was admitted to the hospital for an inguinal hernia repair that could not be done on an outpatient basis because of anticipated extended recovery time required due to his other medical conditions. After being prepared for surgery and taken to the operating room, the patient complained of precordial chest pain. The surgery was cancelled, and the patient was returned to his room. Cardiac studies failed to find a reason for the chest pain, which resolved the same day. The patient's medications for his hypertension and COPD were also administered.

Principal Diagnosis: _____

Secondary Diagnoses: _____

Principal Procedure: _____

Secondary Procedure(s): _____

4

A 70-year-old male who lives in another city and was visiting relatives in the area was brought to the emergency department (ED) by family members. The patient complained of vomiting blood and having very dark stools that appeared to have blood in them as well. The patient had gone out to dinner with relatives for a prime rib dinner. After he came home, he started vomiting and having diarrhea and blamed it on the large meal. He continued to have these symptoms overnight, and his family members insisted he come to the ED. The patient was admitted. The patient is taking Prinivil, Lanoxin, and Lasix for congestive heart failure and atrial fibrillation, and these medications were continued during the hospital stay. The gastroenterologist was called for a consultation and saw the patient. The patient agreed to an upper and lower GI endoscopic examination. The esophagogastroduodenoscopy (EGD) examination included a biopsy and cauterization of a gastric polyp and a biopsy of a pyloric ulcer. The findings of the EGD, confirmed by pathologic studies, were hiatal hernia, acute gastritis with bacteria determined to be helicobacter, gastric polyp, and a chronic deep pyloric ulceration. Hemorrhage was noted in the stomach, coming from the gastritis and the ulcer. The colonoscopy included a cecal polyp at 80 cm that was removed with a hot biopsy forceps. Extensive diverticulosis was present but no areas of bleeding were seen. The attending physician agreed with the findings of the endoscopic examination as reasonable explanations for the patient's symptoms. The serial blood counts did not find any significant anemia. The patient was discharged and given prescriptions and copies of his medical records to take home for his private physician to review.

Principal Diagnosis: _____

Secondary Diagnoses: _____

Principal Procedure: _____

Secondary Procedure(s): _____

5

The patient is an 81-year-old female who was admitted to the hospital for intractable emesis, near syncope, and extreme weakness and fatigue. The patient had been in the hospital two weeks previously for pneumonia, which was treated at that time. A visit in the physician's office five days ago revealed the pneumonia to be resolving. During this hospital stay it was determined the patient had a nonspecific form of gastroenteritis with resulting dehydration. Because the patient had multiple conditions, the physician was queried as to what was the main reason for admission after study, and she stated it was the gastroenteritis. The patient is also known to have a hiatal hernia and reflux esophagitis, which were treated with her usual medications. A chest x-ray still showed the pneumonia to be present, and she was continued on oral antibiotics. The patient was discharged home to continue taking oral antibiotics and her other usual medications.

Principal Diagnosis: _____

Secondary Diagnoses: _____

Principal Procedure: _____

Secondary Procedure(s): _____

6

A 75-year-old male was admitted to the hospital after coming to the emergency department (ED) after having a black melanotic stool the day before and on the day of admission. He had no pain, nausea, or vomiting but felt a little "light-headed." Testing in the ED found grossly guaiac-positive stools. His admitting diagnosis was gastrointestinal bleeding. The patient has an extensive past medical and surgical history, including:

1. Coronary artery bypass graft seven years ago after a myocardial infarction with no symptoms today, but takes one baby aspirin a day

2. Recurrent deep vein thrombosis of lower extremity and recurrent pulmonary emboli; currently taking Coumadin to prevent recurrence

3. History of congestive heart failure; currently taking Lanoxin and Dyazide

4. History of arthritis; currently taking Tolectin

5. History of hyperlipidemia; currently taking Lescol

6. Suspected carcinoma of the pancreas 5 years ago that only proved pancreatitis to be present, no malignancy

7. Appendectomy, colon resection done years before for what sounds like a bowel obstruction and stomach surgery for what the patient calls a "blockage"

8. Large ventral hernia related to his left upper quadrant abdominal incision from past surgery, which is of no consequence at this time

During this hospital stay, he was administered IV medications, vitamin K injection, and two units of nonautologous, fresh plasma was administered intravenously via the peripheral vein to reverse the effects of the Coumadin. Serial CBCs were done, which showed marginally low hemoglobin and hematocrit but nothing requiring treatment for anemia. An EGD was performed by the gastroenterologist, who documented a hiatal hernia with reflux esophagitis, and a bleeding proximal jejunal ulcer. The EGD was simply diagnostic; no biopsies were taken. The private physician used the diagnoses from the EGD and from the past medical and surgical history as the final diagnoses for the case. The patient continued to receive all of his medications while in the hospital and was discharged home for follow-up in the physician's office in one week.

Principal Diagnosis: _____

Secondary Diagnoses: _____

Principal Procedure: _____

Secondary Procedure(s): _____

7

A 60-year-old male was acutely ill when admitted to the hospital for hematemesis. After study, the upper gastrointestinal (GI) bleeding was found to be due to a gastric varix that was caused by alcoholic cirrhosis of the liver and acute alcoholic hepatitis. The patient was known to have long-term chronic alcoholism with which he continues to struggle. The patient was also found to have esophageal varices due to the alcoholic cirrhosis of liver, but these were not bleeding at this time. The surgery performed was the creation of a transjugular intrahepatic portosystemic (venous) shunt (TIPS) performed in the radiology suite. A shunt was passed down via the jugular vein and was inserted between the portal and hepatic veins within the liver to establish communication between these two veins.

The patient was discharged to a skilled nursing facility for surgical recovery and ongoing management of his serious GI diseases.

Principal Diagnosis: _____

Secondary Diagnoses: _____

Principal Procedure: _____

Secondary Procedure(s): _____

8

A 55-year-old male was admitted to the hospital through the emergency department for suspected gallstone pancreatitis. After study it was found the patient had acute pancreatitis, radiologic evidence of gallstones, and possibly stones in the common bile duct. The patient was taken to surgery for an open cholecystectomy and common duct exploration. It was confirmed the patient had chronic cholecystitis with cholelithiasis and choledocholithiasis with obstruction of the biliary system. The physician stated the acute pancreatitis was a consequence of the bile duct stones, but the main reason for the patient's admission to the hospital and the need for surgery were the gallstones and the bile duct stones. The patient had a slow but steady recovery from surgery and was able to return home for further convalescence.

Principal Diagnosis: _____

Secondary Diagnoses: _____

Principal Procedure: _____

Secondary Procedure(s): _____

9

A 40-year-old male was admitted to the hospital through the emergency department for acute abdominal pain. The patient appeared to have alcoholic intoxication. He was treated with nasogastric suction, IV fluids, and pain medications. The patient stated he was told by another physician at another hospital that he had chronic pancreatitis. The diagnosis of acute and chronic pancreatitis was made based on physical findings and laboratory and radiology test results. The patient stated he was supposed to take Dilantin for a "seizure disorder" but stopped taking them because his prescription ran out. He said he had not had a seizure in more than one year. A neurologist was consulted but declined to prescribe the Dilantin again, as the patient had no evidence of seizures while in the hospital. It was determined the patient did have chronic alcoholism. To prevent withdrawal, the patient was administered multiple vitamins and mild tranquilizers and the patient did not experience alcohol withdrawal symptoms during his hospital stay. The patient was discharged and was asked to come to the physician's office for follow-up in five days. The patient was advised to stop drinking and was referred to the outpatient substance abuse treatment center run by the hospital for counseling after discharge, which he agreed to visit.

Principal Diagnosis: _____

Secondary Diagnoses: _____

Principal Procedure: _____

Secondary Procedure(s): _____

10

The patient is a 25-year-old female with moderate mental retardation who needs dental extractions for dental caries on the chewing surface of the tooth penetrating into the pulp and chronic apical periodontitis in three upper right teeth and three lower right teeth. Prior to surgery, the patient was instructed to stop the anticoagulant drug, Coumadin, she is taking and begin taking Lovenox instead. The patient has a history of mitral valve and aortic valve replacements and needs subacute bacterial endocarditis prophylaxis before the surgery. She is taking the anticoagulation therapy because of her past heart surgery. Because the patient needed to be monitored for therapeutic anticoagulant drug levels prior to surgery, she was admitted to the hospital. Management of the anticoagulation was completed in two days, and the patient had the surgical dental extractions of all six diseased teeth on day three. The patient was allowed to return home on day five after the Coumadin was restarted on day four with no ill effects. The patient has follow-up appointments with the oral surgeon and the family physician in the next week.

Principal Diagnosis: _____

Secondary Diagnoses: _____

Principal Procedure: _____

Secondary Procedure(s): _____

11

The patient is an 84-year-old female who was brought to the emergency department by her family upon the advice of the family physician. The patient said she had increasing abdominal pain, nausea, and some vomiting. This condition started two to three days ago, and the patient could not eat due to the nausea. Prior to this episode of illness, the patient had been reasonably well, receiving medications for hypertension and hypothyroidism. The patient was admitted. Overnight the patient appeared to become more acutely ill, developed respiratory distress, and the rapid response team evaluated her and obtained her physician's order to transfer her to the ICU. Soon after, the patient required intubation and mechanical ventilation for acute respiratory failure. The patient had signs and symptoms of septicemia and sepsis, possibly with an intra-abdominal source. Blood cultures grew *E. coli*. She was taken to the operating room, where she underwent an exploratory laparotomy. The surgeons found acute bowel ischemia and gangrene involving 100 percent of the small bowel and the right colon. This was an inoperable condition, and the laparotomy site was closed. The family was advised of the patient's very poor prognosis and offered hospice care, which they accepted. The mechanical ventilation was discontinued after 24 hours in place, and the patient was extubated. She was kept as comfortable as possible overnight and expired in the early morning hours of hospital day four. The physician's final diagnoses were acute ischemic and gangrenous intestine, acute respiratory failure, *E. coli* septicemia, hypertension, and hypothyroidism.

Principal Diagnosis: _____

Secondary Diagnoses: _____

Principal Procedure: _____

Secondary Procedure(s): _____

12

A 39-year-old female patient was transferred from the long-term acute-care hospital to the university hospital for admission. The patient had a four-day history of diffuse and worsening abdominal pain. The patient is ventilator dependent, with a tracheostomy in place for chronic respiratory failure resulting from her severe dermatomyositis. She had evidence of sepsis and was later found to have *E. coli* septicemia with sepsis. She was taken to surgery with the preoperative diagnosis of acute abdomen with free intraperitoneal air. She was found to have a perforated transverse colon with intra-abdominal abscess. The tracheostomy was malfunctioning, too. The surgery performed was an exploratory laparotomy, an entire transverse colectomy with primary end-to-end anastomosis, loop ileostomy, drainage of the intra-abdominal (mesentery) abscess, and open revision of the tracheostomy. After a long stay in the intensive care unit and on the medical-surgical floor, the patient slowly recovered from this major illness. The patient remained on the ventilator for the entire 14-day hospital stay. She was transferred back to the long-term acute-care hospital for extended recovery time.

Principal Diagnosis: _____

Secondary Diagnoses: _____

Principal Procedure: _____

Secondary Procedure(s): _____

13

The patient is a 59-year-old male who was referred to the gastroenterologist by his primary care physician for evaluation of abdominal pain and black stools. The patient said he had acid indigestion and heartburn for many years and took Tums and Pepto-Bismol on a daily basis. Over the past several days, he had been experiencing burning and cramping epigastric pain that was not relieved by the usual medications. He also had noted black tarry stools, which was a new problem for him. His primary care physician had placed the patient on Pepcid. The patient's mother had a history of peptic ulcer disease, but there were no other major illnesses in the family. The gastroenterologist recommended the patient have an upper GI endoscopy to further evaluate the source of the problem, and the patient consented. On an outpatient basis, the physician performed an esophagogastroduodenoscopy at the hospital. The findings included a normal-appearing esophagus. There was a large hiatal hernia pouch extending about 4 cm below the junction to the diaphragmatic closure. The stomach body, angulus, and antrum were normal. The pyloric channel was normal. There was one solitary erosion measuring 3–4 mm in the duodenal bulb, but there was no evidence of recent bleeding. The descending duodenum was normal. No biopsies were taken. The physician's conclusion at the end of the examination was (1) gastroesophageal reflux, (2) hiatal hernia, and (3) small chronic duodenal ulcer. The physician recommended to the patient that he continue to take the Pepcid but discontinue the use of Pepto-Bismol because it possibly could cause the black tarry stools. The patient was to return to the gastroenterologist's office in one month and if symptoms continue and consider an abdominal ultrasound and workup of the large bowel.

First-Listed Diagnosis: _____

Secondary Diagnoses: _____

14

The patient is a 74-year-old male who was admitted for a chronic bleeding duodenal ulcer. Because of significantly abnormal laboratory results, additional studies were performed and it was determined he had obstructive jaundice due to a suspected common bile duct stone. The patient was seen by the gastroenterologist in the hospital and scheduled for an endoscopic retrograde cholangiopancreatography (ERCP). An ERCP with low osmolar contrast was performed with an Olympus video gastroduodenoscope. The duodenum was easily accessed. The ampulla was erythematous and widely patent. The catheter was placed into the pancreatic duct, and a pancreatogram was obtained. The catheter was repositioned into the common bile duct, and a guide wire was passed into the liver. The cholangiogram showed a filling defect within the common bile duct. A double channel papillotome was placed in the common bile duct and a 1 cm sphincterotomy was performed for drainage. The common bile duct was dilated and with an 11-mm balloon, the physician removed a large, hard, yellow stone without difficulty. Using contrast dye injected into the edges of the cut wound, hemostasis was achieved, and the scope was removed. The postoperative diagnoses for the procedure titled ERCP with sphincterotomy and stone extraction were (1) common duct stone obstructed, and (2) chronic duodenal ulcer under treatment.

Principal Diagnosis: _____

Secondary Diagnoses: _____

Principal Procedure: _____

Secondary Procedure(s): _____

15

The patient is a 55-year-old male with a 35-year history of alcohol abuse. He came to the hospital emergency department after having one melenic stool at home. While in the ED, he had another melenic stool. He is known to have esophageal varices secondary to alcoholic liver cirrhosis. He has had sclerotherapy for the varices in the past, but it was noted to be a failure. The patient had attempted to complete alcoholic rehabilitation on three occasions but has been unsuccessful and continues to drink—according to the patient, "only a couple of beers every day." The patient is also known to have thrombocytopenia that may be the result of bone marrow suppressive effect of alcohol but has not been proven, and serial blood counts were performed during this admission. He has had gastrointestinal bleeding investigated during two previous admissions. The patient was admitted and was seen in consultation by a gastroenterologist and a psychiatrist. The day after admission, the patient became increasingly tremulous and anxious, with anticipated alcohol withdrawal occurring. The withdrawal was successfully managed with medications, and the patient stayed in the hospital after threatening to leave against medical advice the evening of day 2. An upper GI endoscopy (EGD) was performed three days after admission. The findings of the exam were two small grade 1 distal esophageal varices 1 cm in length without stigmata. There were no gastric varices. The fundus and body of the stomach were within normal limits. There was mild peripyloric edema but no ulcers in the pylorus or duodenum. No sclerotherapy of the esophageal varices was necessary. It was suspected the GI bleeding had come from the esophageal varices, as there was no other source of bleeding found. The patient was given strong encouragement to continue to work toward his sobriety, especially given the fact he had detoxification therapy while in the hospital to manage his withdrawal. He acknowledged it was a good time to return to Alcoholics Anonymous, which he acknowledged was a good program for him in the past, and to take advantage of other community support systems for recovering alcoholics that the psychiatrist informed him about during this hospital stay, including two visits from gentlemen from the community program. The discharge summary prepared by his attending physician included the final diagnoses and procedures of bleeding esophageal varices in alcoholic liver cirrhosis disease, continuous alcoholism, alcoholic withdrawal, thrombocytopenia, EGD, and alcohol withdrawal treatment.

Principal Diagnosis: _____

Secondary Diagnoses: _____

Principal Procedure: _____

Secondary Procedure(s):   _____

16

A 65-year-old patient had experienced blood in his stools, or melena, for the past several days. Over the past 12 hours, the bleeding had increased, and the patient felt very weak and dizzy. He was admitted to the hospital by his physician. The patient was known to have diverticulosis of the colon, and his physician's first impression was that the bleeding was a result of diverticulitis. The patient was advised to have a colonoscopy and an upper GI endoscopy (EGD), to which he agreed. The colonoscopy was performed, and the patient was found to have diverticulosis, but no inflammation was seen. However, an area of erosion, ulceration, and bleeding was seen in the duodenum during the EGD examination. A biopsy of the duodenum was taken during the EGD. The physician's diagnosis was acute duodenal ulceration with hemorrhage; diverticulosis of colon.

Principal Diagnosis: _____

Secondary Diagnoses: _____

Principal Procedure: _____

Secondary Procedure(s):   _____

17

HISTORY: This patient is a 35-year-old male with a recurrent, reducible right inguinal hernia, noted on examination. He had undergone surgical repair of a right inguinal hernia 2 years ago, so he was familiar with the symptoms and called this surgeon's office for an appointment. The young man works in a health club as a personal trainer of body builders and, therefore, does heavy lifting on a daily basis. Otherwise, he is healthy, well-nourished, and well-built with no other surgical history and no other evident medical problems. Preoperative testing, including a chest x-ray, EKG, and usual laboratory work, were all within normal limits. He is admitted to the hospital for this procedure because it is a recurrent hernia, and the procedure will require that he have highly limited mobility for the next 36–48 hours. He will also stay in the hospital for a short recovery period. He will then be placed on work-related disability and advised to avoid working for a minimum of 4 weeks.

OPERATIVE FINDINGS: A recurrent, reducible right inguinal hernia, direct and indirect, was found. There was no strangulation or gangrene. A right inguinal hernia repair (Bassini) with high ligation was performed.

DESCRIPTION OF PROCEDURE: The patient was taken to the operating room and placed in a supine position on the table. After satisfactory general anesthesia was administered, the right groin was prepped with Betadine scrub and paint and draped in the usual sterile fashion. The skin overlying the groin was incised through the external inguinal ring, exposing the spermatic cord. The cord was then mobilized and a Penrose drain passed around it at the level of the pubic tubercle. The cord was skeletonized proximally, revealing a very small indirect inguinal hernia sac. The sac was dissected away from the remainder of the cord structure, which was left free of injury. The sac was opened and found to contain no contents. There was also a direct inguinal hernia noted but no femoral hernia noted. The sac was twisted and ligated with 3-0 silk suture ligature. The remainder of the sac was amputated. A floor repair was performed as described by Bassini with interrupted 0 Ethibond sutures between the transversalis fascia and the shelving edge of the inguinal ligament. The internal inguinal ring was left to the size of the tip of an adult finger, and the initial suture medially was from the transversalis fascia into the aponeurosis over the pubic tubercle. Upon completion, hemostasis was adequate, and no relaxing incision was necessary. Spermatic cord was returned to the inguinal canal. The ilioinguinal nerve was blocked prior to this procedure and reblocked again with 0.5 percent Marcaine and epinephrine solution. The pubic tubercle, inguinal ligament, and subcutaneous tissue were also anesthetized with 0.5 percent Marcaine and epinephrine solution. The external oblique was then closed with running 3-0 Vicryl. The wound was copiously irrigated and the skin closed with skin clips. A sterile dressing was applied. Gentle traction was placed on the right testicle to fully return it to the scrotum. The patient was transferred to the recovery room in stable condition.

Principal Diagnosis: _____

Secondary Diagnoses: _____

Principal Procedure: _____

Secondary Procedure(s): _____

18

HISTORY: This is a 72-year-old male who presented with a history of epigastric pain for several months. This lasts three to four hours each time and has been occurring every two to three days. He has been nauseated, although there was no vomiting. He has had the urge to go to the bathroom for frequent bowel movements after meals. He has tried to avoid greasy food and has been placed on a prescription antacid, but this only helped to some extent. An ultrasound was performed on the gallbladder, and gallstones were found. An upper GI x-ray showed mild esophageal motility problems with a hiatal hernia. He gets a screening prostate specific antigen (PSA) every year and has had a colonoscopy, which was normal. He consented to a laparoscopic cholecystectomy and was admitted to the hospital.

OPERATIVE FINDINGS: The laparoscopic examination revealed evidence of inflammation of a chronic nature of the gallbladder along with gallstones. There was also a nodule on the liver on the inferior surface on the right lateral aspect of the gallbladder fossa. The rest of the visualized viscera were unremarkable. After pathologic examination, the postoperative diagnoses documented by the provider are cholelithiasis with chronic cholecystitis with a benign right intrahepatic bile duct adenoma.

DESCRIPTION OF PROCEDURE: The patient was prepared and draped in the usual fashion. An umbilical incision was made. A Veress needle was introduced with a sheath, and pneumoperitoneum was established with the usual precautions. Then an 11-mm port was placed. A laparoscope was introduced. Under direct vision, an operative port in the right upper quadrant and two 5-mm lateral ports were placed. A laparoscopic examination revealed evidence of inflammation of a chronic nature of the gallbladder with gallstones. There was also a nodule in the liver. The rest of the viscera visualized were normal. The cholecystectomy was done by gently grasping the fundus. Adhesions were taken down. The neck was then grasped. The Calot's Triangle was then exposed. The anatomy was carefully defined. The cystic duct and the cystic artery were traced up to the neck of the gallbladder. Herein it was secured with hemoclips, divided, and closed to the neck of the gallbladder. Then it was dissected off of the gallbladder bed and retrieved in an Endopouch and removed. Irrigation was carried out. Excellent hemostasis was ascertained. Following this, an evaluation of the nodule was carried out using a hook cautery. The surrounding borders of this nodule, in the area of the right inferior surface of the lobe of the liver, were cauterized. Then a small wedge biopsy of this tissue was taken. The base was cauterized. This tissue was then sent, with the gallbladder tissue, for histopathological analysis. At this point, having ascertained good hemostasis, all the ports were removed under direct vision. The fascia was closed with 0 Vicryl sutures. Subcutaneous tissue was closed with 0 Vicryl sutures. The skin was closed with 4-0 Monocryl. Marcaine 0.5% with epinephrine was injected to achieve postoperative analgesia. The patient tolerated the procedure well and was stable at the end of the procedure and taken to recovery.

Principal Diagnosis: _____

Secondary Diagnoses: _____

Principal Procedure: _____

Secondary Procedure(s): _____

19

HISTORY: The patient is an 85-year-old female who lives independently with her husband in their own home. She has been treated for hypothyroidism, hypertension, and dyslipidemia in the past. Medications for these conditions were continued during her hospital stay. Early this morning she awoke with acute onset of right flank pain. Her husband called 9-1-1, and she was brought to the hospital's emergency department. On examination she was found to be in acute pain with a palpable mass in her abdominal area. Radiologic examination found dilated loops of small bowel trapped between the abdominal wall and the ascending colon and cecum. She was admitted and taken emergently to the operating room for a suspected small bowel obstruction. The patient was found to have elevated blood pressure, which was proven to be due to her acute stress reaction about her condition and impending surgery.

OPERATIVE FINDINGS: The procedure performed was an exploratory laparotomy and release of acute closed loop small bowel obstruction due to adhesions, by lysis of adhesions. Fortunately, the bowel was viable and did not have to be resected.

DESCRIPTION OF PROCEDURE: After routine preparation, the patient was taken to the operating room. A midline incision was made through the scar of previous surgery, which was a hysterectomy. Supraumbilical extension of the scar was performed. Once these minor non-obstructing adhesions were taken down, the abdominal cavity was entered. One loop of small bowel was almost completely obstructed by dense adhesions. These adhesions were carefully lysed, releasing the small bowel from obstruction. The entire small bowel was mobilized and explored from the ligament of Treitz all the way to the ileocecal valve. The wound was irrigated. Hemostasis was obtained after lysis of adhesions that released the acute small bowel obstruction. Lap count and instrument count were correct. Seprafilm adhesion barrier substance was placed in the peritoneal cavity prior to closure. The fascia was closed with PDS loop. The skin was closed with a skin stapler. A dressing was applied. The patient tolerated the procedure well under general anesthesia and was taken to the post-anesthesia recovery area in good condition.

Principal Diagnosis: _____

Secondary Diagnoses: _____

Principal Procedure: _____

Secondary Procedure(s): _____

20

A 63-year-old male was brought to the emergency department (ED) by a fire department ambulance with his family, who reported that he was found unconscious on his front porch. The patient was admitted with a blood alcohol level of 115 mg/100 mL, indicating acute intoxication and intoxication delirium, documented by the ED physician. The family and later the patient confirmed that the man suffered from chronic continuous alcoholism. The diagnostic workup also found evidence of alcoholic liver cirrhosis. The immediate concern was the life-threatening hepatic encephalopathy, which required intensive treatment. The liver cirrhosis was evaluated and treated but will remain a continuing problem for the patient. He recovered from his extreme condition, however, and was able to be discharged. He was strongly advised to stop drinking, and he agreed to attend Alcoholics Anonymous meetings, as he realized the seriousness of his alcoholism.

Principal Diagnosis: _____

Secondary Diagnoses: _____

Principal Procedure: _____

Secondary Procedure(s): _____

21

The patient was a 45-year-old male who was admitted to the hospital by his private physician after vomiting bright red blood during a visit in the office the same day. A consultation with a gastroenterologist was requested. The gastroenterologist recommended an immediate esophagogastroduodenoscopy (EGD) to determine and control the source of the bleeding. The patient consented to the EGD, which revealed an acute, hemorrhaging duodenal ulcer. The bleeding points in the duodenum were controlled endoscopically by cautery. It was also noted that the patient had a sliding hiatal hernia. The patient recovered from the procedure well, suffered no further episodes of vomiting or bleeding, and was discharged with medications. Follow-up appointments with his physicians were scheduled.

Principal Diagnosis: _____

Secondary Diagnoses: _____

Principal Procedure: _____

Secondary Procedure(s): _____

22

The patient is a 60-year-old male who was discharged from the hospital one week ago after being treated for cryptogenic cirrhosis and hepatic encephalopathy. The patient is known to have chronic liver failure as a result of the cirrhosis that was caused by hepatitis the patient had 30 years ago after multiple blood transfusions. The patient is seen in the office today for a post-discharge follow up visit. During the visit it was determined that the patient has felt progressively weaker since coming home from the hospital. The patient also described having polyuria, polydipsia, and diarrhea for the past three days. The patient is also known to have type 2 diabetes requiring insulin. Lab tests done in the office showed the patient had an electrolyte imbalance, probably due to the diarrhea, and a glucose of 300 that is high for the patient. An ambulance was called and the patient was transferred to the hospital for a direct admission with the admitting diagnoses of worsening chronic liver failure. The diagnoses listed for this visit were (1) chronic liver failure, (2) cryptogenic cirrhosis, (3) electrolyte imbalance, (4) uncontrolled (hyperglycemic) insulin requiring type 2 diabetes and (5) diarrhea.

First-Listed Diagnosis: _____

Secondary Diagnoses: _____

23

A 43-year-old male presented to the emergency department complaining of abdominal pain and nausea. The patient says he is unable to keep anything down and was not able to tolerate even water that he tried to drink prior to coming to the hospital. Earlier that evening, the patient had eaten several large servings of steak at a buffet. The patient is admitted and is taken to the operating room for urgent evaluation and removal of a suspected foreign body in the esophagus. The patient undergoes an EGD and an impacted food bolus (a large piece of steak) is found in his lower esophagus. Using rat-tooth forceps, the surgeon dislodges the impacted food and removes it from the esophagus. The patient is kept in the hospital overnight to ensure that he is able to tolerate liquids and food, and is discharged the next day.

Principal Diagnosis: _____

Secondary Diagnoses: _____

Principal Procedure: _____

Secondary Procedure(s): _____

Chapter 12

Diseases of the Skin and Subcutaneous Tissue

Coding Scenarios for *Basic ICD-10-CM and ICD-10-PCS Coding Exercises*

The following case studies are organized following the sequence of the chapters in the ICD-10-CM Tabular List of Diseases and Injuries as published on the Centers for Disease Control and Prevention National Center for Health Statistics website (http://www.cdc.gov /nchs/icd/icd10cm.htm). The objective of this book is to provide the student with more detailed clinical information to code, rather than one- or two-line diagnosis and procedure statements.

ICD-10-CM diagnosis codes are to be assigned to both the inpatient hospital admission and the outpatient visit case studies. In this book, the ICD-10-PCS procedure codes are to be assigned only to the inpatient hospital admission cases. In actual practice, outpatient cases are assigned CPT/HCPCS codes. The ICD-10-PCS codes are only required for inpatient procedures. In the answer key for the exercises, the Alphabetic Index entry is listed after the code to indicate the main terms and sub-terms used to locate the code that must be verified in the ICD-10-CM Tabular List or in the ICD-10-PCS Code Tables prior to assigning the code.

1

A 90-year-old female, a resident of a long-term care facility, was admitted to the hospital with a severe decubitus ulcer on the right buttock described as a stage III pressure ulcer. The patient also had a small chronic ulcer on the right heel, currently limited to the skin. The patient also has generalized atherosclerosis of both extremities. Treatments of the skin conditions were an excisional debridement of the skin of the heel and an excisional debridement into the muscle of the buttock. The wound care nurse closely monitored the patient after surgery and gave detailed instructions to the nurses at the long-term care facility who would be taking care of the patient after discharge. The patient was transferred back to the long-term care facility. The wound care physician and nurse would visit the patient in the long-term care facility within one week to monitor the healing of the pressure and chronic ulcers.

Principal Diagnosis: _____

Secondary Diagnoses: _____

Principal Procedure: _____

Secondary Procedure(s): _____

2

A 20-year-old female was admitted for a procedure to treat a pilonidal cyst that had become abscessed. The procedure performed was an incision and drainage of the pilonidal sinus. The patient will continue to take oral antibiotics to resolve the infection. The patient was discharged home with a follow-up appointment in seven days with the surgeon who performed the procedure.

Principal Diagnosis: _____

Secondary Diagnoses: _____

Principal Procedure: _____

Secondary Procedure(s): _____

3

A 19-year-old female was seen in the dermatologist's office with extensive inflammation and irritation of the skin on her eyelids and under her eyebrows that was spreading to her temples and forehead. Upon questioning the patient, the physician learned that she had recently used new eye cosmetics. The physician had examined the patient during a prior visit for cystic acne. During this visit, the physician also examined the patient's cystic acne on her forehead and jaw line. He advised her to continue to use the medication he had prescribed previously. The physician's diagnosis was contact dermatitis due to cosmetics and cystic acne. He advised the patient to immediately discontinue use of any makeup on the face until the next follow-up visit. The patient was given a topical medication to resolve the inflammation.

First-Listed Diagnosis: _____

Secondary Diagnoses: _____

4

A 50-year-old female was seen in her primary care physician's office complaining of warmth and redness of her left anterior lower leg. Last weekend she was doing yard work and received a small puncture wound on the same area of her leg. She did not think she had a foreign body in the wound. Over the next couple of days the area became red and began to show swelling. Upon physical examination, the physician found a tiny puncture point with obvious cellulitis tracking down her leg from below the knee almost to the ankle. The wound itself required no treatment. The physician recommended the patient take a short-term course of antibiotics and return for a follow-up visit in five days. The diagnosis written on the encounter form was cellulitis of the lower leg from puncture wound.

First-Listed Diagnosis: _____

Secondary Diagnoses: _____

5

A 60-year-old male was seen by a dermatologist at the request of his primary care physician while hospitalized for other medical conditions. The patient states he spends a lot of time outdoors as a mailman and golfing every weekend. The patient expresses the concern that he may have skin cancer. He remembers that his father, a farmer, had many of these same kind of lesions on his arms and neck through the years. After performing a thorough skin examination, the physician finds multiple brown annular keratotic lesions on the patient's arms and lower legs with patchy dry areas around them. The physician performs a skin biopsy by excising a piece of a lesion on his right lower arm and examines the lesion microscopically. No cancer type cells are seen. Given the patient's history of the same lesions in the family and his frequent exposure to ultraviolet sunlight, the physician explains to the patient that he has what is referred to as DSAP, or disseminated superficial actinic porokeratosis. Further, he explains there is no treatment to prevent these lesions from returning once removed. The patient elects not to have any lesions removed at this time but will consider it and make an appointment in the future if he decides to have them removed.

Code only the reason for the consultation and the procedure performed as result of the consultation.

Dermatology Diagnosis: _____

Secondary Dermatology Diagnoses: _____

Dermatology Procedure: _____

Secondary Procedure: _____

6

The 25-year-old patient is seen in the dermatologist's office upon the advice of the family practice physician with the complaint of excessive sweating in particular areas of her body, such as her underarms, soles of her feet, and the palms of her hands. The patient notes that the excessive sweating started when she was a young teenager. She describes this condition as very embarrassing and difficult to manage because nearly every day, she has to take extra clothing with her in order to change her blouse at work. The physician takes a complete history and cannot find any medical condition that might be causing this problem. The physical examination confirms, however, excessive moisture under the arms and on her hands and feet. The physician is certain the patient suffers from primary focal hyperhidrosis. Her primary care physician had given her a prescription for a certain antiperspirant designed for this condition. The patient had tried the antiperspirant but found it to be ineffective as well as irritating to her underarm skin. The dermatologist recommends injections of botulinum toxin at the sites where excessive sweating is occurring. The drug promptly freezes the nerve that would normally stimulate the sweat gland. He had used this therapy for other patients, who were pleased with the results. The patient immediately wants the procedure. The physician injects the subcutaneous tissue of both axillae with the "botox" under sterile technique. The patient is to return in four weeks to report on the results, or sooner if problems are detected. The physician states that if the patient has a positive response, the injections will need to be repeated every six to nine months.

While there is no requirement that ICD-10-PCS procedures are coded on outpatients, code the injection of botulinum toxin for coding practice.

First-Listed Diagnosis: _____

Secondary Diagnoses: _____

Practice Procedure Coding: _____

7

Upon the advice of his family physician, the patient made an appointment with a dermatologist to evaluate an itching, red, blistering condition that recently appeared on his lower arms and lower legs. The patient is a 26-year-old male who works as a salesman in a computer store. The dermatologist asks the patient questions about his recent contact with new soaps, detergents, chemicals, fabrics, fragrances, and outdoor or indoor plants, but the patient reports he has had no new experiences with these items. Upon further questioning, the physician learns the patient had a new roommate move in one month ago with a dog that had taken a strong liking to the patient and follows him everywhere. The physician is then certain the patient's condition is a contact dermatitis resulting from exposure to animal dander. The physician gives the patient samples of a topical ointment and a prescription for a topical corticosteroid medication to reduce the inflammation and relieve the itching. The patient is told this condition is likely to continue as long as the animal resides with him. The patient is advised to return in two weeks for a follow-up visit.

First-Listed Diagnosis: _____

Secondary Diagnoses: _____

8

The patient is a 54-year-old female who has suffered from left-side chronic ulcerative colitis for many years. Today she is seen in her physician's office for a follow-up visit. Of most concern to the patient today are the "red bumps" that are present on her right lower leg. The patient has had similar lesions before now, but the lesions have recently returned and are larger in size than previously. The physician recognizes the lesions as a recurrence of erythema nodosum, which is a complication of her underlying systemic condition. The tender red nodules appear to be coinciding with the worsening of her colitis. The patient thinks she might have bumped her leg against a grocery cart the previous week and blamed that for the tender nodules that appeared first. A topical ointment is prescribed, and the physician advises the patient that the nodules will probably heal as her colitis becomes more controlled with the medication she is currently receiving. The physician treats both the left-sided colitis and the erythema nodosum during the visit today.

First-Listed Diagnosis: _____

Secondary Diagnoses: _____

9

A 60-year-old male returns to the Wound Care Clinic today for a follow-up visit for treatment of his diabetic right heel foot ulcer. The ulcer was present on the right heel with muscle involvement but no necrosis. The patient is a type 1 diabetic with an ulcer attributed to his diabetes. The wound was infected when the patient was first seen in the Wound Care Clinic, but today the ulcer is smaller in size and is not infected. Close surveillance, wound dressings, and the appropriate use of antibiotics were successful in treating this man's foot ulcer and prevented it from becoming gangrenous. The patient receives ongoing education about proper skin and foot care because his diabetic condition makes him at risk for more ulcers. The patient will return in two weeks for a follow-up visit.

First-Listed Diagnosis: _____

Secondary Diagnoses: _____

10

The patient is a 47-year-old female who returns to her dermatologist's office after a one-year absence with pityriasis rosea, a condition she has had several times before. Usually in the spring of the year, the patient suffers from this skin condition. She explains to the physician that she first noticed a 3–4 cm annular or ring-shaped lesion on her trunk that was followed a few days later with many smaller ring-shaped and pustular lesions parallel to the skin folds on her chest and abdomen. The physician notes the red and brown lesions with a trailing scale. Once again, the patient describes the condition as extremely itchy and is seeking another prescription for the topical glucocorticoid cream the physician prescribed in the past. The physician is agreeable to renewing the prescription for treating the pityriasis rosea and offers the patient the option of UV B (ultraviolet light) phototherapy, as the outbreak seems to be more severe this year. The patient states she will try the cream first and make another appointment for the phototherapy if there is no improvement.

First-Listed Diagnosis: _____

Secondary Diagnoses: _____

11

The patient was admitted to the hospital for other medical conditions. The patient was seen in consultation by a dermatologic surgeon at the request of his primary care physician.

The 53-year-old male had two lesions on his scalp. One lesion was 1.2 cm × 1.3 cm × 1.0 cm on the posterior scalp and was slightly raised and slightly erythematous. After injection of local anesthesia in the center of the lesion, a 3-mm punch biopsy was performed. The biopsied tissue was then removed and sent for frozen section to pathology. The frozen section was positive for basal cell carcinoma. A 5-0 Prolene stitch was used to close the defect. The patient had a second lesion about 2 cm away from the first lesion and measuring 0.5 cm × 0.2 cm. The lesion was excised by using a sharpened scalpel to penetrate the skin and dermis on both sides. This lesion was then removed and sent to pathology. The second lesion was reported to be an actinic keratosis and excised in its entirety. It was closed with a 5-0 Prolene stitch times two. Steri-strips were applied. We informed the patient that we will refer him to a plastic surgeon for removal of the basal cell carcinoma, as this may require significant undermining and wound closure may be problematic because of the size of the lesion. There is quite a bit of tension on the patient's scalp, and the excision of the basal cell carcinoma will require the skills of a plastic surgeon. The patient will be seen for follow-up in this surgeon's office in seven days and was given the name and phone number of the plastic surgeon to call for an appointment within the next two weeks.

Code the diagnosis and procedure performed as a result of the consultation.

Dermatology Diagnosis: _____

Secondary Dermatology Diagnoses: _____

Principal Procedure: _____

Secondary Procedure(s): _____

12

The patient is a 56-year-old female admitted to the hospital after being seen in the physician's office for two large draining abscesses on her back. One was on the left-upper back and the other on the right-lower back skin. Both lesions were large, actively draining, and showed some necrotic features to the surrounding tissue. These areas on the back were warm to the touch and tender. Because of the size of the lesions, the patient was admitted as an inpatient for surgery. The surgeon performed an incision and drainage on two areas of the back. The right-lower back actually had two areas of abscess with necrotic tissue present. The cavity was widely opened with an incision that connected the two abscesses. Another incision was made in this area because the fluctuance had penetrated deeper down, and the entire area required drainage and copious irrigation. A Penrose drain was placed to keep the tracks open. The left-upper back had an area of fluctuance of 3 cm × 5 cm. A transverse incision was made deep into the subcutaneous cavity, and all the purulent material was removed from the widely opened area. It was copiously irrigated. Specimens were collected from all these areas for cultures. The fluid cultures grew methicillin-resistant staphylococcus aureus susceptible to Clindamycin. While in the hospital, the patient received intravenous antibiotics. The patient was continued on this antibiotic orally for one more week. The drain was left in for the surgeon to remove about three days after discharge. The patient was known to have hypertension, and it was treated during the hospital stay. The patient had two fasting glucose tests performed in the hospital, and both were significantly elevated at 160 and 180. A hemoglobin A1c was performed with a finding of 9.5. The patient was informed that she had type 2 diabetes, poorly controlled with hyperglycemia. She had a dietary consultation in the hospital and will attend diabetic education classes after discharge. She was discharged with a glucose monitoring kit and a prescription for oral diabetic medication. She will be seen in the primary care physician's office in one week.

Principal Diagnosis: _____

Secondary Diagnoses: _____

Principal Procedure Code: _____

Secondary Procedure(s): _____

13

The patient was a 69-year-old male who had many previous admissions for cellulitis and alcoholic cirrhosis of the liver proven by biopsy. He had hepatic encephalopathy on several occasions and hepatorenal failure two times when he was previously hospitalized. He also has marked exogenous obesity. On this occasion he was admitted for an abrupt elevation of temperature with diaphoresis on the night of admission, following a dinner party. His lower abdominal area was the site of marked reddening and induration at the fold of his panniculus adiposis. His admitting diagnosis was cellulitis of abdominal tissues, and he was started on intravenous antibiotics. He was seen in consultation by an infectious disease physician and a nephrologist. It appeared his cellulitis this time was triggered by edema of the extremities. His abdominal cellulitis responded virtually overnight to the intravenous cephazolin. He also had stasis dermatitis and cellulitis of his legs, but the legs were less red and indurated than his lower abdomen. He was also proven to be hypoalbuminemic. Blood cultures were drawn and *Pseudomonas aeruginosa* was found in his blood. This organism was not susceptible to the antibiotic he received for the first four days of his hospitalization. Because the antibiotics he was receiving would not have been expected to kill the pseudomonas, it was speculated that the process involving the lower abdominal wall was due to gram-positive coccal organisms such as staphylococcus or streptococcus, which is why the abdominal cellulitis responded so quickly to the cephalosporin antibiotics. The organism causing the abdominal cellulitis was not proven. But it was not surprising to find the pseudomonas in his blood by virtue of his anatomic problems as well as his poor hepatic function, which leaves him prone to bacteremia. However, the bacteremia produced no symptoms in this patient with a well-established history of cirrhosis. He was anicteric and did not have any evidence of encephalopathy. He was continued on treatment with the best anti-pseudomonal agent and continued with gentle diuresis to remove the edema fluid in both lower extremities that produce the leg cellulitis. His liver function studies were not any worse than previously noted, but the physicians again encouraged the patient to eliminate alcohol consumption. Because the patient travels extensively for business and pleasure, the physicians emphasized the need to take all of his medications faithfully in order to maintain his apparent resilience in the knowledge of his extensive liver disease and to carry antibiotics with him so that any early onset of cellulitis might be aborted by early treatment. The patient agreed and was discharged after an 11-day hospital stay. His discharge diagnoses were documented as cellulitis, anterior abdominal wall, gram-negative bacteremia (pseudomonas), stasis dermatitis and cellulitis bilateral lower extremities, advanced alcoholic liver cirrhosis with hypoalbuminemia, and morbid obesity.

Principal Diagnosis: _____

Secondary Diagnoses: _____

Principal Procedure: _____

Secondary Procedure(s): _____

14

The 4-year-old female was admitted to the hospital directly from her pediatrician's office because of symmetrical raised red skin lesions over 20 percent of her body. She also has edema of her upper and lower eyelids. The child had been treated with a penicillin-type drug for an upper respiratory infection, and it was suspected the child was having a reaction to that drug. A pediatric infectious disease specialist examined the patient immediately. After reviewing laboratory results, the consultant concluded the patient had Stevens-Johnson syndrome, which is a toxic epidermal necrolysis that produces the skin lesions seen on this child. The consultant attributed the edema of the eyelids to the same syndrome. The patient received a four-day treatment of intravenous immunoglobulin drugs through a peripheral vein and made an excellent recovery. The consultant stated the 20 percent to 25 percent exfoliation of her skin surface caused by the Stevens-Johnson syndrome was an adverse effect of the penicillin this child received for the respiratory infection. The child was discharged home to her parents' care with pediatric home health nursing follow-up.

Principal Diagnosis: _____

Secondary Diagnoses: _____

Principal Procedure: _____

Secondary Procedures: _____

15

The patient is an 89-year-old female admitted to the hospital from the nursing home for surgical treatment of her pressure-induced deep tissue damage of the sacral region over the coccyx. The patient was taken to surgery, and the physician dictated an operative report that described an excisional debridement of the wound over the coccyx with excision through the fascia and into the bone. The patient was transferred back to the nursing home two days later to be visited by the surgeon and the wound care clinical nurse specialist in one week. While the patient was in the hospital, she continued to receive treatment for her chronic diastolic heart failure, coronary artery (native vessel) disease with known total chronic occlusion in at least two coronary vessels.

Principal Diagnosis: _____

Secondary Diagnoses: _____

Principal Procedure Code: _____

Secondary Procedure(s): _____

16

Six months after a house fire in which the patient sustained burns of his right leg, he has developed severe scarring as a result of the third-degree burns. The patient is evaluated in the plastic surgeon's office and scheduled for reconstructive surgery in the near future.

First-Listed Diagnosis: _____

Secondary Diagnoses: _____

17

The patient is a 68-year-old male who is an established patient of the dermatologist who examined the patient today in the dermatology clinic for a flare of lesions of pemphigus foliaceus. The patient has been treated for the condition before by the same dermatologist. The dermatologist updated the patient's history by interviewing the patient. Upon examination, the dermatologist found crusted lesions and soft blisters on the patient's face, scalp, and anterior chest. The sores appeared to be superficial but described by the patient as extremely itchy. The dermatologist stated that a skin biopsy could be taken but doubted it will provide any additional information and, for that reason, the patient declined to consent for a skin biopsy. In the past the patient has been treated with different drugs, specifically corticosteroids and immunosuppressive drugs. Given that this flare-up is the third episode of pemphigus foliaceus for the patient, the dermatologist advised him that it was very important for the patient to follow the instructions to take the prescribed medications exactly as directed. The patient was prescribed Valisone 0.1% topical ointment to be used on his chest and scalp but not on his face because the facial lesions were practically dried up. The patient was also re-started on a low dose of oral Prednisone and again instructed to take the medications as directed. The fact the patient is under treatment for essential hypertension that was acknowledged by the dermatologist as he considered what medications to prescribe.

First-Listed Diagnosis: _____

Secondary Diagnoses: _____

18

The patient is a 55-year-old male with known atherosclerosis of the lower extremities that was worse on the right lower extremity and causing multiple ulcerations of the right calf. For this reason, the patient was seen again in the wound care clinic. The physician examined the non-pressure ulcers on his right calf. The physician updated the patient's history while interviewing him and his wife, and included the fact that the patient has never had vascular surgery or a bypass procedure on his legs. The physician was pleased that the ulcers, that at one time were much deeper into the tissues, were now limited to the muscle without evidence of necrosis and were healing. The physician applied the wound healing dressings to the patient's right lower leg. The patient's wife was again instructed on how to apply the dressings at home. The patient was given an appointment to return to the wound care clinic in two weeks. The patient was known to have type 2 diabetes mellitus that can also cause the skin ulcers, and the physician reviewed the patient's blood sugar result taken during the visit. The patient has taken insulin on a long-term basis. The physician had told the patient that diabetes complicated the healing process, but the ulcerations were caused by the atherosclerosis. The physician concluded the reasons for the visit were (1) atherosclerosis of right lower extremity; (2) non-pressure ulcerations, right calf, with muscle involvement without necrosis; (3) diabetes mellitus, type 2.

First-Listed Diagnosis: _____

Secondary Diagnosis: _____

Chapter 13

Diseases of the Musculoskeletal System and Connective Tissue

Coding Scenarios for *Basic ICD-10-CM and ICD-10-PCS Coding Exercises*

The following case studies are organized following the sequence of the chapters in the ICD-10-CM Tabular List of Diseases and Injuries as published on the Centers for Disease Control and Prevention National Center for Health Statistics website (http://www.cdc.gov /nchs/icd/icd10cm.htm). The objective of this book is to provide the student with more detailed clinical information to code, rather than one- or two-line diagnosis and procedure statements.

ICD-10-CM diagnosis codes are to be assigned to both the inpatient hospital admission and the outpatient visit case studies. In this book, the ICD-10-PCS procedure codes are to be assigned only to the inpatient hospital admission cases. In actual practice, outpatient cases are assigned CPT/HCPCS codes. The ICD-10-PCS codes are only required for inpatient procedures. In the answer key for the exercises, the Alphabetic Index entry is listed after the code to indicate the main terms and sub-terms used to locate the code that must be verified in the ICD-10-CM Tabular List or in the ICD-10-PCS Code Tables prior to assigning the code.

1

A 50-year-old male is treated for severe low back pain and numbness on the left leg over several weeks. The patient thinks the pain is the result of lifting heavy boxes during a recent move to a new residence, but the physician cannot conclude that this was the cause. Diagnostic studies reveal that the patient has a herniated disc. The patient is also found to have osteoarthritis of the lumbar spine with radiculopathy. The patient is admitted for a laminotomy and removal of the nucleus pulpous of the intervertebral disc at L4-L5 to treat the herniated disc but leaving the annulus fibrosus intact. The patient has an uneventful postoperative recovery and is discharged home to begin rehabilitation therapy in the near future.

Principal Diagnosis: _____

Secondary Diagnoses: _____

Principal Procedure: _____

Secondary Procedure(s): _____

2

A 62-year-old female had been treated by her family physician for chronic low back pain. One morning, upon awakening, she could not get out of bed due to severe back pain. She was brought to the emergency department and admitted. X-rays show several severe compression fractures of the lumbar vertebrae as a result of senile osteoporosis. An injection of a steroidal anti-inflammatory agent is administered into the spinal canal to help alleviate her pain from age-related osteoporosis and the pathologic fracture.

Principal Diagnosis: _____

Secondary Diagnoses: _____

Principal Procedure: _____

Secondary Procedure(s): _____

3

This 75-year-old patient is seen again in his primary care physician's office for care of his arthritis. He has generalized degenerative arthritis of the knees, hips, and of the lumbosacral spine. His condition is becoming progressively worse, and different medications have been tried to alleviate the pain and discomfort. Because of his long-standing hypertension, which has not been well-controlled, and angina due to coronary artery disease (with disease in the autologous vein bypass grafts after previous CABG 10 years previously), the patient is not a good candidate for joint replacement surgery. A new arthritis medication is prescribed, and his anti-hypertensive and cardiac medication prescriptions are renewed.

First-Listed Diagnosis: _____

Secondary Diagnoses: _____

4

A 40-year-old female is admitted to the hospital for treatment for systemic lupus erythematosus (SLE). She is going to receive the next course of intravenous infusion of cyclophosphamide, an effective but highly toxic chemotherapy drug, to treat the SLE. The patient currently has a central venous catheter placed in the superior vena cava in which her chemotherapy treatments are administered. The patient has several complications as a result of SLE, including nephritic syndrome, inflammatory myopathy, anemia of chronic disease, and swan-neck deformities of her fingers. During the hospital stay, the patient receives other medications to manage the complications. Intravenous infusion is started on day 1. She is monitored for toxicity, but none is detected and she is able to go home on day 3.

Principal Diagnosis: _____

Secondary Diagnoses: _____

Principal Procedure: _____

Secondary Procedure(s): _____

5

The patient is a 25-year-old female who returns to the orthopedic clinic to see her sports medicine physician. She is complaining of gradually increasing pain in her shinbones that used to abate when she resorted to walking instead of running but now is not relieved by such a walking rest. The woman runs several miles four days a week. Two weeks ago the physician had ordered x-rays of both lower legs. The results were negative for fractures. Because the patient now complained of pain in her right foot, today the physician ordered the x-rays of the legs to be repeated and an x-ray of the right foot to be performed. The radiologist concluded there was a stress reaction in the right and left lower distal tibias and a stress fracture of the second metatarsal of the right foot. Given the patient's history, physical findings, and radiologic evidence, the physician makes the diagnosis of bilateral stress fractures of the tibias and stress fracture of the right second metatarsal of the foot. The patient is instructed to rest and keep off her feet as much as possible for the next eight weeks, specifically with no running or other exercising. Based on her complaints of back pain, the physician also describes the patient as having an acute lumbosacral strain. The patient is to return in four weeks for repeat x-rays. The physician concluded that her injuries were the result of cumulative trauma from the repetitive impact of running on hard surfaces.

First-Listed Diagnosis: _____

Secondary Diagnoses: _____

6

The patient is admitted to the hospital for debridement of the right fibula bone. After multiple outpatient diagnostic tests are performed, the diagnosis of acute osteomyelitis localized in the right fibula due to a staphylococcal infection is made in this 15-year-old male. The child began complaining of pain below the right knee and difficulty walking over the past two weeks. The patient denied any trauma to the leg but, as an active boy who plays soccer and softball, trauma could not be ruled out, although no evidence of an injury was found on the leg. To prevent bone destruction as well as the possibility of the infection spreading to other bones and joints in the lower leg, the child is admitted for surgery. The procedure is an open excisional debridement of the proximal fibula. The patient withstands the procedure well and is discharged to his parents for at-home recovery 1 day after surgery.

Principal Diagnosis: _____

Secondary Diagnoses: _____

Principal Procedure: _____

Secondary Procedure(s): _____

7

The patient is a 30-year-old male who comes to the emergency department complaining of joint pain in his shoulder. The patient, who was a state champion wrestler during his college years, reports that his shoulder has dislocated on several occasions since college, when he had several traumatic dislocations of the same shoulder. On this occasion, the patient was lifting a heavy box overhead to place on a shelf in his mobile home garage. X-rays were taken to examine the shoulder. The ED physician is unable to reduce the dislocation on the initial attempt. With light intravenous sedation, the physician completes a closed reduction of shoulder dislocation. The physician wrote "chronic recurrent dislocation of right shoulder and traumatic arthritis of the right shoulder" as the final diagnosis on the ED record. (While there is no requirement that ICD-10-PCS procedure codes are coded on outpatients, code the closed reduction of the shoulder dislocation for coding practice.)

First-Listed Diagnosis: _____

Secondary Diagnoses: _____

Practice Procedure Coding: _____

8

The patient, a 48-year-old female, was admitted to the hospital for surgical repair of a massive rotator cuff tear of her right shoulder. The patient was known to have hypertension, but it was well controlled and she received medical clearance for surgery. The patient has had pain, weakness, and limited range of motion in her right shoulder, which has been present for several years and has been getting progressively worse. Several years ago she had a fall and injured her right hip but doesn't remember her shoulder being injured at that time. The patient was taken to surgery and placed under general anesthesia. The surgeon found a complete tear of the rotator cuff that appeared nontraumatic and significant tenosynovitis of the shoulder. The surgeon performed a rotator cuff repair, which was accomplished by reattaching the tendon using an arthroscope. A synovectomy of the shoulder was also performed through the arthroscope. The patient was kept overnight in the hospital, received her antihypertensive medication, and was discharged to home on day 2 with a follow-up appointment with the surgeon in 10 days.

Principal Diagnosis: _____

Secondary Diagnoses: _____

Principal Procedure: _____

Secondary Procedure(s): _____

9

The patient is a 56-year-old male with significant hypertensive heart disease who was admitted to the hospital for an arthroscopic partial medial meniscectomy on his right knee. Due to his hypertension and heart disease, the cardiologist advised the orthopedic surgeon to admit the patient to the hospital for at least overnight monitoring after the procedure. During a previous orthopedic surgery, this patient had a hypertensive crisis and was placed in the intensive care unit for monitoring. This surgery was performed uneventfully. The patient had an arthroscopic partial medial meniscectomy of the posterior horn of the medial meniscus, right knee. This was determined to be an old tear, likely from a football playing injury. There were no loose bodies in the medial and lateral gutters. The articular cartilage surfaces were in reasonably good condition. The notches of the anterior cruciate and posterior cruciate ligaments were intact. Within the lateral compartment, the meniscus was intact and the articular cartilage surfaces in good condition. At the conclusion of the procedure, all excess fluid was drained, the portal incisions closed with nylon sutures, an injection of Marcaine was administered for pain control, and sterile dressings were applied. The patient was taken to the recovery room and then transferred to a regular bed. He was discharged the following morning with a follow-up appointment with the surgeon in 10 days.

Principal Diagnosis: _____

Secondary Diagnoses: _____

Principal Procedure: _____

Secondary Procedure(s): _____

10

The patient is a 28-year-old female with severe chronic asthmatic bronchitis and a congenital heart condition—ventricular septal defect—that has been monitored for several years. At this time, the patient has very painful bunions on both feet that make walking increasingly difficult with the fact she is unable to wear a shoe on her left foot. She has acquired this condition rather quickly over the past couple of years. The patient was referred to a podiatrist for evaluation. After taking the patient's history and performing a physical examination of the patient's lower extremities, the physician concluded the patient had hallux abductovalgus, both feet, worse on the left. The patient consented to an outpatient procedure to be performed one week later, specifically, a McBride bunionectomy with soft-tissue correction. The physician also included the diagnoses of chronic asthmatic bronchitis and VSD as secondary diagnoses.

First-Listed Diagnosis: _____

Secondary Diagnoses: _____

11

The patient is a 48-year-old female who was diagnosed with an aggressive form of breast carcinoma in her right breast in the past year and had a radical mastectomy followed by chemotherapy. She has also developed secondary myelofibrosis with therapy-related low grade myelodysplastic syndrome, due to the antineoplastic chemotherapy she has received. On this occasion, the patient called her physician reporting excruciating low back pain that had developed rapidly over the past two days and was told to go to the emergency department. It was feared the patient had a compression fracture or similar condition due to metastatic bone cancer. The patient was admitted and examined by her attending physician, oncologist, and consulting orthopedic surgeon. Imaging of the spine failed to find any pathology, including no metastatic disease, much to the relief of the patient, family, and physicians. The physicians could not explain the rapid onset of low back pain, which was treated with pain medications. On day 3, the patient reported less back pain and better ambulation and was allowed to go home with her family. Chemotherapy will be performed on schedule in the next two weeks, and the patient continued to receive treatment for her myelofibrosis and myelodysplastic syndrome due to the chemotherapy.

Principal Diagnosis: _____

Secondary Diagnoses: _____

Principal Procedure: _____

Secondary Procedure(s): _____

12

The patient is a 19-year-old female college scholar-athlete who is a scholarship basketball player at the state university. She has had repeated injuries to her knees over the past seven years while she has played in competitive sports, including basketball, softball, and soccer. Over the past three months, she had noted a feeling of instability in the left knee, more than usual and with increasing pain over the medial compartment, as a result of these old injuries. The physicians who had treated her over the past year were fairly confident that she had a torn anterior cruciate ligament and suspected possible tears to the medial meniscus and medial collateral ligament from the past injuries and not a new traumatic problem. She was admitted to the hospital for reconstructive surgery, with a planned transfer to a sports rehabilitation unit at the university hospital. At surgery, the orthopedic surgeon found a grossly positive Lachman's sign and anterior drawer in neutral, internal, and external rotation. The medial meniscus was torn at the posterior horn in a complex fashion posteriorly. There was no repairable tissue. The medial collateral ligament was torn; that was probably a new injury. The good news was the surfaces of the patellofemoral joint, medial compartment, and lateral compartments were in good condition. The anterior cruciate ligament was completely torn and was most likely a recent injury just discovered during this procedure. The posterior cruciate ligament was intact, and the patellar tendons rode laterally in the notch. At the conclusion of the procedure, the knee was stable to Lachman and drawer testing. The procedures performed on the left knee were an arthroscopic reconstruction/reinforcement of the anterior cruciate ligament using nonautologous patellar tendon graft, repair of the medial meniscus and medial collateral ligament, also known as the triad knee repair or O'Donoghue procedure that includes a medial meniscectomy. After three days of postoperative recovery, the patient was transferred to the sports rehabilitation unit for a complex rehabilitation program.

Principal Diagnosis: _____

Secondary Diagnoses: _____

Principal Procedure: _____

Secondary Procedure(s): _____

13

A 46-year-old female, a former professional basketball athlete, was admitted to the hospital for hip replacement surgery to treat posttraumatic osteoarthritis that involved both hips.

Her left hip is considerably worse than her right hip. Otherwise, the patient is in good health. Her past medical history included pneumonia three years ago and a hysterectomy for a fibroid uterus at age 40 years. A successful total left hip replacement was performed using a ceramic-on-ceramic hip replacement bearing surface prosthesis cemented in place. The patient was discharged three days later to receive physical therapy at the sports medicine center. She will be scheduled for the right hip replacement at a later date.

Principal Diagnosis: _____

Secondary Diagnoses: _____

Principal Procedure: _____

Secondary Procedure(s): _____

14

A patient comes to the pain clinic for management of chronic neck and shoulder pain that she has suffered since she was the driver in a motor vehicle collision with another vehicle that occurred six months previously. The patient has difficulty sleeping due to the pain and has trouble lifting or moving anything with her left shoulder or arm. After taking a complete history and performing a thorough physical examination, the pain management physician diagnoses the condition as "cervicobrachial syndrome, due to motor vehicle crash 10 months ago and past whiplash injury."

First-Listed Diagnosis: _____

Secondary Diagnoses: _____

15

The patient is seen in the orthopedic clinic for a complaint of muscle wasting or atrophy of the lower legs. In conducting a thorough history and physical examination, the physician learns that the patient had poliomyelitis 50 years previously. The physician determines the muscle atrophy is a result of her old polio and describes it as postpolio syndrome. The physician recommends a trial of physical therapy in the future to prevent further muscular wasting.

First-Listed Diagnosis: _____

Secondary Diagnoses: _____

16

The patient, an active 60-year-old male, who suffered a fracture of the neck of the right femur in an motor vehicle crash 10 years previously when he was a passenger in a car involved in a collision with a pickup truck, is admitted to the hospital for a right total hip replacement. The patient has suffered progressive disability of his hip joint with severe hip pain on standing, sitting, and lying down. Given the patient has no arthritis in any other joint, it is determined that the arthritis in his right hip is a result of the old fracture or trauma. The patient consents to a total hip replacement with an uncemented metal-on-polyethylene bearing surface. The patient is discharged home to be followed up by home health nurses and physical therapists.

Principal Diagnosis: _____

Secondary Diagnoses: _____

Procedure Codes: _____

Secondary Procedure(s): _____

17

The patient is a 70-year-old male who was admitted to the hospital for urology complaints and was found after study to have an enlarged prostate with urinary retention and acute renal failure. While in the hospital, he asked his physician if something could be done for his "sore knees." He stated it was extremely difficult for him to walk and it was limiting his activities of daily living. He was not able to accompany his wife to go shopping or go to church because his knees felt so stiff and painful and he was afraid of falling. An orthopedic surgeon was consulted who examined the patient and ordered radiology examinations of both knees. The orthopedic surgeon concluded the patient's left knee arthritis was worse than in the right knee, but both knees had significant arthritis. The orthopedic surgeon suspected the patella of the left knee could be the main problem and advised the patient to have an arthroscopic inspection of the left knee. The patient consented and was taken to surgery. The operative report documented the following:

OPERATIVE FINDINGS: An arthroscopic debridement of the left patella was performed. The medial meniscus, lateral meniscus, and anterior cruciate ligament (ACL) were normal. The examination of the patellofemoral joint showed the entire surface of the patella had chondromalacia with surfaces graded from 2 to mostly 3. A significant degree of prepatellar bursitis of the left knee was likely the cause of the pain and stiffness. The patient will be given information about a total knee replacement as it is likely he will need the left knee replaced at some time in the future.

DESCRIPTION OF PROCEDURE: The patient was placed under general endotracheal tube anesthesia. The left knee was prepped and draped in the usual manner for arthroscopic surgery of the left knee. After insufflation of lidocaine and epinephrine, three standard ports, two medial and one lateral, were established in the usual manner. There was difficulty in evaluating the suprapatellar pouch as well as the patellofemoral joint initially because of the extensive chondromalacia and synovial reaction. Prepatellar bursitis was present. The medial compartment was first evaluated carefully, and the medical meniscus was found to be normal to observation and probing as were the medial femoral condyle and medial tibial plateau. The ACL appeared to be intact. The lateral meniscus and lateral compartment were normal. In order to see the contents of the femoral-tibial joint, excisional debridement of pedunculated synovial tissue was necessary. On returning to the patellofemoral joint, excisional debridement of synovial tissues was done as well as on the synovial plica material. At this point, the magnitude of the problem on the patella was obvious. The entire surface of the patella was involved with chondromalacia over more of the lateral facet but also on the medial facet with grade-3 chondromalacia. This involved a large portion of the main articular surface of the patella. At the conclusion of this procedure, instrumentation was removed, and sterile dressings applied. The patient was awakened and taken to the recovery room in stable condition.

Directions: Code only the procedure and diagnoses related to the procedure.

Diagnosis Codes: _____

Principal Procedure: _____

Secondary Procedure(s): _____

18

The patient is a 62-year-old male who presents with bilateral knee osteoarthritis confirmed on x-rays and clinical examinations. The patient has severe varus deformities to both knees secondary to his primary localized knee osteoarthritis. He has had two sets of cortisone injections to both knees and hyaluronic acid injections to both knees. He has been prescribed nonsteroidal anti-inflammatory medications, pain medications, and bracing. Despite all of this conservative management the patient continues to have pain and disability, causing severe limitation of his activities of daily living and requiring the use of a walker for ambulation on most days. He was given the options of unilateral or bilateral total knee replacements. He elected to have his left knee replaced first as it was the most painful. It is expected the right knee will be replaced within the next year. He was informed of the risks and complications of total knee replacement including infection, bleeding, neurovascular injury, need for follow-up procedures or operations, deep vein thrombosis, pulmonary emboli, and the remote chance of life threatening conditions, including death. The patient is a robust, healthy man with no medical conditions present other than the osteoarthritis of his knees. The patient is admitted to the hospital for the surgical procedure.

OPERATIVE REPORT

PREOPERATIVE DIAGNOSIS:	Severe osteoarthritis, both knees, worse on left side
POSTOPERATIVE DIAGNOSIS:	Severe osteoarthritis, both knees, worse on left side
PROCEDURE PERFORMED:	Left knee replacement
DEVICES USED:	Smith and Nephew Genesis II system with the OrthoSensor alignment guide. The size was 6 PS femur, size 6 tibia, size 13 constrained polyethylene and a 38 mm anatomic patella.
TOURNIQUET TIME:	Approximately 75 minutes
ESTIMATED BLOOD LOSS:	Approximately 100 mL
ANESTHESIA:	General anesthetic with adductor nerve block and Exparel injection locally into the wound

DESCRIPTION OF PROCEDURE: The patient was taken to the operating room and preoperative antibiotics were administered. Time-out was conducted and the left leg tourniquet was placed. The left leg was marked preoperatively by the patient. The left leg was cleaned and draped in the usual manner. A midline incision was made on the left knee joint followed by medial parapatellar approach to the knee. The patella was everted. The knee was then debrided, at which time, appropriate releases were then performed. The Visionaire cutting block was then placed. Appropriate femoral cut was made for a size 6 femur. We then turned our attention to the tibia. Intramedullary guide was introduced. Appropriate cuts were then made, at which time, trial with a 6 femur, 6 tibia was then performed. Appropriate releases were then conducted using the Orthosensor device with computer assistance. There was found to have a 13-mm poly obtained in excellent stability mediolaterally through a full range of motion. Patella was then cut, a 33-mm patella was placed, obtaining the balanced knee. The trial components were then removed. Pulsed lavage was then used for bony cut surfaces. They were dried. After drying, the three components of femur, tibia, and patella were then cemented in place at the same time. Excess cement was removed. Cement was allowed to harden, at which time, a permanent 13-mm constrained polyethylene was then placed, obtaining excellent medial and lateral stability through a full range of motion and centrally tracking patella. With this, Exparel was injected into the knee joint. The medial parapatella approach was then closed in standard fashion. The subcutaneous tissue was closed in standard fashion. The skin was closed in a standard fashion. The patient had sterile dressing applied to the left knee. In an effort to provide relief and improvement in the right knee, the physician harvests posterior iliac crest bone marrow, centrifuging it to obtain concentrated bone marrow, and then reinjecting it in the muscular area surrounding the right knee. The patient was taken to the recovery area in stable condition.

Principal Diagnosis: _____

Secondary Diagnoses: _____

Principal Procedure: _____

Secondary Procedure(s): _____

Chapter 14

Diseases of the Genitourinary System

Coding Scenarios for *Basic ICD-10-CM and ICD-10-PCS Coding Exercises*

The following case studies are organized following the sequence of the chapters in the ICD-10-CM Tabular List of Diseases and Injuries as published on the Centers for Disease Control and Prevention National Center for Health Statistics website (http://www.cdc.gov/nchs/icd/icd10cm.htm). The objective of this book is to provide the student with more detailed clinical information to code, rather than one- or two-line diagnosis and procedure statements.

ICD-10-CM diagnosis codes are to be assigned to both the inpatient hospital admission and the outpatient visit case studies. In this book, the ICD-10-PCS procedure codes are to be assigned only to the inpatient hospital admission cases. In actual practice, outpatient cases are assigned CPT/HCPCS codes. The ICD-10-PCS codes are only required for inpatient procedures. In the answer key for the exercises, the Alphabetic Index entry is listed after the code to indicate the main terms and sub-terms used to locate the code that must be verified in the ICD-10-CM Tabular List or in the ICD-10-PCS Code Tables prior to assigning the code.

1

An 80-year-old female is admitted to the hospital with fever, malaise, and left flank pain. A urinalysis shows bacteria of more than 100,000/mL present in the urine and a subsequent urine culture shows Proteus growth as the cause of the infection. The patient was treated with intravenous antibiotics through a peripheral vein. Other preexisting conditions of hypertension, arteriosclerotic heart disease (ASHD), previous percutaneous transluminal coronary angioplasty (PTCA) but no history of coronary artery bypass graft (CABG), and long-term chronic obstructive pulmonary disease (COPD) were treated during the hospital stay. The patient also has a history of repeated urinary tract infections (UTI) over the past several years.

Principal Diagnosis: _____

Secondary Diagnoses: _____

Principal Procedure: _____

Secondary Procedure(s): _____

2

A 75-year-old male was admitted to the hospital in acute urinary retention. A transurethral endoscopic resection of the prostate was performed but the entire prostate was not removed. The diagnosis of benign nodular hyperplasia of the prostate was made. The pathologist confirmed the hyperplasia diagnosis and also found microscopic foci of adenocarcinoma of the prostate. The attending physician listed both conditions as discharge diagnoses.

Principal Diagnosis: _____

Secondary Diagnoses: _____

Principal Procedure: _____

Secondary Procedure(s): _____

3

A 52-year-old female was admitted to the hospital with urinary stress incontinence and is scheduled for surgical repair of a paravaginal cystocele. An open anterior colporrhaphy is performed to repair the cystocele that was causing the urinary stress incontinence. The patient has type 2 diabetes on oral anti-diabetic medication and central vertigo that is also treated during the hospital stay.

Principal Diagnosis: _____

Secondary Diagnoses: _____

Principal Procedure: _____

Secondary Procedure(s): _____

4

An 80-year-old male was brought to the emergency department with complaints of lower abdominal pain and the inability to urinate over the past 24 hours. An indwelling urinary catheter was placed in the patient, and he was admitted. After study, it was determined that the patient was in subacute to acute renal failure. The acute renal failure was caused by a urinary obstruction. The urologist concluded the urinary obstruction was a result of the patient's benign prostatic hypertrophy. An intravenous pyelogram of the kidneys, ureters and bladder with low osmolar contrast was performed fluoroscopically and confirmed the physician's diagnoses. The patient was treated with medications, and the acute renal failure was resolved. The catheter remained in place for drainage. The patient would require a resection of the prostate but would return for prostate surgery the following week. The patient was discharged home.

Principal Diagnosis: _____

Secondary Diagnoses: _____

Principal Procedure: _____

Secondary Procedure(s): _____

5

A 60-year-old female patient is brought to the community hospital complaining of flank and back pain, fever with chills, fatigue, and a general ill feeling. The patient was known to have essential hypertension and had a history of renal calculi treated six months ago. The patient was admitted with the diagnosis of possible urinary tract infection. Workup in the hospital showed evidence of acute pyelonephritis. She was treated with intravenous antibiotics via peripheral vein, but while in the hospital the patient had a sudden loss of kidney function. A diagnosis was made of acute renal failure complicating the acute pyelonephritis. The physicians ordered intermittent renal dialysis for the acute renal failure to be performed three times over the next five days, four hours each session, and the hospital arranged for the dialysis service to be performed. The patient was discharged to home care with arrangements for a visit to the nephrologist's office on the second day after discharge to determine if renal dialysis needed to be continued on a temporary basis.

Principal Diagnosis: _____

Secondary Diagnoses: _____

Principal Procedure: _____

Secondary Procedure(s): _____

6

The patient is a 21-year-old male who is known to have polycystic kidney disease, which was diagnosed in the past year after he was found to have hypertension. Upon investigating the cause of hypertension in such a young individual, it was discovered he had polycystic kidney disease, an inherited condition. The hypertension was considered secondary to the kidney disease. On this occasion, the patient was admitted to the hospital because of worsening kidney function. After study, it was determined the patient had chronic kidney disease, stage III, as a result of the polycystic kidney disease that was producing the hypertension. This patient was referred to the university medical center for further management with hopes for better control of kidney function and avoidance of the need for kidney transplant.

Principal Diagnosis: _____

Secondary Diagnoses: _____

Principal Procedure: _____

Secondary Procedure(s): _____

7

The patient is a 46-year-old female, gravida 3, para 3, admitted to the hospital for a scheduled vaginal hysterectomy and bilateral salpingo-oophorectomy. The patient has an extensive gynecologic history and was most recently seen for dysmenorrhea and dyspareunia. She stated she was having prolonged, heavy menses with disturbing premenstrual syndrome that was lasting three to four days before the onset of the menses. Six months ago, an outpatient laparoscopy was performed and extensive endometriosis of the uterus, ovaries, tubes, and pelvic peritoneum was found. Lysis of adhesions and ablation of the endometriosis was attempted, but due to the extensive nature of the disease, it was known the procedure would not be entirely successful. In addition, the patient has been diagnosed and treated for cervical dysplasia described as mild to moderate that was investigated with 11 different biopsies. All subsequent pap smears have been normal. Despite continued treatment, the patient still suffers from chronic pelvic pain, dysmenorrhea, and dyspareunia. After discussing her treatment options, the patient consented to a vaginal hysterectomy and bilateral salpingo-oophorectomy to treat the extensive endometriosis of the various sites previously described. The surgery was accomplished without difficulty, and the patient was able to go home on day three. An additional diagnosis was added to the record when the pathology report was reviewed by the surgeon. The pathologist's report confirmed the endometriosis as well as a small lesion of the cervix that was found to be carcinoma in situ of the cervix.

Principal Diagnosis: _____

Secondary Diagnoses: _____

Principal Procedure: _____

Secondary Procedure(s): _____

8

The patient is a 25-year-old female who is seen in the office today for a follow-up visit for a possible urinary tract infection. Last week the patient was in the office and had complained of pain and burning on urination, frequent urges to urinate, pressure in the lower abdomen, and foul-smelling urine. A urinalysis done last week showed a large number of white blood cells, and a urine culture was collected and sent to the laboratory. The culture confirmed the growth of more than 100,000 *E. coli* organisms. The diagnosis for this visit is more specifically acute cystitis due to *E. coli* organism. The patient has had frequent urinary tract infections in the past, and she is being referred to an urologist for further investigation and possible cystoscopy.

First-Listed Diagnosis: _____

Secondary Diagnoses: _____

9

A 45-year-old male patient is sent to the hospital outpatient radiology department with a physician's order for an intravenous pyelogram. "Renal colic, possible kidney stone" is documented on the physician's order is the reason for the x-ray. The test is performed, and the diagnosis dictated by the physician on the IVP report is "renal colic due to bilateral nephrolithiasis with staghorn calculi." Following hospital and official coding guidelines, the hospital coder is able to use the radiologist's diagnosis as the reason for the outpatient test.

First-Listed Diagnosis: _____

Secondary Diagnoses: _____

10

The 38-year-old male patient is being admitted for the following procedure: transurethral ureteroscopic lithotripsy using high-energy shock waves. The patient is known to have several large bilateral ureteral stones, and other attempts to remove them endoscopically have been unsuccessful. The bilateral lithotripsy procedure is performed without complications, and the surgeon is satisfied that the ureteral stones appeared to be fragmented well and would be eliminated from the body by urination.

Principal Diagnosis: _____

Secondary Diagnoses: _____

Principal Procedure: _____

Secondary Procedure(s): _____

11

The patient is a 75-year-old male who was admitted to the hospital for severe weakness and falling multiple times at home over the past several days. The urinalysis performed in the emergency department showed evidence of a urinary tract infection, and for this reason he was admitted. The patient was also dehydrated. The patient also has bladder neck carcinoma, which has been an aggressive type treated by chemotherapy. He has bilateral nephrostomy tubes in place. There was some suspicion that there might be an obstruction in one of the nephrostomy tubes, but that was not found to be true. The patient also has coronary artery disease and is status post CABG with venous grafts. He has type 2 diabetes on long-term oral anti-diabetic medication and hypercholesterolemia. The patient was seen in consultation by urology, oncology, and cardiology with his current and chronic conditions evaluated and treated with numerous medications, both intravenous and oral. The patient regained considerable strength and was able to return home with follow-up appointments made with four physicians.

Principal Diagnosis: _____

Secondary Diagnoses: _____

Principal Procedure: _____

Secondary Procedure(s): _____

12

The patient is a 45-year-old female, gravida 2, para 2, who was electively admitted for a total abdominal hysterectomy and bilateral salpingo-oophorectomy primarily for her meno-metrorrhagia and severe dysmenorrhea with heavy flow and cramping. She also has uterine fibroids with the uterus being 15 to 16 weeks of gestation size. On the day of admission, a total abdominal hysterectomy, removal of cervix, and bilateral salpingo-oophorectomy was performed. She was found to have massive intraperitoneal adhesions that took an extended period of time to lyse. In the process of removing the adhesions, a small laceration was made in the small bowel. It was quickly repaired. During surgery she had profuse bleeding tendencies, apparently because of the continuous ingestion of ibuprofen she was taking for the pelvic pain she experienced. Bleeding tendencies are known to be an adverse effect of ibuprofen; the physician was not aware of the amount she was taking. After surgery, the patient experienced several complications. First, she was diagnosed with acute blood-loss anemia. She lost about 1,500 mL of blood during surgery, according to the anesthesiologist. She had hypoxemia, which might be attributed to her current smoking of half of a pack of cigarettes per day, even though she tried to quit prior to surgery but was unsuccessful. She developed atelectasis and fever, both postoperative complications. Finally, during the postoperative management of her conditions, she complained of back pain and was found to have hydronephrosis, which may have been caused by the surgery, as so much packing was placed around the ureters to try to protect them. The urologist performed a cystoscopy, retrograde pyelogram of the kidneys, ureters and bladder with low osmolar contrast, and inserted a stent into her right ureter for drainage. Within hours, the patient's problems reverted. She became afebrile, the back pain and atelectasis disappeared. She was able to be discharged home on day 4 postop and has an appointment to see the surgeon in her office in two weeks.

Principal Diagnosis: _____

Secondary Diagnoses: _____

Principal Procedure: _____

Secondary Procedure(s): _____

13

A 46-year-old female was admitted to the hospital through the emergency department feeling tired, weak, and stating that she had not been feeling well for the past three days. She also stated she had diarrhea alternating with vomiting off and on for the past week. Laboratory tests were performed, including an electrolyte panel, BUN, and creatinine, all of which were abnormal. The impression written by the physician on the history and physical examination report was "dehydration with suspected acute renal failure," and intravenous hydration was started. The patient was monitored closely by the nursing staff, including the documentation of fluid intake and output. The patient did not have diarrhea or vomiting. Laboratory tests, including the BUN and creatinine, were repeated over the next 48 hours. Given the patient's general healthy history and the other tests performed, there was no underlying chronic kidney condition. No reason for the patient's diarrhea and vomiting that occurred prior to admission was found. No dialysis was required, as the patient's normal kidney function returned as the patient was rehydrated. The physician concluded the patient's condition was acute renal failure due to dehydration.

Principal Diagnosis: _____

Secondary Diagnoses: _____

Principal Procedure: _____

Secondary Procedure(s): _____

14

The patient is a 68-year-old female who had a hysterectomy 22 years ago and had a cystocele repair eight years ago. Now the patient has had very significant urinary stress incontinence for the past two years and is admitted at this time for surgical treatment. Conservative management with medications provided no improvement of her stress incontinence. The patient required inpatient recovery and monitoring because of her oxygen dependence due to severe COPD. The day of admission the patient was taken to surgery for a suprapubic sling operation. The procedure is a suspension of the urethra using the levator muscle to reposition the bladder neck to restore support to the bladder and urethra. The patient was able to be released from the hospital late in the afternoon on the day after surgery with no complications from the anesthesia, and her lung function returned to her baseline status. Home healthcare services were ordered for the patient, and a follow-up appointment in the urologist's office was scheduled for seven days after surgery.

Principal Diagnosis: _____

Secondary Diagnoses: _____

Principal Procedure: _____

Secondary Procedure(s): _____

15

The patient is a 26-year-old female who is gravida 4, para 3, AB 1 with two past cesarean deliveries and one normal spontaneous vaginal delivery. She had one voluntary interruption of pregnancy at 10 weeks prior to the birth of her children. The patient states she does not want any more children and cannot tolerate oral contraceptives because of the side effects of nausea and vomiting. She also complains of irregular menstrual and intermenstrual uterine bleeding with two periods a month that last between five and seven days. The patient is given the facts about the proposed procedures, the alternatives, risks, complications, and possible failure rate. Nevertheless, the patient consents to the surgery to be performed on an outpatient basis at the hospital. The procedures performed are a dilation and curettage with a diagnostic laparoscopy with bilateral tubal Falope ring application. The pre- and postoperative diagnoses are the same: dysfunctional uterine bleeding and desire for elective sterilization.

While there is no requirement that ICD-10-PCS procedure codes are coded on outpatients, code the diagnostic D&C with laparoscopic bilateral tubal occlusion by Falope ring application for coding practice.

First-Listed Diagnosis: _____

Secondary Diagnoses: _____

First-Listed Procedure: _____

Secondary Procedure(s): _____

16

HISTORY: The patient is a 38-year-old female who gave birth 10 weeks ago. This past week, she developed abdominal pain and symptoms of a urinary tract infection (UTI) and was admitted to the hospital. She was found to have a left ureteral stone, and small bilateral renal stones, as well as bilateral hydronephrosis and UTI. It was recommended that the left ureter be dilated and stented because of the hydronephrosis and the infection. Once the infection has been adequately treated, she will undergo ESWL of the ureteral stone at a later date.

OPERATIVE FINDINGS: The urethra is normal. The bladder is smooth and without stone or tumor. Orifices are in normal location bilaterally. Right retrograde pyelogram showed no evidence of persistent filling defect; however, there is dilation of the collecting system and very mild hydronephrosis on the right side. One the left side, there was a 1-cm stone over the left ureterovesical junction with ureteral dilatation both distal and proximal to this, but especially proximal, and also left hydronephrosis. No other obvious stones were identified.

DESCRIPTION OF PROCEDURE: The patient was taken to the operating area where she underwent IV sedation without problems. Following successful anesthesia, she was placed in the dorsal lithotomy position and prepped and draped in the sterile fashion. A #21 French cystoscopy with lens was introduced into the bladder and thorough inspection of the bladder and urethra was carried out. Following examination, bilateral retrograde pyelograms of the kidneys, ureters and bladder were obtained and reviewed. Next, under fluoroscopic control, a .035 guide-wire was placed up to the left orifice into the renal pelvis. Over this, the left ureter was dilated and a 24 cm × 6 F double-J stent was passed without problems, so that the proximal end curled in the left renal pelvis, and the distal end curled in the bladder. The bladder was then evaluated and the cystoscope was withdrawn. The patient was awakened and transported to the recovery room in good condition, tolerating the procedure well. She will be kept on a course of Ampicillin 500 mg 4 times a day for the next week and will then return at that time for ESWL of her left ureteral stone at a later date.

Principal Diagnosis: _____

Secondary Diagnoses: _____

Principal Procedure: _____

Secondary Procedure(s): _____

17

A 75-year-old male was admitted to the hospital because of refractory temperature elevation, documented as "probable urinary sepsis" that did not respond to outpatient antibiotics. He became more acutely ill the day before admission. He lives alone but was coherent enough to call a neighbor to ask for help. His fever was 104.5°F at home the day of admission. He had been on Ciprofloxacin for approximately 12 hours prior to admission with no change in his fever. He has a history of urinary tract infections (UTI) and was hospitalized six months ago for life-threatening septic shock. He is known to have an enlarged prostate without lower urinary tract symptoms. His only other medical problem is chronic atrial fibrillation, which has been under treatment for several years with an anticoagulant medication that was continued in the hospital. A consultation with a urologist resulted in a nonsurgical workup. After appropriate cultures were drawn, he was started on IV antibiotics and vigorous IV hydration. His blood cultures were returned as negative. His urine culture demonstrated large amounts of a mixed growth that was suggestive of a possible contaminant. This was not unexpected, with the source of his infection considered to be his prostate. He responded dramatically to the IV antibiotics, but it took several days before he became close to afebrile. After four days in the hospital he was well enough to be taken off all IV support and was transferred to a skilled (swing) bed for two more days of observation on oral antibiotics to be sure it is safe to discharge him to home care. His discharge diagnoses were urinary sepsis/UTI due to chronic prostatitis with possible acute prostatitis, BPH, and chronic atrial fibrillation. The physician was queried regarding the diagnosis "urinary sepsis/UTI" and responded to clarify that the diagnosis was "urinary tract infection."

Principal Diagnosis: _____

Secondary Diagnoses: _____

Principal Procedure: _____

Secondary Procedure(s): _____

18

The patient is a 57-year-old male with painful swelling of the right scrotum. The patient also has an elevated PSA that is being monitored. Previous biopsy of the prostate was negative for a malignancy. An aspiration of the hydrocele had been attempted as an outpatient but was unsuccessful as the hydrocele is large and thick-walled. For this reason the patient is admitted to the hospital for surgery, that is, hydrocelectomy by the right tunica vaginalis. The preoperative laboratory tests were all within normal limits and the electrocardiogram result was normal sinus rhythm.

DESCRIPTION OF THE PROCEDURE: The patient was administered general anesthesia and draped in supine position. A right scrotal incision was made and carried down to the tunica vaginalis forming the hydrocele. The hydrocele was dissected free from the scrotal wall back to the base of the testicle and spermatic cord. In this manner the hydrocele was excised and fluid drained. The spermatic cord was infiltrated with 0.25% Marcaine. The edges of the tunica vaginalis adjacent to the spermatic cord were oversewn for hemostasis. The right testicle was replaced into the right scrotal space and affixed to the overlying fascia with sutures through the edge of the tunica vaginalis and the overlying fascia. The right scrotal incision was closed, first closing the fascia, then the skin. A sterile dressing and scrotal support was applied. The patient was transferred to the recovery room in good condition with no apparent complications or adverse reactions to the surgery or anesthesia. The patient will be monitored overnight. Addendum: The patient was examined the morning after surgery and found to be in good condition with minimal scrotal pain and swelling. An appointment was made for the patient to come to the surgeon's office in one week for a postoperative examination.

Principal Diagnosis: _____

Secondary Diagnoses: _____

Principal Procedure: _____

Secondary Procedure(s): _____

Chapter 15

Pregnancy, Childbirth, and the Puerperium

Coding Scenarios for *Basic ICD-10-CM and ICD-10-PCS Coding Exercises*

The following case studies are organized following the sequence of the chapters in the ICD-10-CM Tabular List of Diseases and Injuries as published on the Centers for Disease Control and Prevention National Center for Health Statistics website (http://www.cdc.gov /nchs/icd/icd10cm.htm). The objective of this book is to provide the student with more detailed clinical information to code, rather than one- or two-line diagnosis and procedure statements.

ICD-10-CM diagnosis codes are to be assigned to both the inpatient hospital admission and the outpatient visit case studies. In this book, the ICD-10-PCS procedure codes are to be assigned only to the inpatient hospital admission cases. In actual practice, outpatient cases are assigned CPT/HCPCS codes. The ICD-10-PCS codes are only required for inpatient procedures. In the answer key for the exercises, the Alphabetic Index entry is listed after the code to indicate the main terms and subterms used to locate the code that must be verified in the ICD-10-CM Tabular List or in the ICD-10-PCS Code Tables prior to assigning the code.

1

A 35-year-old female at 22 weeks of her first pregnancy underwent a one-hour glucose screening test that was found to be abnormal, with a blood sugar level reported to be over 200 mg/dL. The patient was sent to the outpatient laboratory for a three-hour glucose tolerance test. The reason for the laboratory test was documented on the physician order as "rule out gestational diabetes; abnormal glucose tolerance on screening during pregnancy."

First-Listed Diagnosis: _____

Secondary Diagnoses: _____

2

The patient is a 26-year-old female, gravida 2, para 1, in her 10th week of pregnancy. While at work, she developed severe cramping and vaginal bleeding. Coworkers brought her to the hospital emergency department, and she was admitted to the hospital. After examination, the physician described her condition as an "inevitable abortion." When the physician was asked to further define her condition, she stated that an inevitable abortion or an incomplete abortion because the cervix was dilated and fetal and placental material probably had already passed from the patient's body. According to the physician, another description of this condition was an incomplete early spontaneous abortion. During this pregnancy the patient had been treated for transient hypertension of pregnancy, for which she was monitored during this hospital stay. She was taken to the operating room where a dilation and curettage was performed to remove the products of conception in order to treat the abortion. There were no complications from the procedure.

Principal Diagnosis: _____

Secondary Diagnoses: _____

Principal Procedure: _____

Secondary Procedure(s): _____

3

A 34-year-old female is admitted in active labor during week 39 of pregnancy. She had a previous cesarean section two years ago as a result of fetal distress and cephalopelvic disproportion (CPD). No fetal distress was found during this admission, but it was determined that the patient still had CPD; therefore, a repeat low cesarean section had to be performed. A healthy 8 lb, 10 oz female was safely delivered.

Principal Diagnosis: _____

Secondary Diagnoses: _____

Principal Procedure: _____

Secondary Procedure(s): _____

4

A 43-year-old female, gravida 1, para 0, was admitted in labor to the hospital obstetrical department. Unexpectedly but happily, this woman found herself pregnant after 15 years of marriage. She had been under the care of a physician who specialized in high-risk pregnancies. Because of her age, the woman was thought to be at higher risk for complications, but her pregnancy was uneventful. The physician described her as an "elderly primigravida, full term 38-week pregnancy, normal delivery with no maternal or infant complications." She had a manually assisted vaginal delivery of a healthy 7 pounds, 5 ounces girl. Mother and infant were able to leave the hospital on day 2 after delivery.

Principal Diagnosis: _____

Secondary Diagnoses: _____

Principal Procedure: _____

Secondary Procedure(s): _____

5

The patient is a 30-year-old female, gravida 3, para 2, in week 40 of pregnancy. The patient is admitted for "induction of labor at term." There is no other reason documented by the physician as the reason for labor induction. The patient was not in labor at the time of admission. The induction is performed by artificial rupture of membranes. Labor proceeds normally, and the woman delivers a healthy male infant vaginally without complications. The mother and infant were able to be discharged from the hospital on day 2.

Principal Diagnosis: _____

Secondary Diagnoses: _____

Principal Procedure: _____

Secondary Procedure(s): _____

6

The obstetrics patient at 15 weeks' gestation (second trimester) is seen for her regular antepartum visit. The woman has confessed to using cocaine both prior to and during her current pregnancy. A drug screen performed during this visit is positive for cocaine. She feels she is unable to quit using the drug on her own, but wishes to become drug-free for the safety of her infant and herself. The patient has consented to admission later today to a specialized antepartum unit at a nearby hospital for drug detoxification and cocaine dependence treatment for pregnant females. The patient will be seen again in the OB clinic in 1 month for continued antepartum care. The patient is also being treated for a urinary tract infection during the pregnancy.

First-Listed Diagnosis: _____

Secondary Diagnoses: _____

7

The patient is seen in her OB physician's office two weeks after a normal vaginal delivery that produced a healthy full-term female infant. The patient has been breast feeding the infant, but over the past two days had developed redness, pain, and swelling of her right breast. Upon examination there appears to be a hard lump in the right breast, and the diagnosis of a postpartum purulent breast abscess is made. The patient is given a prescription for an antibiotic and advised she may take an anti-inflammatory drug to reduce the pain and inflammation. She is also advised to discontinue breast feeding until the infection resolves. The patient will return to the office within seven days for a reevaluation.

First-Listed Diagnosis: _____

Secondary Diagnoses: _____

8

The patient is admitted to the hospital five weeks after delivering a healthy female infant following a full-term pregnancy with the admitting diagnosis of acute cholecystitis with cholelithiasis. The patient was known to have gallstones prior to her pregnancy and had symptoms of the disease recur during the pregnancy and become more serious during the immediate postpartum period. A laparoscopic cholecystectomy is performed without complications. Pathologic examination confirmed the admitting diagnosis. The patient is able to go home one day after the surgery.

Principal Diagnosis: _____

Secondary Diagnoses: _____

Principal Procedure: _____

Secondary Procedure: _____

9

The patient is admitted to the hospital with excessive vaginal bleeding two days following an elective abortion at an outpatient surgical facility. The patient is immediately taken to surgery for a dilatation and curettage. The pathology report describes the tissue removed as "retained products of conception." The previous elective abortion was not completed as expected. At the time of the procedure it was determined the patient had anemia due to the acute blood loss, and it was treated. The physician's final diagnosis is "delayed hemorrhage following elective abortion, now completed, anemia of pregnancy due to acute blood loss." The patient is able to be discharged the next day.

Principal Diagnosis: _____

Secondary Diagnoses: _____

Principal Procedure: _____

Secondary Procedure(s): _____

10

A pregnant female is admitted to the hospital during week 12 of her pregnancy. The patient had called her physician describing vague symptoms, and the physician ordered a complete obstetrical ultrasound. The fetus is seen in utero, but no fetal heart tones are detected and further examination confirms the fetus is dead. The physician describes the condition in one progress note as an inevitable abortion and in the final summary progress note describes the condition as a missed abortion. No medical or obstetrical complication can be found to explain the loss of the pregnancy. A D&C is performed to complete the missed abortion. The mother receives grief counseling and is able to be discharged one day after the procedure.

Principal Diagnosis: _____

Secondary Diagnoses: _____

Principal Procedure: _____

Secondary Procedure(s): _____

11

The patient was admitted from home on May 31 with vaginal bleeding. This is the patient's third admission to labor and delivery during this pregnancy. The patient is 33 years old, gravida 1, para 0, with 34 completed weeks of gestation, with an estimated date of confinement of July 9. She has twin gestation (two placentae and two amniotic sacs) and complete placenta previa. Because of this last episode of bleeding, it was decided to keep her at bed rest in labor and delivery at the hospital so that, should any further excessive bleeding occur, she would be available for emergency cesarean delivery, if necessary. The intent was to keep her until she reached 36 weeks gestation as recommended by the perinatologist in consultation. On June 10 she had bright red bleeding from the vagina. There were contractions of preterm labor noted. Because she was one day short of 35 weeks gestation, it was decided to go forward with a primary low cesarean delivery for the incomplete or partial placenta previa with hemorrhage. She delivered a 4 lb, 9 oz viable female with Apgar scores of 8 and 9 at 16:01 p.m. She delivered a 4 lb, 15 oz viable male with Apgar scores of 7 and 9 at 16:02 p.m. Intraoperative blood loss was approximately 1 liter. She was anemic due to acute blood loss prior to surgery. She had a good recovery from the surgery and her hemoglobin stabilized at 8.2 gm. She was discharged home to follow up in the office in two weeks for an incision check. Her twin infants remained in the premature nursery for further treatment.

Principal Diagnosis: _____

Secondary Diagnoses: _____

Principal Procedure: _____

Secondary Procedure(s): _____

12

The patient was admitted to the hospital from the obstetrician's office at 38 and 3/7 weeks gestation. She came to the office today complaining of not feeling well and noticing a lack of fetal movement over the past day or two. She had been in the office three days ago, and the infant was reactive. The biophysical profile in the office today was 6/8 with no breathing movement. The nonstress test was reactive. The patient also has severe iron deficiency anemia of pregnancy and gestational hypertension complicating her pregnancy. She desires a tubal ligation during this delivery for her grand multiparity. In 2019, she is 38 years old and gravida 6, para 3, AB 2 with an estimated date of delivery of June 30. She has three sons living with two previous cesarean deliveries, one in 2000 and one in 2005. Her oldest son was delivered vaginally in 1999. Because of the decreased fetal movement, a repeat low cesarean delivery was performed on June 19th. A bilateral tubal ligation was also performed by ligation and crushing. Delivered at 4:55 p.m. was a 6 pounds, 2 ounces live female infant with Apgar scores of 7 and 8. The patient had an uneventful recovery from the delivery, was continued on her medications for anemia and gestational hypertension and asked to return to the office in two weeks. Mother and daughter were discharged home together on post-op day 3.

Principal Diagnosis: _____

Secondary Diagnoses: _____

Principal Procedure: _____

Secondary Procedure(s): _____

13

The patient is a 23-year-old female, gravida 2, para 1, AB 0, who was admitted to the hospital in the early morning hours reporting she had sporadic contractions for the past 24 hours. She is 38 and 1/7 weeks gestation. At 2:45 a.m. she had an artificial rupture of membrane, her cervix was 4 to 5 cm dilated and 90 percent effaced. She had variable fetal heart rate decelerations on the external fetal monitoring the fetal heart rate. She was pushing with some of her contractions, and the fetal distress appeared to worsen. Presentation was vertex, and station was minus 1 for most of the morning. The fetal head came down to about zero station. However, since the fetal distress did not abate, a long discussion was held with the patient and her mother about a change in the management of her anticipated delivery. The physician recommended a cesarean delivery for the intrauterine pregnancy be performed because of the fetal distress caused by fetal heart rate decelerations, and the patient consented to it. A low cesarean section was performed at 10 a.m. under spinal anesthesia. A viable male infant with spontaneous respiration and cry was delivered. The cord was doubly clamped and cut, and the infant was placed in the warmer and examined by the pediatrician. The mother's placenta was removed, uterine cavity cleaned, and the uterine incision closed in two layers. Careful inspection of the uterus, fallopian tubes, and ovaries did not reveal any unusual findings or bleeding. The peritoneum was closed vertically, and the fascia was closed. Subcutaneous tissue was closed with plain silk, and the skin was closed with subcuticular sutures followed by staples. The patient received Pitocin and a gram of Ancef, per protocol. The patient's estimated blood loss was about 500 cc with no surgical complications. Postoperatively the patient complained of the typical abdominal discomfort from the incision. The patient was known to have microcytic anemia during her pregnancy, and the anemia was present at the time of delivery and at discharge as well. The anemia continued to be treated. The patient was discharged with her newborn son on day 3 with a follow-up appointment in the obstetrician's office in 10 days.

Principal Diagnosis: _____

Secondary Diagnoses: _____

Principal Procedure: _____

Secondary Procedure(s): _____

14

The 42-year-old female was admitted to the hospital in premature labor at 36 and 4/7th weeks' gestation with 5 cm dilation. The patient is gravida 6, para 5 with five daughters at home ranging in age from 8 to 18 years. This was a "surprise" pregnancy to this elderly multigravida patient and her husband. Two antepartum ultrasounds predicted the birth of a male infant, which has brought considerable excitement to the family. The patient's labor was augmented with Pitocin drip, and she was placed on an external fetal monitor for fetal heart rate monitoring. The patient has a known cystocele that was monitored during the pregnancy and will probably require surgical treatment in the near future. After a short period of labor, the patient had a manually assisted delivery of a healthy male infant at 4 lb 2 oz with Apgar scores of 8 and 9 at one and five minutes. When the patient was visited by the delivering physician in her room later the same day, the patient asked if it was "too late" for tubal ligation, as she and her husband concluded their family was complete and she desired permanent sterilization. The next day the patient was taken to the operating room for a postpartum endoscopic tubal ligation by division and ligation, which was completed uneventfully. The patient was discharged home on day 3, but the male infant remained in the nursery for observation and weight gain. Discharge instructions and a follow-up appointment with her obstetrician were given to the patient.

Principal Diagnosis: _____

Secondary Diagnoses: _____

Principal Procedure: _____

Secondary Procedure Code(s): _____

15

HISTORY: The patient is a 28-year-old, gravida 2, para 1, with complete/total placenta previa with hemorrhage in four bleeding episodes was admitted to the hospital. She has a previous cesarean section for her first child. The patient has received steroids and has consented for a repeat preterm cesarean delivery because of the placenta previa and the threat-to-life hemorrhage that could occur again as the pregnancy continued or during a vaginal delivery. The patient is aware that a hysterectomy may need to be performed if the placenta cannot be removed but will be avoided if at all possible. The patient also is known to have the baby in a double footling breech presentation and had gestational hypertension during this pregnancy. Labor was not allowed to occur in this patient. The patient is a 32 5/7 week gestation.

FINDINGS:

1. Complete placenta previa

2. Viable male infant in double footling breech presentation. Weight 5 lb even. Apgar scores were 6 at one minute, 8 at five minutes, and 9 at ten minutes. The uterus did not have to be removed. There were normal-appearing tubes and ovaries. Of note: the pathologist reported on examination of the placenta that mild-to-moderate amnionitis was present in this mid third-trimester placenta.

DESCRIPTION OF PROCEDURE: The patient was taken to the operating room, where a spinal anesthesia was found to be adequate. She was then prepped and draped in the normal, sterile fashion in the dorsal supine position with a leftward tilt. A Pfannenstiel skin incision was made along the site of the previous scar with the scalpel and carried through to the underlying layer of the fascia. The fascia was incised in the midline, and the incision extended laterally with the use of Mayo scissors. The superior aspect of the fascial incision was then grasped with the Kocher clamps, and the underlying rectus muscles were dissected with the Mayo scissors. Attention was then turned to the inferior aspect of this incision, which in a similar fashion was grasped with the pickups and entered, and the underlying rectus muscles were dissected with the Mayo scissors. The rectus muscle was spread in the midline, and the peritoneum was entered bluntly. The peritoneum was extended superiorly and inferiorly, with good visualization of the bladder, using the Metzenbaum scissors. The bladder blade was placed and the vesico-uterine peritoneum was identified, tented up, and entered sharply with the Metzenbaum scissors. A bladder flap was then created digitally, and the bladder blade was replaced. The uterine incision was made about a centimeter and a half higher than usual due to the placenta previa, and the incision was widened with blunt force. At this time, we were able to reach past the placenta previa and were able to grab both feet. At this point, the bag seemed to rupture. The infant was delivered in double footling breech with the typical breech maneuvers. The head delivered atraumatically. The nose and mouth were bulb suctioned. The cord was doubly clamped and cut. The infant was handed off to the waiting pediatrician. Cord gases and blood were obtained. The placenta was removed. The uterus was exteriorized and cleared of all clots and debris. The uterine incision was then repaired with a 0 Vicryl in a running, locked fashion, and a second layer of the same was used to ensure excellent hemostasis. The uterus was then replaced into the abdomen and the gutters were irrigated and cleared of all clots and debris. The peritoneum was repaired with a 2-0 Vicryl. The 0 Vicryl was then used to reapproximate the rectus muscle in the midline. The fascia was repaired with a 0 Vicryl in a running fashion. The subcutaneous layer was then closed with plain 2-0 silk on a GI needle. The skin was closed with staples. The sponge, lap, and needle counts were correct times two. The patient had been given a gram of Ancef at cord clamp. The patient was taken to the recovery room in stable condition.

Principal Diagnosis: _____

Secondary Diagnoses: _____

Principal Procedure: _____

Secondary Procedure(s): _____

16

The patient is a 25-year-old female, gravida 4, para 3, that was admitted to the hospital for medical induction of labor due to repeated ultrasound findings of oligohydramnios. During her antepartum period, the only medication she took was the prenatal vitamins. The mother was Group B strep negative, HIV negative, and Hepatitis B negative. Given the fact the patient was at 39 weeks 3 days into her gestation and the concern about the oligohydramnios, the patient was admitted. The patient was administered Pitocin 30 units in 500 LR IVPB in a graduated dosage schedule. Following the induction of labor with the Pitocin (oxytocin, hormone), the patient experienced 1 hour and 13 minutes of labor followed by a precipitous vaginal delivery with cephalic, vertex (right occipital anterior) presentation of a male infant, her first son. The patient previously delivered three female infants over the past six years. The baby's birth weight was 3140 grams, and he was 19 inches in length. Apgar scores were 8 and 9 at 1 and 5 minutes after birth. The placenta was delivered spontaneously with the placenta cotyledons and membranes appearing to be intact. The cervix, anterior and posterior fornices, and sidewalls were intact. The patient had no lacerations and did not require an episiotomy. The estimated blood loss was 300 mL. Following the delivery, the pad, sponge, and needle counts were correct. The infant and mother were taken to the recovery area in good condition. Postpartum the patient was given ibuprofen 800mg tab as needed for post-partum cramping that was not severe according to the patient. She was offered Tylenol #3 for post-partum pain but she refused as she felt reasonably well. She did not have complications during her labor, delivery, or postpartum period in the hospital. One day after delivery her vital signs were stable, she had a small to moderate amount of rubra and was voiding without difficulty. She was able to be discharged about 26 hours after delivery with a home health visit scheduled in 48 hours for mother-infant well-being check. She was given an office postpartum appointment for two weeks after delivery.

Principal Diagnosis: _____

Secondary Diagnoses: _____

Principal Procedure: _____

Secondary Procedure(s):   _____

17

The patient was a 21-year-old female who came to the emergency department complaining of vaginal bleeding, low back pain, abdominal cramping mainly on the left side, and pain in the lower pelvic region. A physical examination revealed acute tenderness in the pelvic region, particularly on the left side. The patient stated she missed a menstrual period last month and thought when the vaginal bleeding started she was having a period but the accompanying symptoms were different. She did not think she was pregnant because her menstrual periods were irregular. A pelvic ultrasound identified a mass on the left side probably in her fallopian tube strongly suggestive of an ectopic fallopian pregnancy. Her pregnancy test was positive but the HCG level was not that elevated as would be expected in an 8-week pregnancy. The patient was admitted to the hospital. The physician recommended a D&C to rule out an incomplete or a missed abortion. The physician explained to the patient that she might have an ectopic pregnancy in the left fallopian tube that would require a resection of the ectopic pregnancy if the D&C did not find products of conception in the uterus. The patient consented to the procedure after being informed of the risks and benefits as well as the possible complications. The patient was taken to the operating room.

PREOPERATIVE DIAGNOSIS: Suspected left fallopian tubal pregnancy

POSTOPERATIVE DIAGNOSIS: Confirmed left fallopian tubal pregnancy

PROCEDURE: Diagnostic dilation and curettage to identify the contents of the uterus followed by laparotomy with removal of the contents of the left fallopian tube followed by a left total salpingectomy.

ANESTHESIA: General

FINDINGS: Ectopic pregnancy in the left fallopian tube. Normal right fallopian tube, bilateral ovaries and uterus, no intrauterine pregnancy

DESCRIPTION OF PROCEDURE: The patient was brought to the operating room and placed in the supine position. Following a time-out the patient was identified, the left side of the body that was marked pre-operatively was noted. and the procedure was allowed to continue. General anesthesia was administered. The patient was prepped and draped in the usual sterile manner for both vaginal and abdominal surgery. A single tooth tenaculum was placed through the vagina in the cervix and the cervix was dilated to allow a #9 curetting instrument to be inserted. The uterus was curetted and the specimen removed from the uterus was sent to pathology. The surgeon and staff waited for the diagnostic examination to be performed by the pathologist. The pathologist reported there were no villi in the uterus that indicated there was no intrauterine pregnancy. A laparotomy incision was made. An ectopic pregnancy was identified at the distal end of the left fallopian tube and removed with an attempt to preserve the fimbria. After it was determined the fimbria could not be restored to a normal state, the entire left fallopian tube was dissected off the uterus and removed in total. Hemostasis was performed and the region was copiously irrigated. After confirming there was no bleeding in the area, the fascia was closed using Vicryl sutures. The skin was closed with surgical stapes and sterile dressings were applied. The patient was awakened at the end of the procedure when the anesthesia was discontinued. It appeared the patient tolerated the procedure well with no obvious intraoperative and immediate postoperative complications. The patient was taken to the recovery area in good condition.

POSTOPERATIVE EXAMINATION: The patient was seen by the physician the morning after the procedure and was afebrile with mild abdominal pain and cramping that was relieved by oral pain medication. The patient asked to be discharged and this was agreed to by the physician. The patient was given a prescription for pain control and was given an appointment with the physician seven days after the procedure.

Principal Diagnosis: _____

Secondary Diagnoses: _____

Principal Procedure: _____

Secondary Procedure(s): _____

Chapter 16

Certain Conditions Originating in the Perinatal Period

Coding Scenarios for *Basic ICD-10-CM and ICD-10-PCS Coding Exercises*

The following case studies are organized following the sequence of the chapters in the ICD-10-CM Tabular List of Diseases and Injuries as published on the Centers for Disease Control and Prevention National Center for Health Statistics website (http://www.cdc.gov /nchs/icd/icd10cm.htm). The objective of this book is to provide the student with more detailed clinical information to code, rather than one- or two-line diagnosis and procedure statements.

ICD-10-CM diagnosis codes are to be assigned to both the inpatient hospital admission and the outpatient visit case studies. In this book, the ICD-10-PCS procedure codes are to be assigned only to the inpatient hospital admission cases. In actual practice, outpatient cases are assigned CPT/HCPCS codes. The ICD-10-PCS codes are only required for inpatient procedures. In the answer key for the exercises, the Alphabetic Index entry is listed after the code to indicate the main terms and subterms used to locate the code that must be verified in the ICD-10-CM Tabular List or in the ICD-10-PCS Code Tables prior to assigning the code.

1

A premature female infant was transferred for admission to the high risk neonatal intensive care unit at the university hospital from a smaller hospital for treatment at the age of five hours. The infant weighed 975 grams as the result of a pregnancy that lasted 29 weeks and 5 days. The patient was also treated for neonatal respiratory distress syndrome including nasal CPAP for 72 hours until she stabilized and then spent 10 weeks in the hospital before being discharged to home with pediatric home care services provided.

Principal Diagnosis: _____

Secondary Diagnoses: _____

Principal Procedure: _____

Secondary Procedure(s): _____

2

A 2-day-old full-term male infant was transferred for admission to the high risk neonatal intensive care unit at the university hospital from a smaller hospital for treatment of sepsis due to streptococcus, group B. The physicians concluded that the infant acquired the infection during or shortly after birth from organisms colonizing the maternal genital tract. The mother was found to be a carrier of group B streptococci. The infant had the typical symptoms of neonatal sepsis: respiratory distress, lethargy, and hypotension. Cultures from the infant confirmed group B streptococci found in the blood. The infant was treated with intravenous antibiotics. No complications such as meningitis developed, and the infant was able to be discharged 16 days later and will be followed by pediatric home care.

Principal Diagnosis: _____

Secondary Diagnoses: _____

Principal Procedures: _____

Secondary Procedure: _____

3

An 8-day-old male infant was brought by his mother to his pediatrician's office for his first well exam. The mother told the physician she was concerned about the malodorous discharge from his umbilical stump that she had been cleaning several times a day. Upon examination, the physician found periumbilical erythema and tenderness as well as discharge from the umbilical stump but no hemorrhage from the site. The infant did not have a fever or other signs of systemic infection. The physician prescribed liquid antibiotics to be started the same day and arranged for an appointment with an infectious disease specialist the next day to confirm the antibiotic was appropriate. A culture was taken from the umbilical drainage. The physician's final diagnosis for the office visit was neonatal omphalitis.

First-Listed Diagnosis: _____

Secondary Diagnoses: _____

4

A 2-day-old infant is transferred for admission to the larger community hospital for evaluation and treatment from a small rural hospital where he was born. The infant's mother has type 1 diabetes mellitus. The infant was large at birth (more than 10 pounds) and exhibited hypoglycemia, transient tachypnea, and possibly other endocrine disorders that are character-istic of a syndrome of infants born to diabetic mothers. The infant required special surveil-lance because, as an "infant of a diabetic mother," he was at increased risk for a variety of complications and congenital defects. The infant was also observed for suspected sepsis or other infectious process because of the mother's sepsis. Fortunately, sepsis was ruled out in the infant and no other major problems were found. The infant was discharged to his parents three days after admission to be followed closely by a pediatric specialist.

Principal Diagnosis: _____

Secondary Diagnoses: _____

Principal Procedures: _____

Secondary Procedure(s): _____

5

A 2-day-old female infant was transferred for admission to the Children's Hospital after being noted to be hypoxemic soon after birth. She was a full-term infant from an uneventful pregnancy. A transthoracic contrast echocardiogram of the pediatric heart done on admission did not reveal any major cardiac defects. However, there was right-to-left shunting suggestive of primary pulmonary hypertension in a newborn or persistent fetal circulation. The physicians were concerned about her episodes of significant hypoxemia. During the morning of day 2 the infant required significantly increased inotropic medication support to maintain her hemodynamics. Given the lability as well as the increase in inotropes, it was felt that she would benefit from ECMO support. Neurologically, some movements had been noted earlier today, and the liver function and renal function tests were within normal range, suggesting that there was no significant end-organ injury related to the hypoxia. The infant was taken to the operating room and sedated with fentanyl, Versed, and vecuronium. A transverse skin incision was made 2 cm above the medial aspect of the clavicle and extended down through the subcutaneous tissues and platysma. The internal jugular vein and the carotid artery were identified. Two Ethibond ties were passed proximal and distal around each of the vessels. Intravenous heparin of 50 units/kg was administered. The distal carotid artery was ligated and the proximal carotid cannulated with a 10-French Biomedicus arterial cannula. A longitudinal venotomy was performed, and a 12-French Biomedicus cannula was inserted into the superior vena cava while a 12-French polystan cannula was introduced cephalad, and both were secured to the vessel with a 2-0 tie. The ECMO circuit was brought into the field and tubing divided. The arterial cannula was connected to the arterial end of the circuit, taking care to avoid air entry, and the venous cannulae were connected to the venous end of the circuit. ECMO flows were initiated. The patient tolerated the procedure, and no complications were encountered. The sternocleidomastoid was reapproximated with a 3-0 Vicryl suture and skin was closed with multiple interrupted 3-0 nylon sutures. Dressings were applied in standard fashion. The physicians provided a final diagnosis of persistent fetal circulation or primary pulmonary hypertension of newborn. The continuous veno-arterial extracorporeal membrane oxygenation was successful in treating the patient's symptoms of hypoxemia due to the primary pulmonary hypertension of newborn.

Principal Diagnosis: _____

Secondary Diagnoses: _____

Principal Procedures: _____

Secondary Procedure(s): _____

6

A 12-hour-old infant was transferred for admission to the university hospital neonatal intensive care unit for respiratory problems after being born at a community hospital by vaginal delivery to a woman who had just completed her 39th week of pregnancy. The infant was exhibiting respiratory symptoms consistent with aspiration of meconium at the time of the delivery. The infant had low Apgar scores of 5 and 6 with tachypnea and cyanosis. On admission, the infant was intubated and placed on mechanical ventilation and maintained on it for 48 hours. Within 1 day, the infant's chest x-ray demonstrated patchy infiltrates. The neonatologist diagnosed the infant as having meconium aspiration pneumonia with no signs of pulmonary hypertension as a consequence of the pneumonia. The physician also described the infant as "small for dates," weighing 2,200 grams.

Principal Diagnosis: _____

Secondary Diagnoses: _____

Principal Procedures: _____

Secondary Procedure(s): _____

7

The patient is an infant who was transferred for admission to the university hospital neonatal intensive care unit after being born at a community hospital by vaginal delivery to a woman who had just completed her 38th week of pregnancy. The mother of the infant was addicted to prescription narcotics for back pain from a motor vehicle crash but had switched to prescription methadone during her pregnancy. The infant admitted to the neonatal ICU in narcotic withdrawal after being born addicted to the methadone the mother was taking during her pregnancy. The infant was attached to cardiac and oxygen monitors and exhibited symptoms of drug withdrawal with difficulty sleeping, long periods of crying, diarrhea, and trouble with feeding. A slow process of weaning was started with the infant receiving small doses of methadone to wean her off the drugs. Over time, the infant had fewer symptoms of withdrawal and was gaining weight and sleeping for longer periods of time. On discharge, the physician described the infant as "small for dates," weighing 2,400 grams, and "infant of an addicted mother suffering withdrawal." The infant and her mother will be followed by a pediatric home care team.

Principal Diagnosis: _____

Secondary Diagnoses: _____

Principal Procedures: _____

Secondary Procedure(s): _____

8

A seven-day-old infant was brought by her parents to the university hospital's outpatient high-risk pediatric clinic for her first post-hospital discharge examination. The physician examined the patient and was most concerned about the child's fetal growth retardation. The physician was pleased to see the child had gained weight since leaving the hospital. The physician described the child's condition as premature infant with fetal growth retardation, 36 week 3 day gestation, with a birth weight of 1,600 grams. The parents will bring the child back to the clinic in two weeks.

First-Listed Diagnosis: _____

Secondary Diagnoses: _____

9

A 25-day-old infant is brought to the university hospital's high-risk pediatric clinic by her foster mother for evaluation of her status as a "crack baby." The child's mother was dependent on cocaine, and the infant had a positive drug screen for cocaine at birth and exhibited several symptoms. The infant continues to exhibit transitory tachypnea of newborn. The physician orders a continuation of pediatric home health services to monitor the child's respiratory status and the effect of the noxious substance (cocaine) on the infant. The reason for the clinic visit documented by the physician is "crack baby with continued transitory tachypnea." The infant will be brought back to the clinic in two weeks.

First-Listed Diagnosis: _____

Secondary Diagnoses: _____

10

The parents of a 10-day-old infant bring the newborn to the pediatrician's office to evaluate her slow feeding problems. When the infant was born, the umbilical cord was found loosely wrapped around the newborn's neck. It was quickly removed by the obstetrician, and the infant was observed for respiratory and other difficulties. Slow feeding problems were evident while the infant was in the hospital, and the pediatricians considered the nuchal cord problem as the cause. The physician recommends a change in infant formula and different feeding bottles. The physician also orders pediatric home health services to assist the parents in the child's care at home. A follow-up appointment is scheduled to return to the office in two weeks. The physician's diagnosis is feeding problems in an infant born with nuchal cord around her neck.

First-Listed Diagnosis: _____

Secondary Diagnoses: _____

11

This male infant was born today at 32-3/7th weeks premature weighing 1,920 grams by a repeat cesarean delivery. The infant had Apgar scores of 8 and 9. He had bag-mask inhalation for 30 seconds. His oxygen saturation was then 99 on room air. The infant was admitted to the premature nursery and placed on monitors. He was observed for a suspected infection but found to have none. Otherwise his physical exam showed no abnormalities other than light-for-dates, and he remained in the nursery after his mother's discharge for additional monitoring and weight gain. He was discharged at day 10 to be followed by pediatric home care nurses. No circumcision was performed.

Principal Diagnosis: _____

Secondary Diagnoses: _____

Principal Procedures: _____

Secondary Procedure(s): _____

12

This female infant was born to a 17-year-old mother, gravida 1, para 0, by spontaneous vaginal delivery with vertex presentation. She was born at 38 4/7 weeks gestation and small for gestational age, weighing 2,035 grams (4 pounds, 4 ounces). Her Apgar scores were 6 and 9. The infant required bag-mask inhalation for 2 minutes and 30 seconds, and she was admitted to the neonatal intensive care nursery for continued monitoring and treatment. Initially the infant had transient tachypnea that became respiratory distress and metabolic acidosis. She had hypermagnesemia, as her mother received magnesium therapy. She also had newborn jaundice and was treated with Bili Light or phototherapy. She was observed for possible sepsis, but none was found. The intravenous antibiotics were discontinued after two days. The infant's physical examination on discharge was within normal limits for a premature infant, as her condition improved with laboratory data showing more normal findings. She was discharged at age five days to be followed by pediatric home care nurses with an appointment in the physician's office two days after discharge.

Principal Diagnosis: _____

Secondary Diagnoses: _____

Principal Procedures: _____

Secondary Procedure(s): _____

13

The mother of a 7-day-old infant brought the newborn to the pediatrician's office for her first post-hospital discharge evaluation. Upon examination, the physician noted bilateral conjunctivitis with mild erythema and scant mucoid discharge. A culture was taken from both eyes. Because the mother was diagnosed and treated for a chlamydial infection at the time of delivery, the pediatrician decided the infant had a mild form of neonatal chlamydial conjunctivitis. The infant was prescribed a 14-day course of oral erythromycin. A follow-up appointment is scheduled to return to the office in two weeks.

First-Listed Diagnosis: _____

Secondary Diagnoses: _____

14

A full-term male infant was born at Community Hospital to a mother who acquired a severe case of herpes simplex virus (HSV) during her pregnancy. At the age of one day old, the infant was transferred for admission to University Hospital's special care unit to "rule out HSV visceral and/or central nervous system (CNS) infection." The infant was diagnosed with congenital HSV but did not develop a visceral or CNS-specific infection. The infant was treated with intravenous acyclovir for 10 days. An additional diagnosis of small-for-dates was made for the infant, who weighed 1,990 grams with a gestational age of 38 1/7th weeks. The infant was discharged to his mother's care with neonatal home nursing services to follow the infant's care at home.

Code for the infant at University Hospital only.

Principal Diagnosis: _____

Secondary Diagnoses: _____

Principal Procedures: _____

Secondary Procedure(s): _____

15

A preterm male infant was born at Community Hospital at 33 and 5/7th weeks to a primigravida 30-year-old female. The infant was having respiratory difficulties and was transferred within hours for admission to University Hospital to care for his prematurity and to rule out respiratory distress syndrome. While in the neonatal intensive care unit, the infant's respiratory symptoms abated. A thorough evaluation of the infant included laboratory and imaging studies. One unexpected diagnosis established through the imaging studies was the diagnosis of spina bifida occulta, the mildest form of spina bifida. Only through imaging examinations could the physician see an opening in the vertebrae of the spinal column, with no apparent damage to the spinal cord, which is the definition of spina bifida occulta. The infant remained in the hospital for four weeks gaining weight and maturing. The infant was discharged with the final diagnoses of preterm infant, 33 5/7th weeks gestation, birthweight of 1,600 grams with spina bifida occulta. The infant was discharged to the care of his parents with neonatal home nursing services to follow the infant's care at home. An appointment was made for the parents to return with the infant to see a pediatric neurologist in four weeks.

Code for the infant at University Hospital only.

Principal Diagnosis: _____

Secondary Diagnoses: _____

Principal Procedures: _____

Secondary Procedure(s): _____

16

The patient is a newborn born by cesarean delivery in the hospital during the mother's 38th week of pregnancy and is the mother's first child. The infant weighed 4,559 grams at birth and measured 22 inches in length. The infant's physical examination revealed a healthy, well-developed infant with chubby cheeks and dimpled thighs, but otherwise it was a normal examination. The infant required extra feedings during the four-day hospital stay because the infant's blood sugar dropped without the feedings. The infant's mother did not have diabetes or other medical conditions. However, the parents of the infant were tall and obese, with the mother's height as 6 feet, 2 inches. The mother weighed 250 pounds at the time of delivery having gained 30 pounds during the pregnancy. The infant's father was 6 feet, 6 inches tall and weighed 320 pounds. The pediatrician told the parents that the infant appeared healthy but was an exceptionally large and should be monitored closely for weight changes and will require appropriate feedings. The pediatrician further explained it was not uncommon for large parents to have large babies. The infant was discharged with his mother on the 4th hospital day to be followed up in the pediatrician's office in eight days. A home health visit will be made to the infant's home within two days after discharge to measure the infant's blood sugar and how the infant was taking his feedings. The mother will not be breast feeding the infant. The infant was circumcised during the hospital stay. Discharge diagnoses that were documented by the pediatrician were exceptionally large-for-dates full term infant, 4,559 grams.

Principal Diagnosis: _____

Secondary Diagnoses: _____

Principal Procedures: _____

Secondary Procedure(s): _____

17

A newborn female was born by cesarean delivery to a mother after a gestation of 38 weeks, 1 day. This was the mother's second pregnancy that was uncomplicated other than the fact she had a previous cesarean delivery and went into labor before the date of the scheduled cesarean delivery the following week. The infant appeared normal at birth with a birth weight of 3,150 grams and Apgar scores of 8 and 9 at the one-minute and five-minute mark after birth. Within two hours after birth, the nurses in the newborn nursery noted the newborn had bluish skin and was having noisy breathing, describing it as a grunting sound. The pediatrician on duty examined the infant and concluded she had tachypnea with over 60 breaths per minute. The newborn was transferred to the neonatal ICU and blood tests were ordered. The infant was placed on supplemental oxygen and monitored closely. Within 24 hours after birth, the newborn was breathing quietly at a normal rate with normal measured oxygen levels. The newborn was kept in the neonatal ICU for 12 more hours before being transferred to the normal newborn nursery. The infant was discharged with her mother on the fourth hospital day. The pediatrician documented the final diagnoses for the newborn as full-term with transient tachypnea in a newborn.

Principal Diagnosis: _____

Secondary Diagnoses: _____

Principal Procedures: _____

Secondary Procedure(s): _____

Chapter 17

Congenital Malformations, Deformations, and Chromosomal Abnormalities

Coding Scenarios for *Basic ICD-10-CM and ICD-10-PCS Coding Exercises*

The following case studies are organized following the sequence of the chapters in the ICD-10-CM Tabular List of Diseases and Injuries as published on the Centers for Disease Control and Prevention National Center for Health Statistics website (http://www.cdc.gov/nchs/icd/icd10cm.htm). The objective of this book is to provide the student with more detailed clinical information to code, rather than one- or two-line diagnosis and procedure statements.

ICD-10-CM diagnosis codes are to be assigned to both the inpatient hospital admission and the outpatient visit case studies. In this book, the ICD-10-PCS procedure codes are to be assigned only to the inpatient hospital admission cases. In actual practice, outpatient cases are assigned CPT/HCPCS codes. The ICD-10-PCS codes are only required for inpatient procedures. In the answer key for the exercises, the Alphabetic Index entry is listed after the code to indicate the main terms and sub-terms used to locate the code that must be verified in the ICD-10-CM Tabular List or in the ICD-10-PCS Code Tables prior to assigning the code.

1

A 6-month-old infant, born with a congenital anomaly of the inner ear with impairment of hearing, is admitted for surgery to treat his mixed hearing loss. The patient is taken to surgery to place bilateral single channel cochlear prosthesis (hearing) implants via an open approach. He quickly recovers from the procedure and anesthesia and is discharged home.

Principal Diagnosis: _____

Secondary Diagnoses: _____

Principal Procedure: _____

Secondary Procedure(s): _____

2

A 7-week-old infant was born with a biliary atresia. The patient has severe obstructive jaundice due to the congenital condition. The patient was admitted and the diagnosis is confirmed by surgical exploration with an operative cholangiography done under fluoroscopic guidance with low osmolar contrast (this included views of the gallbladder and bile ducts). The biliary atresia is treated with a Roux-en-Y operation in the hepatobiliary system, also known as the Kasai procedure, where the pediatric surgeon removes blockage in the gallbladder and bile ducts outside the liver and uses part of the small intestine to replace it. As a result, the bile will flow directly from the liver into the small intestine. The surgeon explained to the parents the operation does not cure biliary atresia but it does produce near normal bile flow and corrects problems that result from the bile obstruction. Otherwise, a liver transplant is the only cure for biliary atresia. For this patient, the Roux-en-Y bypass was created from the gallbladder to the small intestine.

Principal Diagnosis: _____

Secondary Diagnoses: _____

Principal Procedure: _____

Secondary Procedure(s): _____

3

A 2-month-old female infant was born with coarctation of the aorta that is a narrowing in a part of the aorta was transferred to this hospital for admission one day after her birth. The narrowing of the aorta forces the heart to pump harder to push blood through the narrowed part and causes many consequences that can be life-threatening including heart failure. The infant was brought to the operating room for excisional repair of the coarctation of the thoracic aorta. The surgeon removed the narrowed portion of the descending thoracic aorta and created an end-to-end anastomosis between the two remaining portions. The procedure was done with the pump oxygenator for circulatory support.

Principal Diagnosis: _____

Secondary Diagnoses: _____

Principal Diagnosis: _____

Secondary Procedure(s): _____

4

The mother of an 8-day-old infant brought the child to the pediatrician's office for the first well-infant checkup. During the physical examination, the femoral head is felt to displace with a jerk, which is repeated as the femur slides back into the acetabulum upon release of the displacing force. The pediatrician is certain the infant has what is called a congenital dislocatable right hip. The mother is requested to bring the infant back to the office in three days. The mother is advised that the condition is likely to resolve within a week or two after birth. If the condition is still present at the next visit, the child will be referred to a pediatric orthopedic physician.

First-Listed Diagnosis: _____

Secondary Diagnoses: _____

5

The patient is admitted to the children's hospital for open heart surgery to repair her congenital heart defects. The patient is a 7-year-old female who was born with Tetralogy of Fallot that was corrected by surgical repair at 2 years of age. She has been seen by the pediatric cardiologist every six months since that surgery, aware of the fact that further surgery would be necessary later in childhood. Since birth, it has also been known that she suffers from the following diagnoses as listed on her discharge summary: "Stenosis of the pulmonary valve with right ventricular outflow obstruction causing pulmonary insufficiency. Stenosis of the left pulmonary artery. Status post previous cardiac surgery with the surgically repaired congenital heart defects performed five years ago." The corrective surgery for these congenital conditions is "1. Right ventricular outflow reconstruction with replacement of pulmonary valve with homograft; 2. Left pulmonary artery reconstruction to hilum with patch arterioplasty; and 3. Right pulmonary artery stenosis arterioplasty." The principal objective is to replace the pulmonary value with a homograft, a nonautologous tissue graft. The right and left pulmonary artery stenosis was corrected with arterioplasty. The surgery is performed under cardiopulmonary bypass and an intraoperative transesophageal echocardiogram of the pediatric heart with no contrast is performed.

Principal Diagnosis: _____

Secondary Diagnoses: _____

Principal Procedure: _____

Secondary Procedure(s): _____

6

A 2-week-old male infant was admitted to the University Medical Center pediatric gastroenterology unit after being seen in the gastroenterology clinic. The infant was full-term when born and fed well after birth but then experienced occasional regurgitation of feedings. Several days later, the vomiting became more frequent and projectile, containing the previous feedings. Shortly after the vomiting, the infant is ready to feed again. The parents were provided information about the child's condition and agreed to surgical correction of the digestive problem.

The operative report is as follows:

PREOPERATIVE DIAGNOSIS: Hypertrophic pyloric stenosis

POSTOPERATIVE DIAGNOSIS: Hypertrophic pyloric stenosis

PROCEDURE: Laparoscopic Pyloromyotomy

INDICATIONS: The infant is a 2-week old male with hypertrophic pyloric stenosis diagnosed based on his history, physical findings and radiographic studies. The patient had metabolic derangements corrected before surgery that was consented to by the parents after receiving full disclosure of the potential risks versus benefits of the procedure.

FINDINGS: The upper abdomen was evaluated and appears normal. There was a hypertrophied pylorus. After the myotomy, no bile staining was found. The stomach was insufflated with air and no bubbles were observed at the myotomy site. The stomach was decompressed prior to the laparoscope's removal.

PROCEDURE: The patient was brought to the operating room and carefully placed and secured on the operating table. A time-out was performed to identify the patient, the diagnosis and the procedure, and anatomical site of the operation to be performed. General anesthesia induction and intubation were performed atraumatically. The stomach was decompressed with suction prior to intubation. Intravenous antibiotics were started. The abdomen was prepped and draped in standard laparoscopic procedure fashion. Marcaine local anesthesia was used at all incision sites. The umbilicus was cleaned with betadine and inverted. The hemostatic forceps was used to spread through the umbilical cicatrix. A 3mm port was introduced and the abdomen insufflated. The vision instrument was inserted and the pylorus was identified. Two incisions were made for the instruments to be inserted in the right upper quadrant lateral to the rectus muscle and the second instrument contralateral to that. The pyloric grasper instrument was placed through the right upper quadrant incision. The electrocautery instrument was inserted through the left upper quadrant incision. The pylorus was grasped and the electrocautery blade was used to incise the serosa. After that, the pyloric spreader was inserted and the pylorus muscle was divided along the length of it to the base of the submucosa. The duodenum was gently clamped and the stomach insufflated with the in-place OG tube. There was no bile leaking or air bubbles noted at the myotomy site. The stomach was decompressed prior to the removal of the instruments. No bleeding was noted from the incisions internally. The optic instrument was removed. The port was removed. The umbilicus opening was closed with 4-0 Vicryl sutures. The upper quadrant skin incisions were closed with 5-0 Monocryl sutures. The wounds were dressed and the patient was extubated and taken to the post anesthesia recovery unit in good condition.

Principal Diagnosis: _____

Secondary Diagnoses: _____

Principal Procedure: _____

Secondary Procedure(s): _____

7

The patient is an 18-month-old male who was born with a complete bilateral cleft lip and palate deformity. He is seen in the University Hospital's outpatient pediatric clinic. The child has had reconstruction surgery to correct the congenital defect. The child continues to have feeding difficulties. While he is free of infection now, he has had a few ear infections. Both the feeding and ear problems are attributed to the cleft lip and palate that appears to be incompletely repaired. The physician recommended to the parents that one more surgery should be performed to improve the symmetry of the palate and lip and alleviate the feeding problems and ear infections. However, it is possible that the child will need ear tubes placed in the future because of the chronic ear infections. A revision of the cleft palate and advancement flap graft is scheduled in the next two weeks.

First-Listed Diagnosis: _____

Secondary Diagnoses: _____

8

The patient is a 21-day-old male who is admitted to the hospital for treatment of Hirschsprung's disease diagnosed by a rectal biopsy three days ago that showed no ganglion cells. He is brought to the operating room where general anesthesia is induced and a left lower quadrant oblique incision was made. Dissection continued with electrocautery until the peritoneal cavity was entered. A stool-filled sigmoid colon was identified and delivered into the wound. A small biopsy was taken from the sigmoid portion of the bowel and sent for frozen section. This was returned normal with normal numbers of ganglion cells. The colon was then tacked to the fascia and peritoneum using interrupted 4-0 silk suture. A #12 red-rubber catheter was placed through the mesentery of the colon and looped upon itself and sutured with 2-0 silk. The colostomy of the sigmoid colon was then opened using electrocautery and both the limbs were found to be widely patent through the fascia. The colostomy was brought to the cutaneous level and a colostomy bag was applied. The sponge, needle, and instrument counts were reported to be correct at the conclusion of the procedure. The child was awakened and taken to the recovery room in satisfactory condition.

Principal Diagnosis: _____

Secondary Diagnoses: _____

Principal Procedure: _____

Secondary Procedure(s): _____

9

A seven-day-old male infant was examined by a pediatric ophthalmologist in the physician's office. The child had been recently discharged from the hospital after birth. He was the product of a full-term gestation and his mother had an uneventful prenatal period. Based on physical findings and testing, the male infant was diagnosed with Trisomy 13. In order to rule out a retinoblastoma, the infant was referred for this examination. The external examination of the lids was normal. There was haziness overlying the limbus superiorly in both eyes, consistent with an anterior embryotoxon, a congenital corneal malformation. The pupils dilated readily. The lenses were clear. The vitreous was clear. Examination of the fundus revealed normal-appearing disks and macular blood vessels with no evidence of any lesion. The consultant wrote the diagnoses on the report returned to the primary pediatrician as "Bilateral anterior embryotoxon, otherwise normal examination with no evidence of retinoblastoma in this newborn infant with Trisomy 13."

First-Listed Diagnosis: _____

Secondary Diagnoses: _____

10

A 1-day-old male infant with a prenatal history of hypoplastic left heart syndrome with ventricular septal defect was transferred for admission to Mid-Size Community Hospital from a smaller regional hospital for evaluation and management. Noninvasive cardiac testing confirmed the congenital cardiac conditions. During the hospital stay the patient was found to have *E. coli* sepsis and received seven days of intravenous antibiotics. The pediatric cardiovascular surgeon from Children's Hospital in the nearby city came to the hospital for a consultation and to meet with the parents to discuss performing a cardiac catheterization and a possible Hybrid Stage I procedure with median sternotomy and bilateral pulmonary artery banding versus a Norwood procedure. The parents agreed with the proposed Hybrid Stage I procedure, and the infant was transferred on day 3 to Children's Hospital for the surgical procedure.

Code for the baby at Mid-Size Community Hospital.

Principal Diagnosis: _____

Secondary Diagnoses: _____

Principal Procedure: _____

Secondary Procedure(s): _____

11

The patient is a 3-week-old female infant who is brought to the pediatrician's office because the mother has observed that the patient appears to be arching her head and neck in an effort to breathe, especially after the child has been sucking on a bottle. The physician examined the infant and was unable to pass a small tube through the right naris to the pharynx, but the left naris was completely open. The physician ordered an immediate CT scan of the nasopharynx to determine the type of occlusion that was producing the complete obstruction of the posterior nares owing to choanal atresia. The physician explained to the mother that the infant had choanal atresia on the left side that is a congenital disorder where the back of the nasal passage is blocked or obstructed by abnormal bone growth or membranous soft tissue. An appointment was made for the mother to take the infant to a consulting physician at the Children's Hospital for evaluation and treatment.

First-Listed Diagnosis: _____

Secondary Diagnoses: _____

12

The patient is 2-year-old male who was brought to the pediatrician's office by his parents for a routine well-child check. During the physical examination, the physician noted the child had an undescended testicle on the right side. No other abnormalities or conditions were found. The parents were given a referral to take the child to a pediatric urologist within the next two weeks to determine the appropriate medical or surgical intervention needed to treat the unilateral cryptorchism.

First-Listed Diagnosis: _____

Secondary Diagnoses: _____

13

A 32-year-old female patient returns to her obstetrician-gynecologist's office to review the findings of her recent transvaginal uterine ultrasound. The patient has been married for three years and has not become pregnant as desired. The physician informs the patient that the ultrasound examination showed that she had a bicornuate uterus, which is sometimes described as a heart-shaped uterus because of the distinct shape of the uterus when viewed externally, for example, on an ultrasound. The physician also explained this is a congenital condition that occurs when the uterine fundus fails to fuse. The patient's condition is a partial bicornuate uterus with an evidenced cleft in the uterine dome. Given the fact that patients with this type of Mullerian abnormality often have a kidney abnormality as well, the patient was given an order to return to the radiology department for a renal ultrasound. The physician's review of the literature about this condition found that reproductive function is generally good in patients with partial bicornuate uteri, but the patient will be referred to a reproductive endocrinologist if she does not become pregnant within the next six months. The patient will return to this physician's office in two weeks to discuss the results of the renal ultrasound if an abnormality is found.

First-Listed Diagnosis: _____

Secondary Diagnoses: _____

14

A 3-day-old female infant was transferred for admission to the city's children's hospital because of noisy breathing, or stridor. The physician who ordered the transfer were concerned about the child having partial respiratory tract obstruction or partial occlusion in the airway. After imaging studies, the pediatrician concluded the infant had laryngomalacia, but not a severe form. After being provided informed consent, the parents consented to the pediatric surgeon to perform an inspection flexible laryngoscopy through a nasopharyngoscope. The surgeon noted in her operative report that no masses or lesions were seen in the nasal cavity. There was a normal hypopharynx. Tonsils were one plus from a superior view. The tongue based was normal and the valleculae are patent. The epiglottis was normal shaped with no redundancy or prolapse. The aryepiglottic folds were not shortened. The vocal cords were bilaterally mobile. The subglottis appeared patent. There was no erythema or edema of the larynx. The posterior pharyngeal wall appeared normal. The physician noted the patient's stridor lessened when the patient was placed in the prone position with head extension. The physicians involved all informed the parents that stridor usually resolves in most infants within two to three months as the child grows. The parents were requested to bring the infant back to the pediatric pulmonary disease clinic in one month. The discharge diagnosis was infantile stridor due to laryngomalacia.

Principal Diagnosis: _____

Secondary Diagnoses: _____

Principal Procedure: _____

Secondary Procedure(s): _____

15

The parents of a one-year-old male brought the child to the pediatric urologist's office for re-evaluation of his coronal, or balanic, hypospadias. The condition was diagnosed at the time of birth. The physician reminded the parents that this urethral anomaly is the most common urethral anomaly that occurs in one out of 300 births. The child's congenital condition is not particularly severe, as his urethra is functional and the child does not have undescended testicles that often accompany hypospadias. Originally the urologist had advised the surgical plastic repair of the hypospadias be completed prior to school age. However, the parents were requesting that the surgery be completed sooner. The parents and physician agreed to wait until the child was at least 18 months old before surgery is scheduled.

First-Listed Diagnosis: _____

Secondary Diagnoses: _____

16

The patient is a 13-year-old female who has complained to her mother about a "sore low back" that she attributed to physical education class at school. The mother brought the young teenager to the physician's office 10 days ago for an examination and returned today for a follow-up appointment to review the results of radiology tests, specifically, a plain diagnostic imaging of the thoracic and lumbar spine and an MRI of the lumbar spine. The MRI had been ordered by the physician after the results of plain films suggested an abnormality of the lumbar area. The MRI of the lumbar spine showed no abnormalities of the vertebrae but the radiologist concluded the patient had spina bifida occulta. The physician explained to the patient and her mother that spina bifida is a congenital neural tube defect in which one or more vertebrae are malformed. The term occulta means it is hidden by the tissue that covers the opening in the vertebrae. The physician also explained this condition commonly goes unnoticed for years after birth because it usually does not produce any symptoms. It is often detected by radiology examination for an unrelated condition. One visible indication of spina bifida occulta is a small dimple or birthmark on the back over the area of the vertebral defect. Upon further examination, the teenager did have a sacral dimple and there was a barely visible skin birthmark over where the spina bifida occulta was seen on the MRI. The physician advised the mother and teenager that the low back pain was not likely related to the spina bifida occulta. The teenager stated the low back pain was no longer present and did not think she needed further physical therapy. The physician examined the teenager again and there was no evidence of back pain today. The diagnoses listed on the patient's record for this visit were (1) Low back pain, cause unknown and (2) Spina bifida occulta, incidental finding.

First-Listed Diagnosis: _____

Secondary Diagnoses: _____

17

The parents of a 3-month-old daughter took their child to the pediatrician's office for a well-child visit. They asked the pediatrician if she thought the infant's head was misshaped and if the infant's nose and eye socket was out of alignment. The pediatrician noted there was no soft spot, or fontanelle, on the child's skull and ordered a CT scan for the child. The parents were referred to the University Cranio-Facial Center for a consultation. At the visit to the center, the child was examined by a pediatric neurosurgeon and cranio-facial surgeon. Based on a physical exam and findings of the CT scan, the surgeons concluded the child had craniosynostosis and explained it was a birth defect that causes one or more of the sutures on a infant's head to close earlier than usual. Further, the skull of an infant is made up of bony plates that allow for growth of the skull. Borders where these plates intersect are called sutures or suture lines. Early closing of a suture causes the infant to have an abnormally shaped head and, in this child's case, a deviated nose and eye socket. The surgeons recommended the parents' consent to an operation on the infant to relieve pressure on the skull to create room for the brain to grow and to avoid damage to it and improve the facial appearance. The parents were given information about traditional open incisional surgery to reshape the affected portion of the skull or an endoscopic surgery with small scalp incisions made over the affected area to open the suture and allow growth to occur naturally and return the infant's head to a normal shape. The endoscopic procedure requires the use of a customized helmet that the infant would wear over the next year to allow the growth of the skull to occur correctly. The parents were asked to consider the options and return to the Cranio-Facial Center the following Monday for another visit to discuss and schedule the surgery if that is their decision. The surgery needs to occur soon because of the infant's age. The parents were also given information about other cranio-facial and pediatric neurosurgeons if they were interested in obtaining a second opinion. The final diagnosis entered in the infant's record for the visit at the University Cranio-Facial Center was craniosynostosis.

First-Listed Diagnosis: _____

Secondary Diagnoses: _____

Chapter 18

Symptoms, Signs, and Abnormal Clinical and Laboratory Findings, Not Elsewhere Classified

Coding Scenarios for *Basic ICD-10-CM and ICD-10-PCS Coding Exercises*

The following case studies are organized following the sequence of the chapters in the ICD-10-CM Tabular List of Diseases and Injuries as published on the Centers for Disease Control and Prevention National Center for Health Statistics website (http://www.cdc.gov /nchs/icd/icd10cm.htm). The objective of this book is to provide the student with more detailed clinical information to code, rather than one- or two-line diagnosis and procedure statements.

ICD-10-CM diagnosis codes are to be assigned to both the inpatient hospital admission and the outpatient visit case studies. In this book, the ICD-10-PCS procedure codes are to be assigned only to the inpatient hospital admission cases. In actual practice, outpatient cases are assigned CPT/HCPCS codes. The ICD-10-PCS codes are only required for inpatient procedures. In the answer key for the exercises, the Alphabetic Index entry is listed after the code to indicate the main terms and sub-terms used to locate the code that must be verified in the ICD-10-CM Tabular List or in the ICD-10-PCS Code Tables prior to assigning the code.

1

A 50-year-old male is an inpatient who is scheduled for a colonoscopy. The reason for the colonoscopy is stated as "change in bowel habits, family history of colon cancer, and possible colonic polyp." A colonoscopy is performed with a biopsy of the descending colon. No polyps were seen in any portion of the large intestine. The pathological diagnosis provided for the biopsy was normal colonic tissue. The physician documents the final diagnosis as (1) change in bowel habits, unexplained, (2) normal colon examination.

Code for only the colonoscopy services performed in the inpatient setting.

Principal Diagnosis (for colonoscopy services): _____

Secondary Diagnoses: _____

Principal Procedure (for colonoscopy services): _____

Secondary Procedure(s): _____

2

A 59-year-old female is referred by her primary care physician to the hospital outpatient radiology department with an order for a CT scan of the abdomen. The patient has been complaining of generalized abdominal pain, fatigue, and nausea but no vomiting over the past several weeks. Previous gastrointestinal imaging studies, including an ultrasound, were abnormal. The physician's diagnosis on the order is "abnormal radiology findings of GI tract, require further definition by CT exam, generalized abdominal pain, fatigue, nausea, rule out abdominal malignancy."

First-Listed Diagnosis: _____

Secondary Diagnoses: _____

3

A patient is admitted to inpatient status for a bronchoscopy with a transbronchial lung biopsy to determine the etiology of a lung mass found on recent x-ray and CT studies. The patient had been complaining of a cough and chest pressure over the past several weeks. The patient is taken to the endoscopy suite. Following administration of conscious sedation, the fiberoptic bronchoscopy is performed. During the process to obtain the transbronchial biopsy, the patient experiences a prolonged episode of bradycardia, and the physician terminates the procedure before the biopsy is obtained. The procedure will be rescheduled after the cardiologist evaluates the patient.

Principal Diagnosis: _____

Secondary Diagnoses: _____

Principal Procedure: _____

Secondary Procedure: _____

4

A 50-year-old male is admitted through the emergency department (ED) with a complaint of chest pain. The EKG and laboratory tests done in the ED are inconclusive, but an acute myocardial infarction is ruled out. During the hospital stay, the cardiovascular function studies could not disprove the existence of coronary artery disease. Results of a nuclear medicine imaging using thallium for the cardiac stress test were mildly abnormal. The patient did not want to have a cardiac catheterization study performed. Gastrointestinal studies, including an EGD with a biopsy of the lower esophagus, were entirely normal with no clinical or pathological evidence of gastroesophageal reflux disease or esophagitis. Given the negative test results, the physician concludes the patient had atypical chest pain, cause undetermined. The patient is requested to make appointments for follow up with both a cardiologist and gastroenterologist for possible additional testing.

Principal Diagnosis: _____

Secondary Diagnosis: _____

Principal Procedure: _____

Secondary Procedure(s): _____

5

A 38-year-old female comes to her physician's office for the results of recent diagnostic studies. The woman had several complaints including numbness of her legs, difficulty in walking, lack of coordination, and trembling in her hands. The symptoms are not present all the time but have occurred more frequently over the past couple of weeks. The patient had also been examined by a neurologist. The patient was told the MRI and neurologic tests, as well as the conclusion of the neurologist, consider her condition to be consistent with multiple sclerosis (MS). When the patient asked whether the physician was certain that she had MS, he said he was not completely certain and made arrangements for her to be examined by physicians in a neurology group that specializes in treating patients with MS.

First-Listed Diagnosis: _____

Secondary Diagnoses: _____

6

A 52-year-old female with known fibrocystic disease of the right breast has an appointment for a diagnostic mammogram at the hospital outpatient department. A screening mammogram done three days previously was abnormal with a suspicious lesion noted in the upper quadrant of the left breast. Findings of fibrocystic disease of the right breast were noted again. The diagnostic mammogram is performed and interpreted by the radiologist. The patient's physician meets with the radiologist to review the findings. The patient's physician agrees with the radiologist's findings of "microcalcifications of breast tissue, left breast" and advises the patient of the benign findings. The status of the fibrocystic disease of the right breast had not changed since last year's mammogram. The patient will have a follow-up diagnostic mammogram in six months.

First-Listed Diagnosis: _____

Secondary Diagnoses: _____

7

A 30-year-old female has a repeat visit in her gynecologist's office to review the results of a recent abnormal Pap smear. Over the past year, the woman had experienced genital warts that appear and disappear on the external areas of her genitals. During the last visit, the gynecologist had performed a colposcopy and a Pap smear. Cells were scraped from the cervix and sent for cytologic and DNA testing. The patient is advised today that the conclusion of the test is "DNA positive for cervical high-risk human papillomavirus (HPV)." The patient consents to a cervical biopsy, which is scheduled for the following week. The patient's genital warts on her external genitalia today were examined and appear to be decreasing.

First-Listed Diagnosis: _____

Secondary Diagnosis Code: _____

8

A mother brought her 7-week-old infant to the pediatrician's office for the stated reason of intermittent diarrhea. The physician examines the infant and takes a comprehensive history, including the infant's food history and eating pattern. The physician considers the possibility that the infant is allergic to the infant formula being fed to the patient, which includes milk products. The physician recommends certain laboratory tests be performed and includes the following diagnosis on the order for the tests "(1) Failure to thrive in newborn, (2) diarrhea, (3) possible milk allergy."

First-Listed Diagnosis: _____

Secondary Diagnoses: _____

9

Family members bring a 19-year-old male to the hospital emergency department. The patient had stated he had a severe headache, fever, and nausea and vomiting. A thorough physical examination and diagnostic imaging was performed. The physician arranges for the transfer of the patient to a larger hospital with the diagnosis of "Rule out meningitis." All records and test results are transferred with the patient. In addition to the physical complaints stated by the patient, the physician adds the diagnosis of meningismus.

First-Listed Diagnosis: _____

Secondary Diagnoses: _____

10

A 56-year-old female is admitted through the emergency department complaining of right upper quadrant abdominal pain. In addition, the patient says she is having nausea and had vomited several times at home. The patient is admitted with the diagnosis of possible cholecystitis. Several tests are performed, and all results are normal, except those of an ultrasound of the abdomen. It is also discovered that the patient has elevated blood pressure readings, but a diagnosis of hypertension is not made. The physician stated "no conclusive diagnosis found." When asked for more documentation concerning the patient diagnosis, the physician stated that the only conclusive findings were the patient's initial complaints, her elevated blood pressure readings, and the abnormal ultrasound of the abdominal area. The patient is discharged for outpatient management.

Principal Diagnosis: _____

Secondary Diagnoses: _____

Principal Procedure: _____

Secondary Procedure(s): _____

11

The patient is a 66-year-old female who was admitted to the hospital after being seen in her physician's office with the complaint of difficulty in swallowing, first solid food and now difficulty with swallowing liquids. She was found to be dehydrated and was admitted. A gastroenterology consult was obtained, and the physician recommended an esophagogastroduodenoscopy to rule out esophageal stricture or obstruction. The patient became very anxious, even with the administration of conscious sedation, during the start of the EGD, and it was postponed. After discussion with the patient and the primary care physician, the gastroenterologist recommended the procedure be performed under general anesthesia, which was accomplished. The EGD was performed, and no obstruction, stricture, lesions, ulcers, polyps, or other disease was found in the esophagus, in the stomach, or small bowel, which was also examined. After being reassured that there was no disease or cancer present in her upper GI tract, the patient appeared very relieved. That evening she was able to eat a soft diet meal and drink liquids. The primary care physician listed the final diagnoses as dysphagia, cause unknown; anxiety disorder; and dehydration.

Principal Diagnosis: _____

Secondary Diagnoses: _____

Principal Procedure: _____

Secondary Procedure: _____

12

The patient is a 15-year-old female who has experienced a fever of 102°F with chills overnight and was brought to the emergency department (ED) by her mother at 5 a.m. Laboratory tests, including a complete blood count and urinalysis, were performed with normal results produced. The patient also complained of body aches and pains, weakness, and fatigue. The patient's family physician was contacted and advised the patient be discharged home and come to his office the same afternoon if she did not feel better. The ED physician wrote the final diagnosis as "fever with chills, possible viral syndrome."

First-Listed Diagnosis: _____

Secondary Diagnoses: _____

13

The patient is a 45-year-old male who was referred by his primary care physician to the cardiologist in his office "to diagnose and treat possible cardiac disease." Three days earlier the patient had abnormal results of a stress test that was done for preventive health purposes. The patient did not have any complaints typical of cardiac disease. When the nurse in the cardiologist's office was taking the patient's history and recording the vital signs, she noted the patient's blood pressure to be 138/88. The patient admitted to being somewhat "stressed-out" by being there, so the nurse waited 10 minutes and took the blood pressure again. This time the blood pressure values were 138/84. After the cardiologist reviewed the patient's history with him and completed the physical examination, the physician personally took the patient's blood pressure and found it to be 136/86. The physician explained to the patient that it was possible that he had hypertension, but he would not make the diagnosis during the first patient visit. The patient was prescribed a mild diuretic and given a follow-up appointment to return in two weeks. The physician completed his progress note about the visit with the impressions of (1) abnormal cardiovascular stress test, (2) elevated blood pressure readings, and (3) rule out hypertension.

First-Listed Diagnosis: _____

Secondary Diagnoses: _____

14

A 58-year-old female requested a same-day appointment with her primary care physician because of recurrent jaw and left shoulder pain that had occurred over the past two days and was increasing in intensity. The physician examined the patient and had the nurse perform an immediate electrocardiogram (EKG) on the patient. The physician recognized these symptoms as a possible acute myocardial infarction (AMI). When the physician noted the EKG was markedly abnormal, he had the staff call for an ambulance immediately and transferred the patient to the nearest hospital's emergency department. The diagnoses recorded by the physician on the progress note for the visit was jaw and shoulder pain, rule out AMI.

First-Listed Diagnosis: _____

Secondary Diagnoses: _____

15

The parents of a 7-week-old female returned to the pediatrician's office for a follow-up visit to examine the infant, who had been previously diagnosed with "colic." Laboratory work performed during the last visit was reported with normal values. The parents stated there had not been much change in the baby since their last appointment, two weeks ago. The infant was inconsolable three or four times a week with symptoms that lasted four to five hours, from the late afternoon through the evening hours. Some of the physician's recommended calming techniques worked, such as the "football hold," placing the infant face down along the length of the father's arm, as well as putting the infant in the car seat and driving around for several hours, but other efforts failed. The breast-feeding mother had eliminated recommended items from her diet, including caffeine, chocolate, and gas-producing foods. The pediatrician encouraged the parents that he had seen many babies like their baby and, fortunately, most of the babies did not experience as much colic after the age of 12 to 14 weeks. The parents made note of additional calming techniques recommended by the physician and his nurse. The physician's examination of the infant during this visit found an otherwise healthy infant. A follow-up appointment was made for three weeks later. The final diagnosis recorded for the visit was full-term female infant with colic.

First-Listed Diagnosis: _____

Secondary Diagnoses: _____

16

The patient is a 25-year-old male Army veteran of the Iraq war, He was in a vehicle that was damaged by an improvised explosive device that did not hit the vehicle directly. However, the four soldiers inside the vehicle had minor injuries. This patient recalls hitting his head on the side door of the vehicle when it crashed but otherwise was uninjured with no loss of consciousness. Since the soldier has been discharged and lives at home, his family describe him as exhibiting irritability and impulsive behaviors that are uncharacteristic of him. Today's visit at the Veterans Administration Outpatient Center is to review test results to explain his behavior change, which the patient also notices but cannot explain. Given the circumstances, the physician concludes the patient has "Late effect symptoms (irritability, impulsiveness) of diffuse traumatic brain injury." The patient was referred to a specialized treatment center that focuses on patients with traumatic brain injury.

First-Listed Diagnosis: _____

Secondary Diagnoses: _____

17

The patient is a 70-year-old male who is seen in his primary care physician's office complaining of nocturia, straining to urinate, and urinary frequency. The patient states he has had these symptoms off and on over the past three years but the symptoms have increased over the past couple of months. He tried an over-the-counter supplement, saw palmetto, but it didn't seem to help. The physician performs a complete physical examination including a digital rectal examination that revealed a mild to moderate enlarged prostate and ordered a PSA screening laboratory test. The patient is also known to have essential hypertension and hyperlipidemia that are under treatment by oral medications. The physician gave the patient a prescription for an alpha blocker medication to hopefully relieve the patient's symptoms. The patient was advised to take the medication faithfully and return to the office in six weeks to evaluate the patient again. At the next visit, the physician and patient will decide if the patient should be referred to a urologist for possible surgical treatment for the enlarged prostate. The physician renewed the patient's usual prescriptions for hypertension and hyperlipidemia. The final diagnoses written by the physician for this visit were enlarged prostate with urinary symptoms of nocturia, straining on urination, urinary frequency, essential hypertension, and hyperlipidemia.

First-Listed Diagnosis: _____

Secondary Diagnoses: _____

18

The parents of a 30-month-old male infant brought the child to the emergency department (ED) of the local hospital stating the child has had a fever between 102- and 103-degrees Fahrenheit over the past 24 hours, seemed tired and was quieter than usual. The child had a mild upper respiratory infection a week ago but the symptoms were no longer present. The child was examined by the ED physician who could not find an obvious infection. The physician noted the patient had a fever of 103°F and exhibited malaise but did not have a toxic appearance. Laboratory tests were ordered including a CBC and a blood culture on two specimens. The child's primary care physician ordered the child to be placed in observation status after the blood culture identified the presence of a bacterial organism and the white blood cell count was reported to be 15,100. The primary care physician concluded the child had bacteremia. The child received an antibiotic intramuscular injection and was closely observed over the next 24 hours. When the child was re-examined by the primary care physician, the child's temperature was 100 degrees Fahrenheit and the child again did not appear toxic. The physician documented there was no obvious evidence of an infection, the child was eating and drinking and appeared more alert. The child was discharged to his parents who were given an appointment with the primary care physician in four days and instructions to call the primary care physician or return to the ED of the fever became elevated again to 102 degrees or more. The final diagnoses documented on the observation records were bacteremia, fever, and malaise.

First-Listed Diagnosis: _____

Secondary Diagnoses: _____

Chapter 19A

Injuries, Effects of Foreign Body, Burns and Corrosions, and Frostbite

Coding Scenarios for *Basic ICD-10-CM and ICD-10-PCS Coding Exercises*

The following case studies are organized following the sequence of the chapters in the ICD-10-CM Tabular List of Diseases and Injuries as published on the Centers for Disease Control and Prevention National Center for Health Statistics website (http://www.cdc.gov /nchs/icd/icd10cm.htm). The objective of this book is to provide the student with more detailed clinical information to code, rather than one- or two-line diagnosis and procedure statements.

ICD-10-CM diagnosis codes are to be assigned to both the inpatient hospital admission and the outpatient visit case studies. In this book, the ICD-10-PCS procedure codes are to be assigned only to the inpatient hospital admission cases. In actual practice, outpatient cases are assigned CPT/HCPCS codes. The ICD-10-PCS codes are only required for inpatient procedures. In the answer key for the exercises, the Alphabetic Index entry is listed after the code to indicate the main terms and subterms used to locate the code that must be verified in the ICD-10-CM Tabular List or in the ICD-10-PCS Code Tables prior to assigning the code.

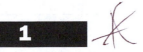

A 16-year-old male is brought to the emergency department with second- and third-degree burns of the chest wall and first- and second-degree burns of the upper arms, above the elbows. The total body surface burn is 25 percent with 9 percent being third-degree. The patient is transferred to the burn unit at the city's university hospital.

*Note: List all applicable codes **excluding** the External Cause codes.*

First-Listed Diagnosis: _____

Secondary Diagnoses: _____

2

The patient, a 22-year-old male, was brought to the emergency department (ED) by friends after being involved in a fight. The patient complains of severe jaw pain, and his face appears asymmetric with the left side of his face appearing out of alignment. The physician obtains x-rays of the man's facial bones and jaw and is advised by the radiologist that a dislocation of the left side of the mandible exists. One 3.0 cm laceration across the metacarpal area of the right hand required skin suturing, which was done in the ED. The patient is admitted to the hospital. The next morning the patient is taken to surgery for a closed reduction of the dislocation of the left mandible. The patient is discharged the next day with a follow-up appointment scheduled with the surgeon in 10 days.

*Note: List all applicable codes **excluding** the External Cause codes.*

Principal Diagnosis: _____

Secondary Diagnoses: _____

Principal Procedure: _____

Secondary Procedure(s): _____

3

A 42-year-old male was in a motor vehicle crash that involved the collision of his vehicle into the expressway median divider. He was brought to the emergency department complaining of leg and foot pain. X-rays showed a displaced left distal or lower femur fracture and a displaced fracture of the neck of the talus (tarsal) bone of the left foot. He was admitted to the hospital and taken to the operating room for an immediate open reduction with internal fixation for both fractures. He was discharged to receive home care and home physical therapy services.

*Note: List all applicable codes **excluding** the External Cause codes.*

Principal Diagnosis: _____

Secondary Diagnoses: _____

Principal Procedure: _____

Secondary Procedure(s): _____

4

The patient is a semiprofessional baseball player who is a pitcher. He is seen in the orthopedic sports medicine physician's office because of a painful right shoulder. The patient felt a pain in his right shoulder while pitching during a game within the past three days. After the game, he felt more severe muscular pain in the shoulder and was unable to use his arm. The physician suspects a severe injury to the biceps tendon and muscles of the shoulder. The patient consents to exploratory surgery and shoulder repair, if indicated. The patient is admitted to the hospital for the surgery. During the open procedure, the physician examines the superior labrum that attaches the biceps tendon to the bones of the shoulder. The physician finds the superior labrum is torn from front to back. An immediate repair or arthroplasty of the shoulder is done to repair the labrum or glenoid ligament and reattach it to the bones of the shoulder joint. The physician describes the injury as a SLAP, or superior glenoid labrum lesion. (This procedure is a repair of the shoulder glenoid ligament also known as the labrum.) The physician advises the patient-athlete that the injury is fairly common among athletes who use their upper extremities in strenuous activities. Physical therapy and athletic training will be the next plan of care for the patient so that he may return to playing baseball.

*Note: List all applicable codes **excluding** the External Cause codes.*

Principal Diagnosis: _____

Secondary Diagnoses: _____

Principal Procedure: _____

Secondary Procedure(s): _____

5

The patient is a 19-year-old male who is brought to the emergency department (ED) by fire department ambulance, which was called by neighbors to the scene of a street fight. Apparently, the patient was beaten by rival gang members. The patient was unconscious when found by the paramedics. The ED physician performs a comprehensive physical examination, and the patient is taken for an MRI of the brain. The patient regains consciousness within 40 minutes of arriving in the ED, less than an hour after being found by the paramedics. The MRI is negative for fractures or internal bleeding. The patient is admitted to the ICU for monitoring. The physician describes the injury as a closed head injury with loss of consciousness of less than one hour. The patient also has multiple lacerations on the face, including his right cheek, forehead, upper lip, and jaw. There are abrasions on both his hands as well as multiple contusions on the abdominal wall and both of the knees and lower legs. The skin lacerations are suture repaired in the ICU after the patient is stabilized. The patient is transferred out of the ICU within 48 hours with no signs of permanent neurologic injury. He is discharged home seven days after his injury occurred.

*Note: List all applicable codes **excluding** the External Cause codes.*

Principal Diagnosis: _____

Secondary Diagnoses: _____

Principal Procedure: _____

Secondary Procedure(s): _____

6

The patient is a 25-year-old male brought to the emergency department (ED) after being shot in the abdomen during a drive-by shooting. The patient was admitted to the hospital with the expectation he would be transferred to the surgical ICU after surgery. The trauma team assembled in the ED, and it was quickly determined the gunshot wound of the epigastric area of the abdomen was complicated by injury to the abdominal aorta, with the retained bullets in the peritoneal cavity. The trauma surgeons attempt to control the bleeding by performing a REBOA procedure. A REBOA is a technique to rescue patients rapidly bleeding to death from injuries to their chest, abdomen or pelvis. The procedure involves placing a flexible catheter rapidly into the femoral artery, advancing to the aorta and inflating a balloon at its tip. This stops blood flow beyond the balloon. This is a temporary procedure as a bridge to get the severely injured patient to the operating room or the angiographic intervention radiology suite for definitive treatment. For this patient, the REBOA procedure was performed in the trauma ER suite. Concurrent imaging suggested the patient had a complete transection of the abdominal aorta. The patient was taken to the operating room for exploration and treatment but suffered cardiac arrest and could not be resuscitated or subjected to surgery. The only procedure performed was the REBOA.

*Note: List all applicable codes **excluding** the External Cause codes.*

Principal Diagnosis: _____

Secondary Diagnoses: _____

Principal Procedure: _____

Secondary Procedure(s): _____

7

The patient is a 44-year-old female who works as a road construction flag holder. The patient was directing traffic on an expressway where road resurfacing was being performed. A truck came too close to the worker and its tires rolled over her left foot. The patient is brought to the nearest hospital's emergency department, where the physician on duty immediately examines the patient and x-rays are performed. The physician describes the patient's trauma as a crush injury of the foot with open fracture. The radiologist's impression documented on the radiology report describes the injury as open fracture of the first metatarsal of the foot. The orthopedic surgeon on call comes to the hospital, and the patient is admitted and taken to surgery for an open reduction and internal fixation of the first metatarsal bone with a fasciotomy. The patient remains in the hospital three days before being discharged to home health services follow-up care, with an appointment to see the orthopedic surgeon in seven days.

*Note: List all applicable codes **excluding** the External Cause codes.*

Principal Diagnosis: _____

Secondary Diagnoses: _____

Principal Procedure: _____

Secondary Procedure(s): _____

8

The patient is a 50-year-old male brought to the emergency department (ED) by fire department ambulance that was called to a restaurant in which the patient was eating dinner with friends. The patient was eating steak when he felt something stick in his chest. He could not dislodge it, and was becoming rather panicky because of the intense epigastric pain. He was still able to breathe unassisted and able to speak. The emergency department physician examines the patient and immediately calls the gastroenterologist for what the ED physician describes as "Steakhouse Syndrome." The patient is examined by the gastroenterologist who suspects the food is lodged in the patient's esophagus. The patient is taken immediately to the gastroenterology procedure suite, and an upper GI endoscopy is performed. The physician finds several large pieces of poorly chewed meat at the level of the lower esophagogastric junction. The physician is able to remove some of the obstruction, but smaller pieces of meat had already passed into the stomach. The physician also documents that reflux esophagitis is present. The physician is able to examine the upper GI tract, including the stomach, and no injury to the mucosa is found. Prior to the procedure, the patient was admitted to the hospital for overnight monitoring and discharged the next morning.

*Note: List all applicable codes **excluding** the External Cause codes.*

Principal Diagnosis: _____

Secondary Diagnoses: _____

Principal Procedure: _____

Secondary Procedure(s): _____

9

The patient is a 15-year-old female who is brought to the emergency department by ambulance from a motor vehicle crash where she was thrown from the vehicle. After a complete history and physical examination, multiple radiologic studies are obtained. The trauma physician determines the patient has an unstable burst fracture of the L2 and L3 vertebrae, but there is no evidence of spinal cord injury. With the parents' consent, the patient is admitted and taken to surgery for repair of her injury. The physician performs an open reduction of the L2-L3 fracture. He also performs a posterior spinal fusion of L2-L3 with an interbody fusion device by posterior approach into anterior column. The procedure also includes L2-L3 interspinous process wiring. Bone is harvested from the right posterior iliac crest for bone grafting. The primary closure includes an L1-L2 laminotomy. The patient tolerates the surgical procedure and is taken to the surgical ICU. Fifteen days later, the patient is transferred to an acute rehabilitation facility for ongoing therapy and recovery.

*Note: List all applicable codes **excluding** the External Cause codes.*

Principal Diagnosis: _____

Secondary Diagnoses: _____

Principal Procedure: _____

Secondary Procedure(s): _____

10

The patient is a 40-year-old male brought to the emergency department (ED) by fire department ambulance after falling off a ladder at home while doing home repairs. Apparently, in an attempt to catch himself, his left hand and wrist broke a window, and he was cut severely by the broken glass. The ED physician examines the patient and orders x-rays of the fingers, hand, and wrist. No fractures are seen. Based on the physical examination, the physician concludes that there is a major injury to the ulnar nerve and also an injury to the tendon in addition to the laceration of the left wrist. The physician repairs the wrist laceration loosely and makes arrangements for the patient to be transferred to another hospital in the city where a hand surgeon waits to examine him and possibly take him to surgery for definitive repair. The patient is transferred by private ambulance to the nearby hospital.

*Note: List all applicable codes **excluding** the External Cause codes.*

First-Listed Diagnosis: _____

Secondary Diagnoses: _____

11

The patient is a 20-year-old male who sustained a drunken fall through a plate-glass window and was cut by the broken glass. He was brought to the Level I trauma emergency department at a local hospital. On examination the patient had a large penetrating wound to the right thoracoabdominal region. The patient had no memory of the event and could not describe how it happened. According to friends, he had been told to leave the bar. They saw him leave alone and agreed he was "drunk." The fall through the glass window of a store occurred about a half a block down on the same street. The patient was hemodynamically stable in the ER, but the CT scan revealed several retained objects in the right upper quadrant that had violated the liver, as well as possible violation of the right kidney. The patient was admitted and taken by the trauma surgeons to the operating room for an exploratory laparotomy. The injuries found during the procedure were a major laceration through and through of the liver, a laceration of the jejunum, and a hematoma of the right kidney. Exploratory laparotomy was performed with repair of the liver laceration, repair of the jejunum laceration, examination of the right kidney, and removal of three fragments of leaded glass from the abdominal wall and fascia. Examination of the colon revealed no injuries. A #10 JP drain was placed into the abdomen at the operative site for postoperative drainage. The fascia, subcutaneous tissue, and skin edges were closed with sutures and staples. The patient was taken to the recovery area in stable condition. In addition to the injuries described with the operative findings, the patient was treated for acute alcoholic poisoning and multiple small skin lacerations (that did not need repair) of the right shoulder and right lower leg. After an extended hospital stay that included physical therapy, antibiotic and postoperative treatment, wound care management, and substance abuse preventative counseling, the patient was discharged home.

*Note: List all applicable codes **excluding** the External Cause codes.*

Principal Diagnosis: _____

Secondary Diagnoses: _____

Principal Procedure: _____

Secondary Procedure(s): _____

12

Fire department ambulance and paramedics brought a 14-year-old male to the Level I trauma emergency department after he was shot in the head by a drive-by shooter while standing with some friends on a neighbor's porch. The entrance was into the right posterior parietal area of the skull, and the bullet was lodged in the occipital area. The inlet gunshot wound was hemorrhaging. The injury traumatized a major portion of the brain. When the patient arrived at the hospital, he was deeply comatose with cerebrate rigidity. His pupils were fixed and dilated with severe respiratory compromise. He was intubated and placed on a ventilator and admitted to the pediatric ICU. After discussing his condition with his parents, consent was obtained and the patient was taken to surgery, even though everyone understood the patient was in extremely critical condition. The following procedures were performed: decompressive craniotomy of the right parietal bone, duraplasty, and insertion of an intracranial pressure (ICP) monitor. The objectives of the procedure were to drain blood from beneath the skull bone and to repair the dura. Massive injuries to the brain were found as a result of the gunshot wound: comminuted skull fractures of the parietal bone, cerebral contusion, subdural hemorrhaging, diffuse cerebral edema, and herniation of the brainstem. The patient never regained consciousness. It became evident the patient could not recover from these injuries, and the family consented to organ donation of his lungs, liver, kidneys, skin, and other tissue. The family did not consent to donating his heart. A flexible fiberoptic bronchoscopy was performed to examine the lung to determine the suitability for donation, and no injury or inflammation was found. The patient was pronounced dead approximately 50 hours after the original injury.

*Note: List all applicable codes **excluding** the External Cause codes. Do not code the surgeries required for the organ donations.*

Principal Diagnosis: _____

Secondary Diagnoses: _____

Principal Procedure: _____

Secondary Procedure(s): _____

13

The patient is a 21-year-old male who was found by a passing police vehicle sitting on the side of a city street with a bleeding face and dazed appearance. A fire department ambulance brought the patient to the emergency department. The patient claimed to have no memory of what happened or chose not to tell the healthcare providers the circumstances that caused his injury. He did remember being on the street, walking home from a friend's house. Alcohol and drug screens were negative, but the patient was extremely quiet and sleepy. He did not complain of the amount of pain the physicians would have expected in a patient with the injuries found, which were bilateral mandibular angle fractures, laceration of the skin of the jaw, and a fractured tooth. The patient was admitted and taken to surgery the following morning and administered IV antibiotics to prevent infection. The procedures performed were an open reduction and internal fixation of the mandibular fractures, a repair of the jaw laceration, and forceps extraction of one fractured tooth of the lower jaw. The patient had no complications during or after the procedure. The preoperative urinalysis and subsequent urine culture showed a urinary tract infection, which was treated. X-rays of his skull and neck showed no fractures or injuries.

The patient also had abrasions on the right hand that were cleaned and bandaged. At the time of discharge, the patient still claimed to have no memory of what happened to him but otherwise appeared to be alert, cooperative, and thinking clearly. City police interviewed the patient during the hospital stay to investigate a possible crime but were unable to gain any information and found no witnesses to the event. He was discharged to the care of his older sister, with whom he lives, and follow-up appointments were given, primarily for care of his fractured mandible.

*Note: List all applicable codes **excluding** the External Cause codes.*

Principal Diagnosis: _____

Secondary Diagnoses: _____

Principal Procedure: _____

Secondary Procedure(s): _____

14

The patient is a 30-year-old male brought to the emergency department by his mother after being injured in an argument with a male neighbor two days ago. The patient fell down his front steps at this home trying to grab the neighbor, who had come to the patient's home complaining of loud music. The patient complained of pain and significant swelling of his right leg, near his knee, which had been replaced two years ago. Neither the patient nor the mother could tell the physician the reason for the knee replacement other than it "collapsed" and had to be replaced. The patient also has had hemophilia A disease since birth and was diagnosed as HIV positive 10 years ago. He is asymptomatic related to his HIV status and has had no infections or consequences of it. X-ray of the leg showed a right tibia fracture at the upper or proximal end. Because of his hemophilia, the fact the patient had a replaced joint near the site of the fracture, and the potential complications of an open reduction type treatment, the patient was admitted to the hospital. The leg was splinted and elevated for 48 hours until the swelling was under control. He was taken to the operating room on day 3, and a closed reduction, closely monitored under imaging, was performed, and an excellent reduction was achieved. A cast was applied. He complained of severe pain from the time of admission, and this was managed fairly well with injectable and oral analgesic medications. He was also administered intravenously via a peripheral vein a total of 3,000 units of Factor VIII on a daily basis for the hemophilia status. The patient and his mother were instructed that the patient was to use the wheelchair they had at home to get around and not to put any weight on the right leg. Home healthcare services were ordered, and a medical vehicle was arranged to take the patient home and get him into the house. A follow-up appointment with his orthopedic surgeon for fracture care was given to the patient, and he was encouraged to contact his hematologist at University Hospital as soon as possible. Copies of the patient's record were given to him.

*Note: List all applicable codes **excluding** the External Cause codes.*

Principal Diagnosis: _____

Secondary Diagnoses: _____

Principal Procedure: _____

Secondary Procedure(s): _____

15

The patient is an 80-year-old female who fell out of bed and injured her left ankle. Examination in the emergency department revealed pain, swelling, and deformity around the left ankle. The patient denied any other pain or injury. She was admitted to the orthopedic floor and seen promptly by an orthopedic surgeon and her attending physician. X-rays were taken that showed a trimalleolar fracture of the left ankle with displacement. The patient had a significant past medical history with a previous cerebral infarction last year in this right-handed woman. The left hemiplegia was due to an old cerebral infarction of the distribution of the right middle cerebral artery. She had vigorous physical therapy following this and had been doing well with ambulation and self care since that time. She also has type 2 diabetes of long standing and ischemic heart disease that continues under treatment. While she was in the hospital, she continued to receive her oral diabetic medication. An EKG showed inferior lateral ischemia that was not a new finding. The day after admission, the orthopedic surgeon performed a closed reduction and casting of the left tibia. X-rays taken following the reduction revealed alignment to be in good position. The patient tolerated the procedure well and had no intra- or postoperative complications. A slight urinary tract infection was noted, and an antibiotic was prescribed. The patient was discharged home with home health services ordered.

*Note: List all applicable codes **excluding** the External Cause codes.*

Principal Diagnosis: _____

Secondary Diagnoses: _____

Principal Procedure: _____

Secondary Procedure(s): _____

16

HISTORY: The patient is an 11-year-old male who was riding his bicycle in front of his home, hit a bump in the pavement, and fell off his bicycle. Because of severe wrist pain, he was taken to the emergency department, where x-rays confirmed displaced right distal radius Salter-Harris type I fracture and right distal Salter-Harris type I ulna fracture. The patient was seen by an orthopedic surgeon, who advised admission and a closed reduction of the fractures that was agreed to by the patient and his parents.

OPERATIVE FINDINGS: The right wrist has a deformity with some expected level of swelling. His fingers are moving, and he is neurovascularly intact. The skin is intact. Contra-lateral wrist is nontender. Fingertips are pink with good capillary refill. Lower extremities are nontender. X-ray films have been reviewed, which reveal fractures of both the distal radius and distal ulna with 100 percent displacement.

DESCRIPTION OF PROCEDURE: The patient was taken to the operating room and placed supine on the table with all of his extremities adequately padded. The patient was administered laryngeal mask anesthesia. A closed reduction was performed. The fractures were found to reduce. Fluoroscopy was used to view the fractures in multiplanar views. Given the nature of the fracture pattern, it was deemed appropriate to pin the radius to increase stability. Two K-wires were then placed percutaneously under direct fluoroscopic guidance across the fracture site. The growth plate was avoided. The fracture and pins were then visualized in multiplanar fluoroscopy, and the fracture and pins were noted to be in good position. The pins were bent and cut. Final films were obtained. Sterile dressings followed by a sugar tong type of splint were then applied. The patient tolerated the procedure well, was awakened in the operating room, and was taken to recovery. There were no complications of this procedure.

*Note: List all applicable codes **excluding** the External Cause codes.*

Principal Diagnosis: _____

Secondary Diagnoses: _____

Principal Procedure: _____

Secondary Procedure(s): _____

17

HISTORY: The patient is a 79-year-old retired female from Iowa, in general good health, brought to the emergency department (ED) with the complaint of acute pain in her right hip. The patient is on a bus trip vacation with a senior citizen's group, with the destination Nashville, Tennessee and the Grand Ole Opry. After the group stopped at a restaurant en route, she fell off a curb in the parking lot while walking back to the bus. She was able to be helped up and got back on the bus and rode on to their hotel in Nashville. Someone got a wheelchair from the hotel, and she was able to be pushed around, including to the show at the Opry's Ryman Auditorium. After the show, she told her companion that she thought she should go to the emergency department because the hip was hurting more than earlier in the day. Radiographs in the ED revealed a subcapital impacted right hip or upper femur fracture. Emergent orthopedic consultation was obtained, and the patient was admitted. The patient's physician in Iowa was contacted, and he provided her medical history including the type of medication she received for her essential hypertension, which was her only medical problem. She continued to receive her Lisinopril for blood pressure control while admitted. The day after admission, the patient was taken to the operating room, where the fracture was noted to be already well reduced. A 3-pin fixation utilizing cannulated screws to the right hip was performed without difficulty. A day after surgery, physical therapy was started and by discharge on day 3, the patient was able to ambulate with a walker. Her son and daughter came to Nashville with a rented motor home to transport the patient back to Iowa. Access to the patient's electronic health record was provided to her physician in Iowa for continuation of care.

DESCRIPTION OF PROCEDURE: The patient was taken to the operating room, placed in the supine position on the fracture table for an open internal fixation. Once adequate anesthesia was obtained, the right hip girdle was sterilely prepped and draped. The hip was well-aligned, and no traction was required. Image intensification was brought into appropriate position, and the AP and lateral projections were obtained. This showed the fracture to be well reduced on its own. A 3-cm incision was then made just distal to the greater trochanter and carried down to the level of the subcutaneous tissues. Small bleeders were cauterized along the way. Great care was taken to ensure no harm came to any significant neurovascular structures. The iliotibial band was identified, incised in line with its fibers, and gently retracted. Access was gained to the lateral femoral cortex. A guide pin was placed without difficulty into the femoral head and neck. AP and lateral projections revealed adequate guide pin placement. Then an appropriately sized 16-mm thread 7.0 cannulated screw was placed over the guide pin. Image intensification revealed adequate screw placement. Two additional screws were then passed in a parallel fashion into the inferior and posterior portion of the femoral head and neck. Once the 3-pin fixation was completed, AP and lateral projections revealed adequate fracture stabilization and hardware placement. The wound was irrigated with copious amounts of normal saline solution. The iliotibial band was reapproximated with 0-Vicryl suture in an interrupted fashion. Subcutaneous tissues were closed with 2-0 Vicryl sutures, the skin was closed with clips, and a sterile dressing was applied. The patient was taken to the recovery room by the anesthesiologist and nursing staff in stable condition.

*Note: List all applicable codes **excluding** the External Cause codes.*

Principal Diagnosis: _____

Secondary Diagnoses: _____

Principal Procedure: _____

Secondary Procedure(s):   _____

18

The patient is a 50-year-old female who was previously treated by closed reduction and external fixation of a fracture of her right tibia, distal medial malleolus, which she suffered as the result of a fall downstairs. During follow-up care, it becomes evident the fracture is not healing. X-rays demonstrate a nonunion of the distal tibia. The patient is admitted for surgical repair of the nonunion. The surgery performed is an open reduction of the tibia with bone grafting. Bone for the grafting is harvested from the patient's left iliac crest. The distal medial malleolus tibial bone, at the site of the non-union, is osteotomized and repositioned. The harvested bone graft is packed into the fracture site to replace the missing bone, and three screws are inserted to secure the area. The patient is discharged the day after surgery for recovery at home.

*Note: List all applicable codes **excluding** the External Cause codes.*

Principal Diagnosis: _____

Secondary Diagnoses: _____

Principal Procedure: _____

Secondary Procedure(s):   _____

19

The patient fell out of a chair at the nursing home and was previously treated by closed reduction with external fixation for a fracture on the surgical neck of the right humerus. There was a malunion of the fracture in the 80-year-old female patient, and she was admitted for an open reduction of the humerus with bone grafting. During the surgical procedure, the orthopedic surgeon harvested bone from the patient's left iliac crest. The humeral fracture site was opened and the area of malunion was osteotomized, cleaned, and repositioned. Internal fixation was accomplished with screws and the harvested bone was packed into the fracture site at the humeral head to replace the missing bone segment. The patient recovered from the procedure uneventfully and was discharged on the second hospital day. Other chronic conditions treated in the hospital were arteriosclerotic heart disease, chronic renal insufficiency, and type 2 diabetes mellitus on oral anti-diabetic medication. The patient was given an appointment to see the orthopedic surgeon in his office in five days and was going to be followed by home health nurses for post-operative care.

*Note: List all applicable codes **excluding** the External Cause codes.*

Principal Diagnosis: _____

Secondary Diagnoses: _____

Principal Procedure: _____

Secondary Procedure(s): _____

20

The patient is a 40-year-old chef at a local restaurant who was burned while at work two weeks ago and was treated by a trauma physician in the emergency department of the hospital. Today she is being seen by the same trauma physician in the trauma clinic as an outpatient to examine the healing of the burns she sustained on her right hand and wrist, right forearm, and right side of the neck. The burn dressings were removed and the burn sites were examined for evidence of healing and lack of infection. No debridement was required. Medicated ointments were applied to the burn areas and new burn dressings were applied to the three sites. The final diagnoses were documented by the physician for this follow up visit:

1. First- and second-degree burns, multiple sites on right hand and wrist, normal healing

2. First- and second-degree burns, neck, normal healing

3. First-degree burns, right forearm, normal healing

*Note #1: List all applicable codes **excluding** the External Cause codes.*

Note #2: Assign the ICD-10-PCS procedure codes for the dressing change for practice purposes as this procedure could occur in the inpatient setting. The ICD-10-PCS procedure codes are not required to be reported for outpatient visits.

First-Listed Diagnosis: _____

Secondary Diagnoses: _____

First-Listed Procedure: _____

Secondary Procedure(s): _____

Chapter 19B

Poisoning by, Adverse Effects, Underdosing, Toxic Effects of Substances, Other Effects of External Causes, Certain Early Complications of Trauma and Complications of Surgical and Medical Care

Coding Scenarios for *Basic ICD-10-CM and ICD-10-PCS Coding Exercises*

The following case studies are organized following the sequence of the chapters in the ICD-10-CM Tabular List of Diseases and Injuries as published on the Centers for Disease Control and Prevention National Center for Health Statistics website (http://www.cdc.gov /nchs/icd/icd10cm.htm). The objective of this book is to provide the student with more detailed clinical information to code, rather than one- or two-line diagnosis and procedure statements.

ICD-10-CM diagnosis codes are to be assigned to both the inpatient hospital admission and the outpatient visit case studies. In this book, the ICD-10-PCS procedure codes are to be assigned only to the inpatient hospital admission cases. In actual practice, outpatient cases are assigned CPT/HCPCS codes. The ICD-10-PCS codes are only required for inpatient procedures. In the answer key for the exercises, the Alphabetic Index entry is listed after the code to indicate the main terms and subterms used to locate the code that must be verified in the ICD-10-CM Tabular List or in the ICD-10-PCS Code Tables prior to assigning the code.

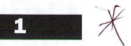

1

A 25-year-old female was found unresponsive in her apartment by her roommate and brought to the hospital by fire department ambulance paramedics. She had recently been treated for depression, and her roommate found the patient's prescription bottle of antidepressant medication empty. The patient's other prescription bottle of lorazepam was also empty. The emergency department (ED) staff talked to the patient's psychiatrist and confirmed these medications had been prescribed for depression. An empty bottle of vodka was found in the bedroom near the patient's body. The ED examination and toxicology studies confirm a drug overdose of these two medications and alcohol. Another friend received a suicide text message from the patient the same afternoon. While the patient was receiving treatment in the ED, she suffered a cardiopulmonary arrest and died. Physician documented poisoning in a suicide attempt with antidepressant, lorazepam, and vodka.

First-Listed Diagnosis: _____

Secondary Diagnosis: _____

2

A patient with congestive heart failure and six weeks status post-acute MI had been prescribed and was correctly taking Lanoxin (digoxin). She began to experience nausea and vomiting with extreme fatigue. She was admitted to the hospital. Blood drug levels are taken and it is determined the patient is experiencing a side effect of the medication. A different medication is prescribed for her heart disease to avoid these symptoms. The patient's cardiac conditions are evaluated and found to be stable.

Principal Diagnosis: _____

Secondary Diagnosis: _____

Principal Procedure: _____

Secondary Procedure(s): _____

3

The patient had surgery one week previously for acute appendicitis with a peritoneal abscess. She is admitted now for fever, pain, and redness at the operative site. There is evidence of cellulitis of the operative wound, and cultures of the abdominal wall wound drainage confirm *Staphylococcus aureus*, methicillin resistant, as the cause. She receives intravenous antibiotics for the infection and also receives oral antidiabetic medication for type 2 diabetes mellitus. The physician's diagnoses on discharge were: post-operative wound infection at the incisional surgical site, superficial, with MRSA (methicillin resistant staphylococcus aureus); type 2 diabetes.

Principal Diagnosis: _____

Secondary Diagnosis: _____

Principal Procedure: _____

Secondary Procedure(s): _____

4

An 80-year-old male was brought to the emergency department (ED) by his family with the chief complaint of "nose bleed." The patient is taking Coumadin under prescription by his internist for chronic atrial fibrillation. The patient is also known to have congestive heart failure. The patient said his nose began bleeding about two hours ago and he was unable to stop the bleeding with other methods he had used in the past. He reported that he had these nose bleeds before today. However, today the bleeding is more pronounced and could not be stopped at home. In the ED, the physician is able to control the bleeding somewhat but recognized that an ENT physician should be called in for consultation. The patient's laboratory work revealed anemia and an EKG showed the existing atrial fibrillation. Because of his various conditions, his internist admitted him to the hospital. He was seen by the ENT physician, who was able to stop the bleeding with an anterior and posterior packing. The packing was removed on day 2, and the epistaxis had stopped. Repeated laboratory work confirmed the physician's diagnosis of "chronic blood loss anemia." The patient continued to receive medications for the chronic atrial fibrillation and congestive heart failure, and new medications were started to treat the anemia. The patient's Coumadin was continued, but the dosage was lowered. In the physician's discharge progress note, he wrote "Epistaxis due to Coumadin therapy with resulting chronic blood loss anemia in a patient with chronic atrial fibrillation and congestive heart failure."

Principal Diagnosis: _____

Secondary Diagnosis: _____

Principal Procedure: _____

Secondary Procedure(s): _____

5

A 12-year-old female is brought to the primary care physician's office by her mother. The mother states that she had taken the child to the urgent care center five days previously because the child had acute otitis media. The urgent care physician had prescribed azithromycin. The child's condition did not improve, and, in fact, she developed red spots and itchiness on her arms and chest. The primary care physician examines the patient and concludes that the child has an allergy to the medication. The acute otitis media is still present as the medication seemed to have no effect on the infection. The physician tells the mother to discontinue the azithromycin medication and a new prescription is given. On the encounter form the physician writes "pruritus due to drug allergy to azithromycin and acute otitis media."

First-Listed Diagnosis: _____

Secondary Diagnosis: _____

6

The patient, a 35-year-old male, is brought to the emergency department (ED) by friends who report that the patient has chest pain. Upon questioning, the patient admitted to being a cocaine addict and to having used cocaine several times over the past 24 hours. The patient stated "maybe I overdosed," as he experienced chest pain on a previous occasion when he used more cocaine than he normally used. The patient is placed on telemetry in the ED and is later admitted to a telemetry bed on a nursing unit. Further cardiovascular testing finds no evidence of an acute myocardial infarction or respiratory disease. However, it is determined that the patient has hypertension that had never been treated. The physician determines that this event is a cocaine overdose that occurred with the consequence of chest pain. The patient is also treated for hypertension and is strongly advised to continue the antihypertensive medications and to seek help to overcome the cocaine addiction, as the two conditions have serious consequences on his long-term health. A referral is given to the local community mental health center, which offers a drug counseling service. The patient agrees and is discharged accompanied by his brother.

Principal Diagnosis: _____

Secondary Diagnosis: _____

Principal Procedure: _____

Secondary Procedure(s): _____

7

The patient is a 67-year-old male who comes to his cardiologist's office with complaints of pain and warmth around the pacemaker generator pocket in his left upper chest wall. The physician examines the patient and determines the patient has cellulitis of the chest wall due to an infected pacemaker pocket and needs to have the pacemaker generator moved to a different location of the chest wall to allow the infected pocket to heal. The patient has a history of a MRSA infection being treated in the past. The type of infection that appears present at this time will be investigated to check for a recurrence. The physician makes arrangements for the patient to have outpatient surgery the next day.

First-Listed Diagnosis: _____

Secondary Diagnosis: _____

8

The family practice physician examines a 56-year-old male established patient who comes to the office with his wife. The patient states that he has felt dizzy and lightheaded over the past three days. The patient is on medications for hypertension and states he has been taking all as prescribed. The physician and the physician's nurse take the patient's blood pressure and find it to be 100/70 mm Hg, which is much lower than the patient's pressure as normally recorded. The patient had been taking antihypertensive medications of irbesartan (Avapro) and metoprolol (Toprol) with a low-dose diuretic. The physician is unable to determine which medication was the cause but is certain the patient's symptoms of vertigo and light-headedness are more likely the side effects of the Avapro or the antihypertensive medications. New prescriptions are issued for adjusted dosages of the medications, and the patient is advised to go to the emergency department and call this physician if the symptoms get worse over the next 24 hours.

First-Listed Diagnosis: _____

Secondary Diagnosis Code: _____

9

The patient is a 25-year-old female who was prescribed ciprofloxacin by her family physician for an *E. coli* urinary tract infection and advised to take one 250-mg tablet every 12 hours for 10 days. Because she was leaving on a vacation trip on Saturday, the patient doubled up the dosages and for the past three days had taken two 250-mg tablets every 12 hours. During the past 24 hours, the patient had diarrhea severe enough for her to come to the emergency department (ED). A urinalysis shows bacteria still present to support the diagnosis of UTI. The physician recognizes these symptoms as not only side effects of the medication but, in this patient's situation, an accidental overdose of ciprofloxacin, as she had not followed the physician's directions in the amount of the medication she was to take. The ED physician advises her to continue taking the medication as prescribed without alterations.

First-Listed Diagnosis: _____

Secondary Diagnosis: _____

10

The patient had surgery two weeks previously for insertion of a central venous vascular catheter for infusion to treat colon carcinoma. The patient is admitted to the hospital extremely ill with the admitting diagnosis of "sepsis." The patient's signs and symptoms include elevated temperature, rapid heart rate and respirations, and elevated white blood cell count. After study, the physician determines that the patient has sepsis due to the peripherally inserted central catheter (PICC) that apparently is the source of the infection. The physician and consultants further describe the patient's condition as systemic inflammatory response syndrome, or sepsis, in a patient with an infection. Blood cultures show evidence of methicillin susceptible staphylococcal aureus (MSSA) organisms as the cause of the sepsis. Intravenous antibiotic medications and other therapy are administered for the infection and the carcinoma. The PICC line is removed at bedside by the infusion center nurse who had been monitoring the infusion site. The patient recovers and is discharged home in 10 days to be followed in the oncology clinic in 1 week.

Principal Diagnosis: _____

Secondary Diagnosis: _____

Principal Procedure: _____

Secondary Procedure(s): _____

11

The patient is an 80-year-old male with multiple medical problems: Parkinson's disease, glaucoma, total blindness in the right eye (category 4) and low vision in the left eye (category 1), old MI six months ago, recent abnormal cardiac stress test, status post right total knee replacement, and primary generalized osteoarthrosis. On this occasion he is admitted to the hospital for a planned revision of his right total knee arthroplasty. The patient has been evaluated by cardiology and cleared for surgery. He had been seen by the orthopedic surgeon several weeks ago and scheduled for this revision arthroplasty. About 10 to 12 years ago the patient had a total knee replacement on the right side for osteoarthritis. He developed increasing pain in his knee, and the orthopedic evaluation found aseptic loosening of the tibial surface or component of his knee. The patient was taken to surgery on the day of admission and had a revision right knee arthroplasty of the tibial surface. The surgeon found femoral and patellar surface components of the previous knee replacement to be stable and in good working order. The tibial surface component was found to be grossly loose and was able to be removed with little effort. The tibial tray had divided completely from the cement mantle. The orthopedic surgeon proceeded to replace it with a new tibial surface component only using cement. The patient recovered well from surgery without complications and was transferred to a skilled unit facility for rehabilitation and to increase his ability to perform activities of daily living independently. All of his medical conditions were monitored and treated while he was in the hospital for this surgery.

Principal Diagnosis: _____

Secondary Diagnosis: _____

Principal Procedure: _____

Secondary Procedure(s): _____

12

One year ago, this 40-year-old female received a left kidney transplant from an unrelated donor to treat her end-stage renal disease. The physicians were notified by the transplant network that the donor was diagnosed with low grade lymphoma, and the transplant patient was tested for any evidence of the lymphoma in the donated kidney. Unfortunately, the transplanted kidney was proven by a previously performed biopsy to have non-Hodgkin's lymphoma. The patient was admitted to the hospital. A nephrectomy was performed to remove the transplanted kidney. The patient received one four-hour session of hemodialysis for the end-stage kidney disease still present. The patient had an uneventful recovery and was discharged home with home health services and to continue to receive hemodialysis as an outpatient at the dialysis center.

Principal Diagnosis: _____

Secondary Diagnosis: _____

Principal Diagnosis: _____

Secondary Procedure(s): _____

13

The patient is a 24-year-old male who received an orthotopic liver transplant two months ago to treat his primary biliary cirrhosis. The patient was admitted at this time after a transplant clinic visit on the same day because of a generalized macular rash on his chest. The patient also complained of diarrhea and an enlarging abdomen that the physicians identified as ascites. A skin biopsy of the chest was performed and revealed a significant number of donor lymphocytes due to acute graft-versus-host (GVH) disease. The physicians informed the patient that his acute GVH disease is a complication of his liver transplant but can be treated with medications such as corticosteroids, immunosuppressants, antibiotics, and immunoglobulins. The patient remained in the hospital for five days and started on a medication regimen with relief of his diarrhea and lessening of the symptoms of the ascites and the rash. The patient was discharged home with home health services and an appointment with the transplant clinic in two weeks.

Principal Diagnosis: _____

Secondary Diagnosis: _____

Principal Procedure: _____

Secondary Procedure(s): _____

14

The patient is a 7-year-old male who was brought to the emergency department (ED) by his mother because of a suspected allergic reaction. The patient was experiencing wheezing, urticaria, and itching and tingling on his lips and in his mouth. The patient was at a party at school and ate cookies that contained small bits of peanuts, unknown to him at the time. The mother states he has a known allergy to peanuts and has had reactions in the past when exposed to peanuts, even without eating them. The physician described the patient's condition as a relatively mild anaphylactic reaction to food (peanuts), and the patient received an injection of epinephrine. He was observed in the ED for another three hours and had a complete resolution of his symptoms.

First-Listed Diagnosis: _____

Secondary Diagnosis: _____

15

A 30-year-old male was brought to the emergency department (ED) by a fire department ambulance that was called by police to a building where suspected drug sales and use were occurring. The patient was found minimally unresponsive on the floor in the apartment where other individuals were arrested for solicitation and illegal possession of narcotics, including cocaine and heroin. The patient was later identified by his sister, who stated that he is a chronic heroin addict. Upon arrival to the ED, the patient was found to be combative and in acute respiratory failure. He required immediate intubation and was placed on continuous mechanical ventilation and admitted to ICU. The drug toxicology screening test later returned the finding of a high level of heroin that coincided with the patient's heroin dependence with intoxication and delirium on admission. The patient's respiratory function continued to worsen. He developed acute renal failure and became unresponsive to treatment. The patient expired within 72 hours of admission.

Principal Diagnosis: _____

Secondary Diagnosis: _____

Principal Procedure: _____

Secondary Procedure(s): _____

16

The patient is a 60-year-old female who came to the emergency department with a variety of complaints, including diarrhea, swelling of her face, weakness, and fatigue. Given the variety of her complaints and her extensive medical history, the patient was admitted to the hospital. The emergency department physician was most concerned with her facial swelling and documented it as the admitting diagnosis.

The patient is known to have multiple primary and secondary malignancies for which she is currently receiving outpatient chemotherapy and radiation therapy. She has primary carcinoma of the right kidney with metastasis to the intra-abdominal lymph nodes, primary non-small-cell carcinoma of the lung, left upper lobe, with metastasis to the anterior mediastinum, and a past history of carcinoma of the anal canal, which was cured surgically. She is also under treatment for hyperthyroidism. She has had diarrhea for two days and was found to be severely dehydrated. She has been at home receiving antibiotic therapy through a peripherally inserted central catheter (PICC), placed prior to this admission, for a staph aureus septicemia infection from an implanted chemotherapy port that was removed. The antibiotic treatment via the PICC was continued this admission. She has significant swelling of her face and neck. Upon further investigation, it was thought that she had angioneurotic edema as a result of an allergic reaction, possibly to one or more of the medications she was taking or possibly as a result of a food allergy. The patient also presented with cellulitis of the face. She received her ongoing antibiotic therapy for the septicemia, additional antibiotic therapy for the facial cellulitis, which did not involve the orbits themselves, intravenous therapy for her dehydration, and medications for the diarrhea and hyperthyroidism. She was seen by oncology to assess the progression of her renal and pulmonary malignancies and metastases. The oncologist requested a consultation with a urologist to evaluate the patient for any ureteral malignancy or obstruction. The urologist performed a cystoscopy with a diagnostic biopsy of the right ureter. No obstruction was found and the biopsy found benign tissue from the ureter. The patient was relieved of most of her distressing symptoms and allowed to go home to continue receiving antibiotic therapy through her PICC. She was discharged with home healthcare services.

There were three final diagnoses that appeared to meet the definition of principal diagnosis: angioneurotic edema, cellulitis of the face, and dehydration. The attending physician was queried to determine the principal diagnosis and together with the coder decided the main circumstance of the admission and most extensive therapy was directed at diagnosing and treating the angioneurotic edema.

Principal Diagnosis: _____

Secondary Diagnosis: _____

Principal Procedure: _____

Secondary Procedure(s): _____

17

The patient is a 53-year-old male with end-stage renal disease and chronic glomerulonephritis. He has been dialyzed through an arteriovenous (AV) fistula (radial artery to cephalic vein) in his left arm for two years, most recently two days ago. His end-stage renal disease is the result of his long-standing hypertension. When he went for his dialysis treatment this morning, it was noted that the access was clotted, and he was taken to an emergency department for direct admission for inpatient care. Because of his urgent need for dialysis, a central venous (Quinton) catheter was placed percutaneously in the left internal jugular vein, and four hours of dialysis was accomplished on the day of admission. He was placed on antibiotics and taken to surgery on day two for an open thrombectomy of the right AV fistula. The clot was located in the cephalic vein. The AV fistula did not have to be revised. The patient had no complications from the procedure or during his six-day hospital stay. The Quinton catheter that was used for his dialysis access while in the hospital was left in place for the physician at the renal dialysis center to evaluate at his next dialysis appointment in order to determine whether it can be removed, and when the AV fistula will be available for access for dialysis. His discharge diagnoses were written by the physician as (1) end-stage renal disease, (2) chronic glomerulonephritis, (3) hypertension, (4) clotted obstructive AV fistula. The procedures performed were dialysis, insertion of the left internal jugular vein catheter, and arteriotomy of the right AV fistula with thrombectomy.

Principal Diagnosis: _____

Secondary Diagnosis _____

Principal Procedure: _____

Secondary Procedure(s): _____

18

The patient is a 22-year-old female who returns to her primary care physician's office complaining that the acute cystitis she was diagnosed with two weeks ago has not improved. During the first visit the patient described her symptoms as painful, burning, frequent urination. A urinalysis performed at the first visit revealed the presence of white cells, blood, and bacteria. The primary care physician had prescribed a ten-day dose of ciprofloxacin 250 mg. Upon questioning, the patient admitted that she took the drug as prescribed for five days and felt better. On the sixth day she left on a cruise vacation and decided to leave her medications at home because she thought she could not drink alcohol with the medication and she knew she was going to drink alcohol on vacation. During her seven-day cruise her symptoms returned and she made an appointment with the physician when she got home. The primary care physician advised the patient that her acute cystitis was not properly treated without taking the full ten-day supply of the medications. The patient was again given a ten-day dose of ciprofloxacin and strongly encouraged to take all the medications as prescribed. The conditions documented by the physicians for this office visit was acute cystitis with medication noncompliance in a patient who intentionally discontinued the ciprofloxacin as originally prescribed.

First-Listed Diagnosis: _____

Secondary Diagnosis: _____

Chapter 20

External Causes of Morbidity

Coding Scenarios for *Basic ICD-10-CM and ICD-10-PCS Coding*

Note: Assign only External Cause of Morbidity codes (V01–Y99) for the following scenarios.

Reminders from the ICD-10-CM guidelines for external cause codes:

- An external cause code may be used with any code in the range of A00.0–T88.9, Z00–Z99, classification that is a health condition due to an external cause. Though they are most applicable to injuries, they are also valid for use with such things as infections or diseases due to an external cause, and other health conditions, such as a heart attack that occurs during strenuous physical activity.

- Assign the external cause code with the appropriate 7th character (initial encounter, subsequent encounter, or sequela) for each encounter for which the injury or condition is being treated.

- An external cause code can never be a principal or first-listed diagnosis.

- No external cause code from chapter 20 is needed if the external cause and intent are included in a code from another chapter, for example, poisoning codes.

- When applicable, place of occurrence, activity, and external cause status codes are sequenced after the main external cause code(s). Regardless of the number of external cause codes assigned, there may be only a rare instance that more than one place of occurrence code is used, for example, when a new injury occurs during a hospitalization, but usually there would be only one place of occurrence code, one activity code, and one external cause status code assigned to an encounter.

- A place of occurrence code, Y92, is generally used only once, at the initial encounter for treatment. Do not use place of occurrence code Y92.9, Place of occurrence of the external cause, unspecified place or not applicable, if the place is not stated or is not applicable.

- An activity code, Y93, is used only once, at the initial encounter for treatment. The activity codes are not applicable to poisonings, adverse effects, misadventures, or sequela. Do not assign Y93.9, Activity codes, unspecified activity, if the activity is not stated.

- An external cause status code is used only once, at the initial encounter for treatment. A code from category Y99, External cause status, indicates the work status of the person at the time the event occurred. The external cause status codes are not applicable to poisonings, adverse effects, misadventures, or late effects. Do not assign code Y99.9, unspecified external cause statue, if the status is not stated.

- There is no national requirement for mandatory ICD-10-CM external cause code reporting. Unless a provider is subject to a state-based external cause code reporting mandate or these codes are required by a particular insurance payer, the reporting of ICD-10-CM codes in Chapter 20, External Causes of Morbidity, is not required.

- Read the entire set of chapter-specific coding and reporting guidelines for ICD-10-CM Chapter 20, External Causes of Morbidity, codes V00–Y99, from the ICD-10-CM Official Guidelines for Coding and Reporting

INSTRUCTIONS:

For this chapter, follow the instructions and reminders below for coding the exercises number 1 through number 22.

1. Code ONLY the external cause codes for each exercise
2. Do not code the injury or medical condition for each exercise
2. Code each exercise as an "Initial Encounter"
3. A coding reminder: When assigning an external cause code, remember "E-P-A-S." For each exercise provided with the necessary information, use the External Causes Index assign a code for

    a. **"E"** for the event,
    b. **"P"** for the place of occurrence,
    c. **"A"** for the patient's activity status, and
    d. **"S"** for the patient's work status of external cause

EXERCISES:

1. Injury in a fight between spectators at a football game, location was a sports stadium. Patient is a student and was a spectator at the sports event.

   External cause code(s): _____

2. Self-inflicted gunshot wound using a handgun, stated to be intentional; location was his garage at home, a single-family house. Patient is an unemployed worker.

   External cause code(s): _____

3. Driver injured in a motor vehicle collision with another vehicle on a highway. Patient is an employed driver for a delivery company.

    External cause code(s): _____

4. Patient is a construction worker who fell off scaffolding at a building construction site. Patient is an employed construction worker.

    External cause code(s): _____

5. Homeowner fell off a ladder in his yard while washing exterior windows at his home, a single-family house. Patient is an unemployed homeowner.

    External cause code(s): _____

6. Patient was the driver of a motor vehicle that struck a bridge abutment on a highway. Patient is a student driving his vehicle while talking on a handheld cellular phone.

    External cause code(s): _____

7. Patient was a passenger on a commercial (fixed wing) airplane flight who was injured when the plane experienced a forced hard landing at the city public airport. Patient was flying to a vacation destination.

    External cause code(s): _____

8. Patient was a vacationer who stepped on broken glass in the sand while walking on the beach at the oceanside resort. Patient was on vacation and walking on the beach.

    External cause code(s): _____

9. Child was injured when he dove into the swimming pool at the next-door neighbor's home, a single-family residence, and struck the side of the pool with his leg. Patient was a student and diving off a springboard platform.

    External cause code(s): _____

10. Patient was brought to the emergency department with wounds suffered in a drive-by gang shooting using a handgun, which appeared to be a homicide attempt. Shooting occurred on a local residential street. Patient was riding a bike and is a high school student.

    External cause code(s): _____

11. A hospital patient fell out of his bed and injured his hip while in the hospital. Patient was a retired individual in the hospital.

    External cause code(s): _____

12. A patient was assaulted by an acquaintance and was stabbed in the abdomen with a knife during the argument, which occurred in a parking lot. Patient was an unemployed worker.

    External cause code(s): _____

13. The patient has a closed head injury as result of a tree falling on him in the front yard of his home, a single-family residence, during a tornado. Patient was off work on vacation at home.

    External cause code(s): _____

14. The child was scalded with hot tap water while in the bath in his mother's apartment bathroom. This was confirmed as child abuse. The abuser was the boyfriend of the child's mother, and the incident occurred in the home. Patient was a student.

    External cause code(s): _____

15. The patient was overcome by heat exhaustion while working near a blast furnace in a steel mill. Patient was an employed steel worker in the mill.

    External cause code(s): _____

16. The patient was working as a paid landscaper and injured his back by straining to lift excessively heavy stones being placed for a decorative border around the entrance to a city park.

    External cause code(s): _____

17. A teenager was brought to the emergency department with an injured right wrist that was the result of the patient running and falling off his skateboard. The accident occurred in a parking lot. The patient was a student in high school.

    External cause code(s): _____

18. A 30-year-old male was brought to the emergency department complaining of back and neck pain from a fall that occurred after he collided with another player while playing basketball at the local outdoor basketball court. The patient was spending leisure time playing basketball.

    External cause code(s): _____

19. A 50-year-old male was brought to the emergency department and diagnosed with a right hip fracture that was a result of a fall off his skis while snow skiing downhill on a mountain at a local ski resort. Patient was on vacation at the ski resort.

    External cause code(s): _____

20. A child was struck by a vehicle and dragged several feet when he ran across the residential street in front of his home. He sustained head injuries and multiple fractures and was admitted to the trauma intensive care unit at the hospital after being brought to the emergency department by fire ambulance. Patient was a student who was running across the street.

   External cause code(s): _____

21. The patient is an express delivery company driver who was bitten by a family's dog when he walked up on the house porch at a single-family residence to deliver a package. The dog was on the house porch and attacked the driver by biting him on his right ankle. The patient was a paid employee of the delivery company.

   External cause code(s): _____

22. The patient is a paid auto mechanic working for a commercial vehicle repair garage and burned his hand when he touched a hot engine part while doing repairs on a customer's vehicle.

   External cause code(s): _____

Chapter 21

Factors Influencing Health Status and Contact with Health Services

Coding Scenarios for *Basic ICD-10-CM and ICD-10-PCS Coding Exercises*

The following case studies are organized following the sequence of the chapters in the ICD-10-CM Tabular List of Diseases and Injuries as published on the Centers for Disease Control and Prevention National Center for Health Statistics website (http://www.cdc.gov /nchs/icd/icd10cm.htm). The objective of this book is to provide the student with more detailed clinical information to code, rather than one- or two-line diagnosis and procedure statements.

ICD-10-CM diagnosis codes are to be assigned to both the inpatient hospital admission and the outpatient visit case studies. In this book, the ICD-10-PCS procedure codes are to be assigned only to the inpatient hospital admission cases. In actual practice, outpatient cases are assigned CPT/HCPCS codes. The ICD-10-PCS codes are only required for inpatient procedures. In the answer key for the exercises, the Alphabetic Index entry is listed after the code to indicate the main terms and subterms used to locate the code that must be verified in the ICD-10-CM Tabular List or in the ICD-10-PCS Code Tables prior to assigning the code.

1

A 27-completed-week gestation infant is delivered by cesarean section. The infant weighs 945 grams. The infant's lungs are immature, and she subsequently develops respiratory distress syndrome, requiring a long inpatient stay in the neonatal intensive care unit. The infant was placed on CPAP, continuous positive airway pressure, for greater than 96 hours, almost five days. The infant eventually is able to go home with her family. The physician's diagnosis is "liveborn infant, delivered by cesarean section, extreme immaturity with a birth weight of 945 grams at 27 weeks of gestation, with resulting respiratory distress syndrome."

Principal Diagnosis: _____

Secondary Diagnoses: _____

Principal Procedure: _____

Secondary Procedure(s): _____

2

While an inpatient in the hospital for chronic persistent atrial fibrillation, the 60-year-old male patient is scheduled for a cystoscopy. This is a follow-up examination because the patient has a history of bladder carcinoma that was resected seven years previously. At that time, the patient received chemotherapy but has not been treated for the cancer for nearly six years. He has had yearly cystoscopic examinations, and no recurrence of the bladder cancer has been found. The cystoscopy and biopsy of the bladder is performed by the urologist who documents as the postoperative diagnosis "history of transitional cell carcinoma of the bladder with no recurrence found, follow-up examination, mild benign prostatic hypertrophy evaluated."

Principal Diagnosis: _____

Secondary Diagnoses: _____

Principal Procedure: _____

Secondary Procedure(s): _____

3

While the 35-year-old patient, gravida 6, para 6, is in the hospital for newly diagnosed uncontrolled hypertension, she requests a tubal ligation/sterilization to be performed by her OB-GYN physician as she does not want to have more children. Once her hypertension was controlled, the procedure was scheduled. The physician performs the following procedure with the following diagnosis: laparoscopic tubal ligation using Falope rings, admission for desired sterilization and multiparity.

Principal Diagnosis: _____

Secondary Diagnoses: _____

Principal Procedure: _____

Secondary Procedure(s): _____

4

A full-term, 38-week gestation, infant is born by vaginal birth in the hospital to a 35-year-old female who develops gestational diabetes during the pregnancy. The mother required close monitoring during the pregnancy because of rather severe fluctuations in blood glucose level. The infant, weighing 8 pounds, 5 ounces, appears normal and healthy. However, because of the mother's gestational diabetes, the infant is kept as an inpatient in the hospital two days longer than usual to observe for possible metabolic disorders as a result of his mother's condition. No symptoms are exhibited by the infant, and the results of diagnostic studies performed are negative. The pediatrician writes the discharge diagnosis as normal, full-term infant, observed for possible effects of mother's gestational diabetes, no disease found.

Principal Diagnosis: _____

Secondary Diagnoses: _____

Principal Procedure: _____

Secondary Procedure(s): _____

5

A 75-year-old retired nun has a total hip replacement for localized osteoarthritis of the right hip. After surgery, she experiences significant difficulty in ambulating, along with gait abnormalities. Physical therapists treat the patient while she is in the hospital, but on day 6, she is discharged to home to be followed up by home health services.

The patient is seen three times a week by a nurse and physical therapists. The patient receives an anticoagulant drug to prevent clots. This requires the nurse to draw blood for a PT/PTT laboratory test weekly. Physical therapists treat the patient for her gait abnormality and difficulty in walking as part of her aftercare following the hip joint replacement. Physical therapy performed includes gait training and strengthening exercises to increase the patient's mobility.

Code for the home health services received.

First-Listed Diagnosis: _____

Secondary Diagnoses: _____

6

A premature twin infant with a liveborn mate is admitted to the special care nursery after the cesarean delivery during which he was delivered. The infant is treated for his prematurity and low birth weight as well as neonatal jaundice associated with the preterm delivery. The infant receives ultraviolet light phototherapy to the skin over multiple days for the jaundice and is discharged to his parents after one month in the hospital. The pediatrician's discharge diagnoses were premature twin infant, result of a 34-week pregnancy, with a birth weight of 1,800 grams, with newborn jaundice of preterm delivery.

Principal Diagnosis: _____

Secondary Diagnoses: _____

Principal Procedure: _____

Secondary Procedure(s): _____

7

The fire ambulance brings a family to the hospital emergency department (ED) after a serious motor vehicle crash when their vehicle collided with another vehicle on the interstate highway. The father and mother were seriously injured and are admitted to the hospital with multiple fractures and head trauma. During the crash, the 10-month-old infant was secured in a rear-facing child seat in the backseat. The ED physicians examine the infant carefully and request several x-rays to be performed. All x-rays are negative, but the physicians are still particularly concerned about the infant given the serious nature of the crash. They decide to admit the infant to the hospital for monitoring and further testing for undetected injuries. After day 2, no injuries can be found in the infant, and he is discharged to the care of his maternal grandparents.

Note: Assign codes only for the infant.

Principal Diagnosis: _____

Secondary Diagnoses: _____

Principal Procedure: _____

Secondary Procedure(s): _____

8

The patient is a 32-year-old female who is 24 weeks pregnant. She is being followed up by her physician as a high-risk pregnancy because of her history of having a hydatidiform mole 10 years previously. The patient is considered to have a history of infertility as the patient has not been pregnant since she was treated for the hydatidiform mole with surgical evacuation. The physician orders ongoing laboratory testing for monitoring of the current pregnancy, and no problems have been detected. The patient will return for her next prenatal visit at 27 weeks.

First-Listed Diagnosis: _____

Secondary Diagnoses: _____

9

The first visit of the day for this pediatrician in her office is a 2-week-old infant who was born by vaginal delivery to a woman during the 39th week of pregnancy. All laboratory tests done in the hospital were normal and the infant was discharged with her mother on day 2. The mother reports that the infant has been nursing well and has generally been a delight. The pediatrician examines the infant at the age of 14 days. The only abnormal finding was the presence of prickly heat on the infant's trunk that was due to the hot weather present in the past week and the infant might have been overly dressed. The mother is counseled regarding the prickly heat, general infant care, nursing, and the recommended infant vaccinations to be performed during the follow-up visits.

First-Listed Diagnosis: _____

Secondary Diagnoses: _____

10

The patient admitted to the hospital is a 28-year-old female who is a third-grade school teacher. She is donating her left kidney for a young boy in her class who has polycystic kidney disease and is in need of a kidney transplant. The donor has a history of an allergy to latex, so she was protected from any exposure to latex supplies during her hospital stay. This allergy did not prevent her from being a donor. The teacher's surgery, a unilateral open nephrectomy, is performed uneventfully, and she is discharged to her home to recover.

Principal Diagnosis: _____

Secondary Diagnoses: _____

Principal Procedure: _____

Secondary Procedure(s): _____

11

The 30-year-old male patient was seen in the physician's office for change of the dressings on both hands. The patient is a construction worker who was injured on the job seven days ago. He was handling a rope used to pull up a heavy metal structure when the rope began to run through his gloved hands. He tried to stop the rope and states that his gloves actually caught fire. He developed painful abrasions to both of his hands. He was brought to the emergency department (ED) of the hospital near the construction site. The ED physician applied cool dressings to the hands and removed some avulsed skin from several fingers. During this office visit, the patient's dressings were changed, and Silvadene was applied to the fingers. The wounds did not appear infected. The reason for the visit documented by the physician was "Change of dressings to protect the healing deep abrasions on both hands."

First-Listed Diagnosis: _____

Secondary Diagnoses: _____

12

The 60-year-old male patient was seen in his primary care physician's office for routine fracture healing. The patient suffered traumatic fractures of his pelvis that occurred four weeks ago. The patient was walking across a street when he was hit by a vehicle, knocked down, and the vehicle ran over his pelvis. The fractures did not require surgical treatment. After the hospital stay, the patient was transferred to an acute rehabilitation facility, and he improved dramatically over the past four weeks. He was discharged from the rehabilitation facility two days ago and will begin outpatient physical therapy tomorrow. During this office visit, his fracture was evaluated. The physician also reviewed and signed the physical therapy plan of treatment and orders for the patient to continue to receive fracture aftercare.

First-Listed Diagnosis: _____

Secondary Diagnoses: _____

13

The patient, a 70-year-old male, was seen in his cardiologist's office for a report of the echocardiogram that was performed on the patient within the past week. The man had the mitral valve in his heart replaced about 20 years ago and has had some vague symptoms that led the physician to order the echocardiogram. Based on the physical examination and the report of the echocardiogram, the cardiologist concluded the synthetic heart valve was near the end of its life and needed to be replaced. The physician informed the patient that this was an expected event, that valves do not last forever, and that the need to replace it did not mean the valve was defective or causing a complication. To prevent the patient from experiencing serious problems by delaying the inevitable replacement, the physician arranged for the patient to be admitted to the hospital the same evening, with consultation with the cardiothoracic surgeon immediately. One day later the patient had the previous mitral valve removed and replaced with a new synthetic prosthetic valve by thoracotomy and had an uneventful recovery.

Note: Assign codes only for the inpatient services.

Principal Diagnosis: _____

Secondary Diagnoses: _____

Principal Procedure: _____

Secondary Procedure(s): _____

14

The patient is a 17-year-old high school senior who was in his chemistry laboratory when another student spilled a non-medicinal chemical during a lab assignment. Other students in the classroom complained of nausea and shortness of breath and all students were taken to the emergency department (ED) for examination. This patient had no symptoms or complaints. The student was examined by the ED physician and found to be well. The diagnosis written by the infant on the record was "Well adolescent, exposed to non-medicinal chemical, no injury or disease found."

First-Listed Diagnosis: _____

Secondary Diagnoses: _____

15

A five-month-old female was brought by her mother to the pediatrician's office for her scheduled "Synagis" shot. Synagis is a medication given prophylactically to high-risk infants to protect them from acquiring the respiratory syncytial virus (RSV) and avoid an acute respiratory illness. The physician's progress note for the visit concludes with his impression of "Ex-30 week premature infant here for Synagis injection, subcutaneous, completed."

First-Listed Diagnosis: _____

Secondary Diagnoses: _____

16

The patient is a 35-year-old female who is admitted for prophylactic robotic-assisted laparoscopic total abdominal hysterectomy (TAH) and bilateral laparoscopic salpingo-oophorectomy (BSO). She is having this elective removal of her uterus, cervix, tubes, and ovaries because she has a strong history of ovarian cancer in her family, including her grandmother, aunt, sister, and cousin. She has three healthy children. The surgery was performed without complications, and the patient had an uneventful postoperative period. After surgery, the gynecologic oncologist who performed the surgery informed the patient that a tiny area of malignancy, Stage 1 ovarian carcinoma, was found in the right ovary. The patient was discharged for recovery at home with the assistance of a home health agency and will return to her oncologist's office in two weeks to discuss further treatment.

Principal Diagnosis: _____

Secondary Diagnoses: _____

Principal Procedure: _____

Secondary Procedure(s): _____

17

The patient is a 50-year-old female who is being seen today in the transplant clinic to monitor her status as a live-donor kidney transplant recipient. She received a right kidney transplant six months ago. The patient also has chronic kidney disease, stage 4, in her left kidney and continues to receive medications as treatment for her kidney disease but does not require renal dialysis treatments at this time. The diagnoses listed in her medical record by her transplant surgeon for this visit is (1) Status post right kidney transplant and (2) Chronic kidney disease, stage 4.

First-Listed Diagnosis: _____

Secondary Diagnoses: _____

18

The reason for the visit today at the oncologist's office is to perform a yearly follow-up examination following cancer treatment. The patient is a 60-year-old female who is a cancer survivor and has no evidence of cancer present. The patient was diagnosed with right breast cancer 10 years ago and had a right mastectomy, totally removing her right breast. The patient's mother, aunt, and sister also had breast carcinoma treated over the past 30 years. The conditions listed by the oncologist to summarize this visit were (1) Follow up on mastectomy for breast malignancy, no recurrence identified, (2) History breast carcinoma, (3) Surgically absent right breast, (4) Strong family history of breast cancer.

First-Listed Diagnosis: _____

Secondary Diagnoses: _____

19

The patient is a 75-year-old male who is seen in his primary care physician's office for a screening examination to rule out prostate cancer. The patient does not have any prostatic or urinary system symptoms. As part of the physical examination, the physician performs a digital rectal examination on the patient. The physician also writes an order for the patient to take to the laboratory for a screening prostatic specific antigen (PSA) test. A complete skin examination was performed as well because of the patient's past skin malignancy. The final examination written by the physician in the office record is screening for prostate cancer, no symptoms and personal history of melanoma in-situ, no symptoms found.

First-Listed Diagnosis: _____

Secondary Diagnoses: _____

20

The patient is a 26-year-old G1 P0 patient who is being seen in the obstetrician's office during the patient's 38th week of pregnancy in anticipation of a normal delivery following an entirely normal pregnancy. The patient is scheduled for a return visit to the obstetrician's office during the 39th week of pregnancy. The final diagnosis documented was primigravida patient, 38th week of gestation, supervision of normal pregnancy.

First-Listed Diagnosis: _____

Secondary Diagnoses: _____

Chapter 22

Advanced Coding Scenarios for *Basic ICD-10-CM and ICD-10-PCS Coding Exercises*

The following are advanced case studies meant to provide the student with more detailed clinical information to code, requiring ICD-10-CM diagnosis codes and ICD-10-PCS procedure codes. In the answer key for the exercises, the Alphabetic Index entry is listed after the code to indicate the main terms and sub-terms used to locate the code that must be verified in the ICD-10-CM Tabular List or in the ICD-10-PCS Code Tables prior to assigning the code.

1

The patient is a 56-year-old male who was admitted with a history of hematemesis for the past 36 hours. He also had some tarry black stools. The patient shared that he was under a great deal of stress dealing with his wife who is a known prescription pain medication addict. He was recently diagnosed with hypertension and attributes that to the stressful home situation. After admission, the patient's blood pressure was 180/110 and the urgent hypertensive condition had to be controlled prior to additional testing which determined him to have an acute, giant gastric ulcer that was actively bleeding. It was also noted that the patient was taking Pradaxa for longstanding persistent atrial fibrillation. He was administered Idarucizumab, a reversal agent for Pradaxa, through a peripheral vein and taken for immediate surgical intervention. The patient was then scheduled for surgical intervention.

PROCEDURE PERFORMED: Subtotal gastrectomy with Billroth II anastomosis

OPERATIVE PROCEDURE: The patient was brought to the operating room and placed on the table in a supine position, at which time general anesthesia was administered without difficulty. His abdomen was then prepped and draped in the usual sterile fashion. An upper midline incision was made. The peritoneum was then entered using the Metzenbaum scissors and hemostats. A retractor was placed, and he was noted to have a cirrhotic liver with micronodular cirrhosis. The left lobe of the liver was mobilized at that point, and the retractors were placed. On palpation of the stomach along the lesser curvature at approximately the mid portion, there was a large gastric ulcer located in the body of the stomach. At this point, the gastrocolic omentum was taken off the greater curvature of the stomach to the level just above the pylorus. Additionally, the lesser omentum was taken down off the lesser curvature of the stomach just above the level of the pylorus. The body of the stomach was then transected approximately 3 cm above the ulcer. At that point, the stomach was reconstructed in a Billroth II fashion by bringing the jejunum through the transverse colon mesentery. Two stay sutures were placed to align the jejunum along the posterior wall of the stomach, and a GIA stapler was used to create the anastomosis without difficulty. The stomach and jejunum were then pulled below the transverse colon mesentery, and this was tacked in several places using 3-0 silk sutures. A feeding tube was then placed in the jejunum using the feeding tube kit without difficulty. The abdomen was then irrigated thoroughly using normal saline solution. Hemostasis was achieved using Bovie electrocautery. The midline incision was then closed using #1 PDS in a running fashion. The skin was closed using skin staples. A sterile dressing was applied. The patient was extubated in the operating room and returned to the intensive care unit in guarded condition.

The patient showed continued improvement over the next four days with controlled blood pressures and minimal pain following the procedure. Physician discussed the micronodular cirrhosis and the patient admitted to alcohol dependence, despite multiple attempts at AA. The patient was not exhibiting any withdrawal symptoms, and was agreeable to pursuing outpatient treatment to refrain from drinking. The patient was then discharged and urged to attend a community resource group such as NAR-ANON to help with coping strategies for dealing with his stressful home situation.

Principal Diagnosis: _____

Secondary Diagnoses: _____

Principal Procedure: _____

Secondary Procedure(s): _____

Source: Adapted from AHIMA *ICD-10-PCS Coder Training Manual* 2016.

2

The patient is a 33-year-old male steelworker who suffered a full thickness burn two months ago from molten iron splashing onto his right foot. He also has pure hypercholesterolemia and hypertension. There is a 40-pack-a-year smoking history but the patient did quit 10 years ago. The patient presents for elective debridement of the healing wound and split thickness skin graft.

OPERATION: Split thickness skin graft from right thigh to right foot

OPERATIVE DESCRIPTION: The patient was taken to the operating room and placed supine on the operating table. After adequate IV sedation was provided, the right lower extremity was prepped and draped in the standard sterile fashion. Sharp debridement of the ulcer was carried out. The ulcer was approximately 4 × 5 cm in area in the lateral dorsum of the right foot. Debridement was carried down to viable tissue. A 4 × 5 cm split thickness skin graft was harvested from the upper aspect of the right thigh. The graft was then meshed and applied to the right foot wound. The graft was secured with a running locked #3-0 chromic suture. Two centrally located chromic sutures were placed for further support. Attention was placed to the donor site, which was dressed with Xeroform and 4 × 4 gauze. The right lower extremity was then wrapped in Kerlix dressing. Sponge and instrument counts were correct at the end of the case. The patient tolerated the procedure well and was transported to the recovery room.

Principal Diagnosis: _____

Secondary Diagnoses: _____

Principal Procedure: _____

Secondary Procedure(s): _____

Source: Adapted from AHIMA *ICD-10-PCS Coder Training Manual* 2016.

3

The patient is a 57-year-old female who was admitted from the emergency department with chronic skin ulcer on the mid-back calf accompanied with fever and lethargy. Initial inspection of the ulcer found it to extend deep to the bone, where it was obvious that necrosis was occurring. Due to the extensiveness of the necrosis and the patient's overall deteriorating condition, she reluctantly agreed to a below-the-knee amputation in an attempt to eliminate the infectious source. Prior to surgery, her comorbid conditions that include Graves' disease, multiple sclerosis, hypertension, and cotton wool spots were monitored and medicated as necessary.

PROCEDURE: Right below-the-knee amputation

DESCRIPTION OF PROCEDURE: The patient was brought to the operating room and placed supine on the operating room table. The patient was placed under general endotracheal anesthesia. A tourniquet was placed on the right proximal thigh and the right lower extremity was prepped and draped in a standard sterile fashion.

A below-the-knee amputation was carried out directly below the tibial tubercle with a posteriorly based flap. The skin and soft tissue were cut sharply to bone along the line of the skin incision. Once the soft tissue was incised the tibia and fibula were provisionally cut with an oscillating saw and the remainder of the right lower extremity was removed and sent to pathology. Next, the tibia and fibula were dissected out subperiosteally proximal to the anterior portion of the skin incision and re-cut with the oscillating saw. The anterior portion of the tibia was beveled again with the oscillating saw and smoothed with a rasp. The fibular cut was beveled in a lateral to medial direction while extending posteriorly.

The nerves and blood vessels were then addressed. The anterior tibial and posterior tibial arteries, as well as the peroneal artery and attendant veins were suture ligated with #1 Vicryl suture. The anterior and posterior tibial nerves and peroneal nerve were also identified, pulled out of the wound, cut short, and allowed to retract back into the soft tissue. In addition, large veins were identified and ligated. The tourniquet was then released for a total tourniquet time of 32 minutes and minimal bleeding was encountered. Several smaller bleeders were ligated. There was some clotting observed, which was important as the blood clotting was of significant concern preceding this operation. The wound was closed over a medium Hemovac drain with 2 limbs, with the posterior flap brought anteriorly. The fascia was closed using interrupted 1 Vicryl suture, and the subcutaneous tissue was closed using interrupted 3-0 Monocryl suture in a simple buried fashion. Staples were placed at the level of the skin in the interest of time.

After a sterile compressive dressing was placed and Hemovac drain extension and reservoir were attached and activated, the patient was awoken from anesthesia and sent to the ICU in unchanged condition.

Unfortunately, after surgery, the patient continued to deteriorated. Blood cultures returned as *E. coli* positive with the sepsis becoming severe when the patient went into acute, hypoxic respiratory failure. Within 36 hours of surgery the patient expired.

Principal Diagnosis: _____

Secondary Diagnoses: _____

Principal Procedure: _____

Secondary Procedure(s): _____

Source: Adapted from AHIMA *ICD-10-PCS Coder Training Manual* 2016.

4

This 54-year-old male presented to the emergency department with unrelenting abdominal pain of both the lower left quadrant and the entire right side. He relates a previous history of Crohn's disease for which he has been hospitalized multiple times. During his examination, a left midfoot ulcer that exposed the tissue of the hypodermis was identified. The patient indicated multiple treatments, including debridement and grafts (which failed) had been tried but the condition persists. GERD, OSA, and dyslipidemia were current conditions for which the patient was receiving treatment. The patient has COPD attributable to smoking a pack of cigarettes per day, which he continues to do despite the breathing issues. Prilosec, Crestor, and Humalog (administered daily for his type 1 diabetes) are the current medications for him. An x-ray indicated the patient had extensive diverticulitis of the sigmoid colon with perforation. There was evidence of Crohn's disease with obstruction of the right colon and the proximal transverse colon. It was decided the patient needed emergent surgery to attend to these conditions.

PROCEDURES: Exploratory laparotomy; sigmoid colectomy; extended right hemicolectomy; colostomy

PROCEDURE DESCRIPTION: After consent was obtained for the procedure, risks and benefits were described at length. The patient was taken to the operating room and placed supine on the operating room table. Preoperatively, the patient received 3 g of IV Unasyn. The patient was placed under general endotracheal anesthesia. PAS stockings were applied to both lower extremities. The patient's abdomen was then prepped and draped in the standard surgical fashion.

A midline laparotomy incision was made from just around the umbilicus to the pubic symphysis. The midline of the fascia was divided, and the abdomen was entered. With exploration of the abdomen, extensive diverticular disease of the distal sigmoid colon was noted.

First order of business was to mobilize the sigmoid colon for a sigmoid colectomy. The left ureter was identified and was far from the area of the sigmoid colon. The sigmoid colon was mobilized laterally to include the area of the diverticulitis. The sigmoid colon was mobilized down to the peritoneal reflection. The medial aspect of the sigmoid colon was also mobilized. The colon was then completely mobilized. A point of transaction was chosen at the proximal sigmoid colon. The mesentery was then taken down across the sacrum. The vessels were tied with 2-0 silk sutures. The sigmoid colon was mobilized down to the proximal rectum. Once the proximal rectum was identified, the sigmoid colon was again transected, this time using a contour Ethicon stapler with a blue load. Both the right and left ureters were identified prior to any transection of the sigmoid colon. A 3-0 Prolene suture was then tagged to either edge of the rectal staple line. The specimen was then passed off the field.

The right colon was then inspected. Multiple perforations with sites of deserosalization with exposed mucosa were identified in the right colon. The right colon was mobilized by taking down the white line of Toldt all the way up to and including the hepatic flexure. The omentum was taken off the transverse colon with electrocautery. Once the colon was completely mobilized and became a medial structure, the terminal ileum was transected, this time also using a 45-mm GIA stapler with a blue load. A point of transection was chosen in the mid transverse colon just proximal to the middle colic artery where the last site of deserosalization was identified. The mid transverse colon was divided with a GIA 45-mm stapler with a blue load. The mesentery to the right colon and transverse colon were then taken down with Pean clamps and tied with 2-0 silk sutures. The specimen was then passed off the field.

The abdomen was then irrigated. Hemostasis was assured. The ileocolic anastomosis was then created between the terminal ileum and the mid transverse colon. The bowels were positioned to lie alongside each other, and a side-to-side functional end-to-end anastomosis was created using a 45-mm GIA stapler with a blue load. The enterostomies were then closed together with a running 3-0 PDS suture followed by interrupted 3-0 GI silks in a Lembert fashion. A stitch was placed at the crotch of each of the bowel connections. A finger was palpated at the anastomosis, and it was widely patent. Mesenteric defect was then closed using 3-0 Vicryl suture in a running fashion.

Attention then turned toward formation of the end-descending colostomy. The descending colon had already been mobilized enough to make it to the anterior abdominal wall without any difficulty. A point on the anterior abdominal wall on the left-hand side just below the umbilicus was chosen for the colostomy. A small 1.5 to 2-cm circular incision was made on the anterior abdominal wall midway through the rectus muscle. The anterior fascia was divided in a cruciate fashion. The rectus muscles were split, and two fingers were palpated through the defect into the abdominal cavity. The descending colon was then grasped with an Allis clamp and passed through the defect and exteriorized. There was no tension on the colon. On the undersurface of the peritoneum, the colon was tagged with 3-0 GI silk sutures ×2.

The midline fascial incision was then closed with a running #1 looped PDS ×2. The surgical incision was then irrigated with copious saline. The skin was then closed with surgical staples. The ostomy was then matured by removing the staple line and sewing the ostomy in place with 3-0 Vicryl sutures. The sutures were sewn in circumferentially. An ostomy appliance was applied.

Sterile dressings were applied, and the patient was awakened from general anesthesia and transported to the recovery room in stable condition.

Four days later, the patient returned to surgery to address the non-healing midfoot ulcer. This time the physician has chosen to use Miroderm, a wound matrix derived from porcine liver as the skin substitute. Once the patient was sedated, debridement of the wound was performed leaving a 4 × 6 cm area over which the Miroderm was placed. The patient was taken to PACU in stable condition. The wound was monitored over the next several days and initial healing was promising.

Five days later, the patient was recovered enough for discharge to be followed by home health for the next three weeks.

Principal Diagnosis: _____

Secondary Diagnoses: _____

Principal Procedure: _____

Secondary Procedure(s): _____

Source: Adapted from AHIMA *ICD-10-PCS Coder Training Manual* 2016.

5

This 72-year-old female comes to the emergency department with inability to walk. She complains of low back pain that has been ongoing for years, but has recently become much more severe, to the point today of not being able to walk. She is accompanied by her daughter, who provides further history of a CVA twelve months ago, with the patient still experiencing difficulty with attention and concentration as a result. Her mother has hypothyroidism after irradiation for thyroid cancer. Her diabetes, type 2, has been uncontrolled recently, and BGMs on admission was 398. This hyperglycemic condition will need brought under control and consult to neurosurgery regarding the patient's lumbar DDD.

Neurosurgery determined that due the patient's multiple medical conditions it would be prudent to obtain glycemic control and then proceed to surgery for the back issues as it was apparent after testing that the patient was in need of a fusion.

PREOPERATIVE DIAGNOSIS: Degenerative disk disease, L3-4, L4-5

OPERATION: Posterior lumbar interbody fusion, anterior column, L3-4 and L4-5, using nanoLock fusion devices and Danek pedicle screws with autogenous bone graft

PROCEDURE DESCRIPTION: Patient was brought to the operating room and after induction of satisfactory general endotracheal anesthesia, was placed in the prone position on the spinal frame. Back prepped and draped in the usual sterile fashion.

A #18 gauge needle was used to identify the posterior spinous process of L3-4, L4-5, marked with Indigo Carmine stain and substantiated by x-ray. Just to the left of the midline, an incision was made and the incision was carried down through the skin and subcutaneous tissue and fascia. The tissues just under the skin were separated and the left and right lower back muscles were moved aside, exposing the back of the spinal column.

Using the same lumbar incision, dissection of a suprafascial plane was made to identify the posterior superior iliac spine (PSIS). Using an osteotome, the cortical bone of the PSIS was chipped off to expose the cancellous undersurface. A large bone gouge was utilized to harvest the cancellous bone from left iliac crest. The bone was morselized and stored for use later in the procedure. The graft site was then irrigated with antibiotic irrigation and packed with Gelfoam. The fascial opening was then closed. Laminectomy was then performed.

The fusion was completed using the posterior lumbar interbody technique utilizing a nanoLock interbody fusion device. The L3-L4 level was addressed first. An alignment guide was placed over the L3-L4 disk space and the disk was incised with a knife. A drill was used to make a hole into the disk space and spacers were put in sequentially up to a size #11. Cross-table lateral x-rays were taken of the lumbar spine. A C-ring retractor was placed over the spacer on the left side and the locking tube sleeve was inserted into the body of L3 and L4. The hole was drilled and loose fragments were moved with the straight pituitary. The nanoLock device was then selected and packed with bone graft obtained earlier from the iliac crest. The bone graft was packed into the device at the distal end and the device was inserted on the left side. The proximal end of the device was packed with bone. The same technique was completed on the right hand side. After completion of the procedure at the L3-L4 level, the same technique was done at the L4-L5 level. Because this was a two-level device procedure, the pedicle screw instrumentation was used to augment the stabilization. The pedicle screw was put into the L3 vertebral body by making a burr hole at the junction of the facet joint and transverse process on the left. The curette was used to make an entry hole into the pedicle and the screw was inserted. The same technique was done on the contralateral side and at the L5 level bilaterally. The screw from L3-L5 was connected to the other L5 screw with a rod on both sides, and then the rods were locked into place with the locking nuts, and the rods were then connected with a transverse connector piece. Final x-rays were taken. The wound was then closed in anatomic layers using interrupted Vicryl suture for the deep layer and staples for the skin. Sterile dressing was applied and the patient was taken to the recovery room in satisfactory condition.

Principal Diagnosis: _____

Secondary Diagnoses: _____

Principal Procedure: _____

Secondary Procedure(s): _____

Source: Adapted from AHIMA *ICD-10-PCS Coder Training Manual* 2016.

6

The following documentation is from the health record of a cardiac service patient.

DISCHARGE SUMMARY

Admit Date: 1/9/XX

Discharge Date: 1/12/XX

FINAL DIAGNOSES: Coronary artery disease (CAD)

Long QT syndrome

Hypertensive heart disease

History, family, sudden cardiac death

PROCEDURES: Percutaneous transluminal coronary angioplasty with stent insertion (1/10/XX)

Permanent dual chamber pacemaker insertion (1/9/XX)

HISTORY OF PRESENT ILLNESS: The patient is a 50-year-old female who was admitted to another hospital on 1/8/XX after experiencing unexplained fainting and a fluttering feeling in his chest. She thought his heart was "beating too fast." Her father died of sudden cardiac death at age 52. This family history may indicate a genetic characteristic of her heart disease. At the first hospital, the patient was found to have an abnormal EKG with a long QT syndrome demonstrated and an abnormal results of a Holter Monitor study. There she underwent a cardiac catheterization, showing the presence of severe two-vessel coronary artery disease. The patient does not have any history of a CABG in the past. The patient also is known to have hypertensive heart disease. She was transferred to our hospital to undergo a percutaneous transluminal angioplasty and further diagnosis and treatment of the Long QT syndrome.

PHYSICAL EXAMINATION: Vital signs were abnormal with a pulse of 50 and blood pressure 100/85. HEENT: PERRLA, faint carotid bruits. Lungs: Clear to percussion and auscultation. Heart: perceived rhythm was abnormal. Extremities and abdomen were negative.

HOSPITAL COURSE: To manage the patient's Long QT syndrome, a permanent dual chamber pacemaker with atrial and ventricular leads was implanted on 1/9/XX. An incision was made into the left chest wall with the dual chamber pacemaker being placed in the subcutaneous pocket. Next, a small incision was made in the skin, and the leads were percutaneously passed into the right ventricle and right atrium.

On 1/10 the patient underwent a PTCA of both the left anterior descending artery (LAD) and the right coronary artery (RCA.) Before the PTCA but during the same procedure, she was found to have severely calcified arteriosclerotic plaque in the LAD. An atherectomy was performed in the LAD using the new technology Diamondback orbital atherectomy system. When the lesion was removed, a drug-eluting stent was deployed in the LAD without complications and good results were obtained. The second vessel (RCA) did not require a stent as part of its PTCA.

Postoperatively, the patient was stable and was subsequently discharged. The patient's hypertensive heart disease was managed and monitored during the hospital stay and the patient continued taking her normal medications for her conditions. (Code for the second hospital stay.)

Principal Diagnosis: _____

Secondary Diagnoses: _____

Principal Procedure: _____

Secondary Procedure(s): _____

Source: Adapted from AHIMA *ICD-10-PCS Coder Training Manual* 2016.

7

PREOPERATIVE DIAGNOSIS: Bronchial alveolar cell carcinoma of the left lung, upper lobe; history of non-Hodgkin lymphoma previously treated; past history of smoking; suspected lymph node metastasis

POSTOPERATIVE DIAGNOSIS: Same with mediastinal lymph node metastasis proven

OPERATION: Video-assisted thoracoscopic (VATS) left pneumonectomy, uniportal with excision of subcarinal/mediastinal lymph nodes

INDICATIONS: The patient is 60-year-old male with a 30 pack-a-year past history of smoking cigarettes (quit 2 years ago), who was diagnosed with bronchial alveolar cell carcinoma of the left lung. After consultation with surgical oncology, pulmonology, critical management and radiation therapy, the patient was offered the risks and benefits of various cancer treatment. After much discussion about the extent of his disease, prognosis and treatment options, the patient elected the VATS pneumonectomy with a single portal approach. After surgery, the pathologist reported the presence of bronchial alveolar cell carcinoma in the left lung and metastatic carcinoma in the mediastinal lymph nodes in the final report.

PROCEDURE: This patient was operated on under general endotracheal anesthesia. We used a double lumen tube where we could selectively ventilate both lungs. He was in the lateral decubitus position. A 5–6 cm incision was made in the 5th intercostal space and the thorascope was placed in the posterior aspect of the incision. The instrumentation and staplers were inserted through the anterior aspect of the incision. There was a large diffuse lesion in the left upper lobe periphery. The lesion had previously been biopsied, and we were dealing with a bronchial alveolar cell carcinoma. The man did have a past history of non-Hodgkin lymphoma years ago, which was presumably cured. The mediastinum was approached on the lateral aspect. The pneumonectomy procedure involves the examination of the main pulmonary artery, superior and inferior pulmonary veins, subcarinal lymph nodes and the left mainstem bronchus. The lung was retracted posteriorly and inferiorly. The dissection is started by opening the mediastinal pleura. The left main pulmonary artery was divided with an endostapler. The inferior vein is divided with an endostapler after retracting the lung upward. The subcarinal or mediastinal lymph nodes were excised in the area of the superior and posterior main bronchus. The bronchus is divided after all the vascular elements were divided by retracting and elevating. The lung is pulled through the endostapler to create a bronchial short stump. This completed the pneumonectomy. A single chest tube for drainage is required in the left pleural space for this type of disease and treatment and is placed at the end of the procedure. The area was inspected meticulously for hemostasis and the presence of any incidental adverse events of which none were found. The thoracoscope and the instrumentation were removed. The small incision was sealed and dressed. He tolerated the procedure well. He had some expected hypotension throughout the entire procedure. Blood gases were satisfactory during the procedure and he seemed to be responding to the withdrawal of the anesthesia well. The patient was taken directly to the surgical ICU for recovery.

Principal Diagnosis: _____

Secondary Diagnoses: _____

Principal Procedure: _____

Secondary Procedure(s): _____

Source: Adapted from AHIMA *ICD-10-PCS Coder Training Manual* 2016.

8

PRE-OPERATIVE DIAGNOSIS: Severe peripheral arterial disease, arterial insufficiency due to aorto-iliac occlusive disease or atherosclerosis

POSTOPERATIVE DIAGNOSES: Atherosclerosis of native arteries, bilateral legs, with intermittent claudication

OPERATION: Open aorto-bifemoral bypass graft

INDICATIONS: The patient is a 78-year-old male who has complained of muscle aches, cramping and pain in his legs from his thighs to his feet for several years and he states it is getting worse. He has limited mobility as the cramping in his legs prevent him from walking more than a block. On physical exam, he has diminished pulses in his legs with very faint pulses in his feet. He underwent an abdominal aortogram plus bilateral iliofemoral angiography of the lower extremities as an outpatient a month ago and was found to have severe aorto-iliac occlusive disease due to atherosclerosis. The patient was treated for carcinoma of the small bowel over 10 years ago with no recurrence. The patient has also been under treatment in the hospital for essential hypertension that he has had for many years. He also quit smoking 20 years ago. The patient was given the risks and benefits of an aorto-bifemoral vascular graft and he consented to the procedure with the hope of eliminating the pain and cramping in his legs that will allow him to become more active again.

PROCEDURE: The patient was prepped and draped, and groin incisions were opened. The common femoral vein and its branches were isolated, and rubber loops were placed around the vessels. At the completion of this, the abdomen was opened and explored. The patient was found to have evidence of radiation therapy in the abdominal wall and some of the small bowel due to his past treatments for history of carcinoma of the small intestine. The remainder of the abdominal exploration was unremarkable.

After the abdomen was explored, a Balfour retractor was put in place. The abdominal aorta and iliac vessels were mobilized. Bleeding points were controlled with electrocoagulation. The tapes were placed around the vessel. The vessel was measured, and the abdominal aorta was found to be a 12-mm vessel. An 11 × 6 bifurcated micro-velour graft was then pre-clotted with the patient's own blood.

An end-to-end anastomosis was made on the aorta and the graft using a running suture of 2-0 Prolene. The limbs were taken down through tunnels, and an end-to-side anastomosis was made between the graft and the femoral arteries with running suture of 4-0 Prolene. The inguinal incisions were closed with running sutures of 2-0 Vicryl and steel staples in the skin. The subcutaneous tissue was closed with running suture of 3-0 Vicryl, and the skin was closed with steel staples. A sterile dressing was applied. The patient tolerated the procedure well and returned to the recovery room in adequate condition.

Principal Diagnosis: _____

Secondary Diagnoses: _____

Principal Procedure: _____

Secondary Procedure(s): _____

Source: Adapted from AHIMA *ICD-10-PCS Coder Training Manual* 2016.

9

DIAGNOSES: Sustained ventricular tachyarrhythmia; survivor (history) of sudden cardiac arrest; ischemic cardiomyopathy; history of myocardial infarction three months ago; status post PTCA for coronary artery disease still present

PROCEDURE: Placement of a dual chamber implantable pacing cardioverter defibrillator (AICD)

INDICATIONS: The indications for the placement of the dual chamber AICD in this 67-year-old male are based on his complex cardiac conditions and history. Within the past month, he survived sudden cardiac arrest and was hospitalized after being resuscitated in the emergency department. Three months ago, he had a serious acute myocardial infarction followed by a three vessel PTCA for coronary artery disease that we expect is still present. The placement of the dual chamber AICD is to manage and control his recurrent ventricular tachyarrhythmia present with the ischemic cardiomyopathy.

DESCRIPTION OF PROCEDURE: After informed consent was obtained, the patient was brought to the cardiac catheterization procedure suite. The procedure was done under conscious sedation with fluoroscopic guidance. One percent Lidocaine was used to anesthetize the skin in the left abdominal area and a skin incision was made. A pocket was made in the subcutaneous tissue of the abdomen for the ICD generator, securing good hemostasis. The left subclavian vein was easily cannulated twice using a pediatric set, which was upsized to regular 037 wires, the position that was checked under fluoroscopy.

I then dilated the access volts with 9-French dilators and used 7-French access sheaths through which a 7-French right ventricular lead was advanced and placed under fluoroscopic guidance. It was an active fixation lead. The numbers looked good, and the lead was sutured down.

A 7-French lead was then advanced under fluoroscopic guidance and placed in the right atrial appendage. The numbers looked good. There was no diaphragmatic stimulation and the lead was sutured down. The leads were then attached to the generator, which was tested and sutured down in the pocket. The wound was irrigated several times with antibiotics at the end of the procedure. Wound was closed with layers. The patient tolerated the procedure well without any complications. (The ICD is Model Virtuoso DRD 154AWG. Atrial and ventricular leads are Medtronic.) (Note: Do not code the fluoroscopy.)

Principal Diagnosis: _____

Secondary Diagnoses: _____

Principal Procedure: _____

Secondary Procedure(s): _____

Source: Adapted from AHIMA *ICD-10-PCS Coder Training Manual* 2016.

10

PREOPERATIVE DIAGNOSES: Symptomatic severe aortic stenosis, coronary artery disease, status post CABG, hypertension on metoprolol, chronic kidney disease stage 3, hypothyroidism on synthyroid, congestive heart failure on bumex, familial hypercholesterolemia on statins, chronic atrial fibrillation, rate controlled, not on anticoagulation, and anemia due to chronic disease.

POSTOPERATIVE DIAGNOSES: Same as above

INDICATIONS: The patient is an 87-year-old female with extensive medical history with increasing symptomatic aortic stenosis. The lady is of sound mind and cognition and fully understands her disease processes as well as the risks and benefits of a transcatheter aortic valve replacement (TAVR) procedure. Her estimated ejection fracture is 60–65%, but she had decreased left ventricular diastolic compliance and/or increased left atrial pressure. She has been managed medically for several years by her primary care physician, cardiologist, nephrologist, endocrinologist and now by her interventional cardiology physician and cardiovascular surgeon. She was evaluated and approved by two cardiologists for the new technology Edwards device TAVR procedure and is considered a good candidate based on her current medical conditions and treatments but would be unable to withstand an open thoracotomy for an aortic valve replacement.

PROCEDURE(S) PERFORMED: Transcatheter aortic valve replacement with Edwards Intuity Elite Valve System using rapid deployment technique through a minimally invasive surgical approach. (Bovine pericardial aortic bioprosthetic valve, zooplastic.) Preceded by the placement of the new technology cerebral embolic protection system (Claret Medical Sentinel) for the prevention of a stroke as a complication of the TAVR procedures. TAVR includes an aortic valve balloon valvuloplasty, insertion of Swan-Ganz catheter, and placement of temporary ventricular pacing wire.

DESCRIPTION OF PROCEDURE: Within the operating room, the patient induced to general anesthesia, positioned, draped, and prepped sterile. Two left subclavian introducer sheaths inserted. Swan-Ganz catheter as well as temporary right ventricular pacing lead placed. Next, a left femoral arterial venous access was obtained percutaneous. A right common femoral artery was identified and accessed percutaneous, and 2 Perclose devices placed. Next, a single deflection filter was placed in the aortic arch to reduce the risk of an ischemic stroke from the release of vascular debris during the TAVR procedure. The wire was then placed to the aortic arch and following dilation, a 14-French sheath inserted centrally following systemic heparinization. The aortic valve was crossed and the delivery system comprised of a balloon expandable stent that permitted the new valve to be precisely placed under rapid deployment. A balloon aortic valvuloplasty performed. An Edwards Intuity Elite bioprosthesis valve was then implanted and secured in place with three Ethibond stitches. This was completed under rapid ventricular pacing with contrast aortography identifying the aortic annulus and delivered through this location. Additional 2 mL of contrast was used to facilitate expansion of the valve, which resulted in a well-seated valve with trivial residual paravalvular insufficiency. Catheters were extracted and hemostasis was achieved with closure of the Perclose device following removal of sheaths and catheters within the right groin. Effects of heparin reversed with protamine. An additional Perclose device was used to facilitate hemostasis at the left femoral arterial access site. With assurance of hemostasis, the patient awoke in the operating room, transferred to the cardiac intensive care for recovery and care.

Principal Diagnosis: _____

Secondary Diagnoses: _____

Principal Procedure: _____

Secondary Procedure(s): _____

11

Indication for Surgery: Right shoulder symptomatic rotator cuff arthropathy

Preoperative Diagnosis: Right should rotator cuff tear complete

Postoperative Diagnosis: Same with morbid obesity with BMI of 44

Operation: Right reverse total should replacement including biceps long head biceps tendon, also included repair of rotator cuff, tenodesis and latissimus dorsi transfer

Assistant Surgeon: Necessary for careful retraction of neuro vasculature during component implantation and fixation

Findings: Total cuff tear arthropathy

Specimens: None

Complication: None apparent

Technique: The patient is a 61-year-old female who has continued shoulder weakness and pain. She has complete, end-stage rotator cuff tearing on her MRI. After discussion of the risks and benefits, she will proceed with the above-mentioned procedure. She understands risks may include but are not limited to infection, bleeding, injury blood vessel/nerve, blood clot, stiffness, failure of the prosthesis, fracture, dislocation, need for further surgery and other perioperative medical and surgical complications. Medical comorbidities are morbid obesity and a BMI of 44 that makes the surgery more difficult.

   After informed consent, the patient was brought to the operating room, placed in a well-padded beach chair position. All bony prominences were well-padded. Preoperative 3 g of IV Ancef had been administered within 1 hour of the skin incision. Timeout occurred identifying correct patient, site and procedure. Standard deltopectoral approach was performed to the shoulder. Full-thickness skin flaps were created. The cephalic vein was identified and protected. The biceps tendon sheath was opened and a tenodesis was performed to the superior border of the pectoralis major tendon with 0 Vicryl stitches. The remaining subscapularis was taken down anteriorly. The retractors were used to protect the surrounding neurovasculature and the humeral head cut was performed. There was minimal supra and infraspinatus remaining attached. The protection cap was placed on top of this and then the glenoid was exposed. The remnant of the labrum was excised. The long head biceps was released and a tenodesis was performed to the superior border of pectoralis major tendon. We placed her central guide-pin and over-reamed this on the glenoid. There was significant glenoid anteversion. We needed to augment this deformity. We prepared her glenoid for implantation size this to be a small and then implanted her actual glenoid with bone filling the central vault. Peripheral screws were also drilled measured and placed. We then placed our glenosphere. We then prepared our humerus. We used a canal finder followed by broached until we had appropriate fill and then trialed. We had the appropriate verse. We felt that the ten was most appropriate. We had difficulty initially reducing the should more proximal in order to do so. We then trialed and it had excellent range of motion of the construct, no impingement, and was stable. We then thoroughly irrigated the canal and implanted the actual prosthesis. We then re-trialed the poly and felt the +0 was most appropriate. We then cleared this and implanted her actual poly. We have performed a final reduction. The shoulder was then taken through final range of motion. The shoulder was quite stable with full flexion abduction external rotation. The axillary nerve was palpated and intact with tug test. There is no obvious impingement. The deltopectoral interval was closed with a running 0 Vicryl stitching. The subcutaneous was closed with inverted 2-0 Vicryl followed by a running 4-0 Monocryl and prineo for the skin. The wound was re-dressed with Telfa, gauze, foam tape and the arm was placed in the abduction pillow sling and the patient was transferred to the post anesthesia recovery unit in stable condition. Postop plan is the patient will follow up in the clinic in two weeks for anticipated wound check and x-rays. The patient is admitted to the floor and receive 24-hour prophylactic IV antibiotics with 3 g IV

Ancef every 8 hours. We will use aspirin 325 mg po daily for one month for DVT prophylaxis as well as SCDs and early mobilization.

Grafts/Implants: ExacTech equinoxe reverse total shoulder arthroplasty, 10mm press fit preserve humeral stem, 38 mm glenosphere with +0 liner.

Principal Diagnosis: _____

Secondary Diagnoses: _____

Principal Procedure: _____

Secondary Procedure(s): _____

12

Preoperative Diagnoses: 1. Large right renal pelvic stone. 2. Multiple medium-to-large non-obstructing calyceal stones.

Postoperative Diagnoses: Same

Procedure Performed: Renoscopy with pyelotomy, extraction of renal calculi

Indications for Procedure: A 68-year-old female who had presented with complaints of right flank pain. CT imaging had revealed a large stone obstructing the right renal pelvis. In addition to that, she had multiple stones in the mid-to-lower calyceal structures. The stones in the calyces were nonobstructing. She presents today for extraction of her large right renal pelvic stone. Additionally, renal endoscopy is being performed to remove her additional renal stones.

Procedure and Findings: The patient was brought to the operating room, received general anesthesia via an endotracheal tube, placed in a modified left flank position. Her lower chest and abdomen were prepped and draped in a sterile fashion. Abdomen was insufflated with CO2 via Veress needle. Laparoscopic robotic trocars had been placed. The assistant surgeon reflected the right colon exposing the right kidney. Dissection was carried out on the ureter and traced to the renal pelvis. Renal pelvis was opened and the assistant surgeon had extracted a large stone. Via this pyelotomy, a 16-French flexible cystoscopy was advanced across our laparoscopic trocar and into the renal pelvis. Under direct vision, the various infundibular and calyceal structures were inspected. Several medium stones were identified. These were snared within a stone basket and extracted. I noted there were additional stones in the lower pole, infundibulum and calyx. Again, the basket was used to extract the stones. At the conclusion of the renoscopy, it appeared that the patient was stone free. The assistant surgeon closed the pyelotomy. The patient was removed from anesthesia and transferred to the post anesthesia care unit. The patient will be admitted and evaluated in the morning for possible discharge.

Principal Diagnosis: _____

Secondary Diagnoses: _____

Principal Procedure: _____

Secondary Procedure(s): _____

13

Preoperative Diagnoses: History of perforated sigmoid diverticulitis

Postoperative Diagnoses: History of perforated sigmoid diverticulitis

Procedure Performed: Exploratory laparotomy, reversal of Hartmann's colostomy

Anesthesia: General

Indications: The patient is a 67-year-old female, who approximately four months ago, had perforated sigmoid colon requiring Hartmann's procedure. She now presents to the operating room for Hartmann's colostomy reversal. I have discussed this with the patient preoperatively and she understands and wishes to proceed.

Description of Procedure: The patient was brought to the operating room and placed on the operating table in supine position. General endotracheal anesthetics administered. Foley catheter was placed. The patient was placed in the Allen stirrups in the lithotomy position. There the abdomen and perineum were exposed, prepped and draped in sterile fashion. Midline laparotomy was re-incised from umbilicus down to pubis. Incision was carried through skin and subcutaneous tissue, as well as through midline fashion in the abdominal cavity. There is a mild amount of adhesions in her abdominal cavity, but these were taken down using sharp dissection. The area of the tissue leading up to the colostomy from inside the abdomen is freed up sharply. The skin level of the colostomy was incised circumferentially around the skin with skin around the colostomy and this tissue separate free from the subcutaneous tissue, muscle and fascia and the colostomy is reduced in the abdominal cavity. This does not require any additional mobilization of the more proximal descending colon, as this portion of colostomy was easily down at the pelvis and were actually able to resection about 8 cm of her colon going up into the colostomy. This portion of colon was cleaned up, transected, and then secured with purse string suture of 2-0 Prolene suture. The anvil of a 28 EEA device was delivered through this opening limb of the descending colon to prepare for anastomosis.

There the pelvis was then addressed. The rectal stump was easily seen as it had been tagged with Prolene sutures. The rectal stump was freed up. Mesorectum was freed up and ad additional portion of the most distal sigmoid at the end of the upper rectum was taken to ensure that we were in to the upper rectum. This was transected with a TA-60 stapler.

The EEA device was delivered trans-anally in the rectal stump. The spike was delivered through the rectal stump and secured to the anvil. The EEA device was closed down and fired creating 2 full-thickness donuts of tissue. This lays without undue tension. We actually insufflated air into the rectum with saline in the pelvis. There was no evidence of leak.

The areas of dissection were inspected. There were no bleeding points noted. After counts were correct, the abdominal contents replace and the midline fascia was closed. Prior of note is that prior to closing the midline fascia, the fascia, the ostomy site was closed by using figure-of-eight interrupted #1 Vicryl sutures. The midline fascia was closed using running #1 Vicryl sutures. Skin and subcutaneous tissue of the midline incision was closed. We irrigated and closed using surgical staples. The area of the ostomy site was packed with iodoform gauze.

Sterile dressings were applied. The patient was then extubated without difficulty and transferred to recovery room in stable manner. The patient tolerated the procedure well.

Principal Diagnosis: _____

Secondary Diagnoses: _____

Principal Procedure: _____

Secondary Procedure(s): _____

14

Preoperative Diagnoses: Loop ileostomy, status post sigmoid resection and status post closure of colo-vesical fistula

Postoperative Diagnoses: Same

Procedure Performed: Closure of loop ileostomy

Anesthesia: General

Indications: The patient has a transverse loop colostomy done after sigmoid resection for diverticulitis with an abscess and colo-vesical fistula. The conditions have healed and the patient consented to the closure of the loop ileostomy to return the GI tract to its normal state.

Description of Procedure: Under general anesthesia with the patient in supine position, the area was prepped and draped in the usual manner. An elliptical incision was made around the colostomy. This was carried through the subcutaneous tissue. The segment of the colon was excised and dissected free all the way down to the fascia. The ileum and colon were separated from the fascia and the peritoneum ant the adhesions were lysed under the peritoneal surface. After the loop was excised completely freed, a side-to-side anastomosis of the ileum and colon using the GIA 80 was done. Hemostasis was secured and the end was closed with TA 60. The closer was reinforced with 3-0 silk and the bowel was placed in the abdomen. The fascia was closed with continuous #1 PDS. The skin was packed open. The patient tolerated the procedure well and was sent to the recovery room in good condition.

Principal Diagnosis: _____

Secondary Diagnoses: _____

Principal Procedure: _____

Secondary Procedure(s): _____

15

Preoperative Diagnoses: Staph epidermis bacteremia, urinary tract infection,

Postoperative Diagnoses: Same

Procedure Performed: Remove right-sided Mediport, implantable VAD, with culture

Anesthesia: Local with IV sedation

Complications: None

Estimated blood loss: Minimal

Indications: This is a very pleasant patient with multiple medical morbidities who has had a recent stroke as the reason for a prior hospitalization. The patient has had a Mediport, that is a totally implanted VAD for long-term access for IV procedures. The patient at presentation to the hospital has had several sources of infection found, including urinary tract infection, but also has a Staph epidermis bacteremia. This made her Mediport suspect as the source of infection. She was started on IV antibiotics but after several days the blood cultures are still positive for Staph Epidermis. Therefore, we will remove the port. Procedure and risks are reviewed and informed consent obtained.

Description of Procedure: The patient was brought into the operating room on her bed. She was not moved as she has significant pain issues. Therefore, intravenous sedation was administered to the patient on her hospital bed. Broad-spectrum antibiotics were administered per Infectious Disease and then the right neck and chest were prepped and draped in a sterile fashion. The site of the right internal jugular Mediport was noted with the reservoir in the subclavicular area. This was infiltrated with 0.5% Marcaine with epinephrine. An elliptical incision was used to cut out the old scar. Dissection was carried down to a well-incorporated incorporating Mediport. This was removed in its entirety, intact, with the catheter intact as well. The tip of the catheter was cut off and placed in a sterile specimen cup and forwarded to Pathology for culture. The pressure was held in the area of the internal jugular entrance of the catheter for 10 minutes. Excellent hemostasis was achieved. Then, the site was irrigated and closed in two layers. Steri-strips and sterile dressings were applied. The patient was awakened and taken to the recovery room in stable condition. She tolerated the procedure well.

Code the diagnoses and procedure for this operative report

Principal Diagnosis: _____

Secondary Diagnoses: _____

Principal Procedure: _____

Secondary Procedure(s): _____

16

Preoperative Diagnoses: Limited motion of left knee due to postoperative adhesions in a patient status post left knee replacement. Mild joint effusion.

Postoperative Diagnoses: Same

Procedure: Manipulation of the left knee under anesthesia, followed by aspiration of the knee and injection of left knee with 10mL of 0.5% Marcaine solution

Anesthesia: General

Description of Procedure: With the patient under general anesthesia, the left knee was manipulated. Prior to manipulation the range of motion was from 0 to about 85 degrees. Following manipulation, the range of motion had improved from 0 to 120 degrees of flexion. With manipulation audible tearing of the scar tissue was noted. He tolerated the procedure well.

Then using aseptic technique, the left knee was aspirated with removal of 10 mL of blood tinged fluid. Then the left knee was injected with 10ccs of 0.5% Marcaine solution. Then sterile bandage was applied. He was lightened from anesthesia and transported to the recovery room. The patient had been admitted to inpatient care for recover and physical therapy prior to discharge. Blood loss was minimal.

Principal Diagnosis: _____

Secondary Diagnoses: _____

Principal Procedure: _____

Secondary Procedure(s): _____

17

Preoperative Diagnoses: History of bilateral breast carcinoma. Right central breast carcinoma excision two weeks ago, current condition, with positive margins. History of left breast carcinoma ten years ago.

Postoperative Diagnoses: Same

Procedure: Bilateral simple mastectomy

Anesthesia: General

Brief Operative History: The patient is a 68-year-old female who has been followed by our service for a number of years. She was diagnosed 10 years ago with a carcinoma in situ of the left breast. She underwent a wide excision and radiation therapy and has done well until a recent office visit revealed a palpable mass in the right breast. Core biopsy proven to be a carcinoma. MRI showed only the known tumor and we took her to surgery for a lumpectomy and a wide excision, re-excise the margins, and the final pathology came back positive margins and possibly 3 orientations. So, after a long discussion, she has elected to undergo bilateral simple, skin-sparing mastectomy to treat the bilateral problem. We are taking her to the operating room now. She has elected to not to undergo a reconstructive procedure at this time.

Description of Procedure: The patient was taken to the operating room. General anesthesia was induced. Her arms and legs were padded appropriately. SCDs applied, lower body Bair Hugger placed, and her entire upper torso was sterilely prepped and draped in usual fashion. Beginning on the left breast, an elliptical incision incorporating the nipple-areolar complex and the prior excisional scar was performed. Flaps were raised superiorly to the clavicle, medially to the midline, inferiorly to the inframammary fold, and laterally out to the latissimus dorsi muscle. The breast was then removed from the pectoralis major muscle incorporating the fascia, reflected laterally and truncated, marked for orientation, sent to patient for permanent section. Irrigation was performed. Hemostasis extensively achieved where necessary using electrocautery. There was no evidence of bleeding at the end of the case. Two drains were brought in through separate incisions. These were 10mm channel drains secured in place with silk suture. Subcutaneous tissue closed with 2-0 undyed Vicryl suture. Skin closed with monofilament self-locking Quill type suture.

We then went to the right breast and an elliptical incision incorporating the prior excisional biopsy scar in the nipple-areolar complex was performed. Again, flaps were raised superiorly to the clavicle, medically to the midline, inferiorly to the inframammary fold, and laterally out to the latissimus dorsi muscle. The breast was then removed from the pectoralis major muscle incorporating the fascia, reflected laterally and truncated. It was marked for orientation and taken to pathology where gross inspection demonstrated the cavity in the central aspect of the breast and the cavity was on the pectoralis major fascia. We took the fascia as the deep plane to the biopsy cavity. Irrigation was performed. Hemostasis was achieved where necessary using electrocautery. There was no evidence of bleeding at the end of the case. Two drains again were brought in through separate incisions. Again, 10 mm channel drains secured in place with silk suture. The subcutaneous tissue was closed with 2-0 undyed Vicryl suture. Skin closed with a monofilament Quill type suture. Benzoin, Steri-Strips and sterile dressings were applied and the patient was transferred to the recovery room in stable condition.

Principal Diagnosis: _____

Secondary Diagnoses: _____

Principal Procedure: _____

Secondary Procedure(s): _____

Answer Key

Chapter 1

Certain Infectious and Parasitic Diseases

1. **First-Listed Diagnosis:** **A56.09** Cervicitis, chlamydial

   Secondary Diagnoses: None indicated by the documentation provided

   Rationale: ICD-10-CM has a combination code that includes the diagnosis of cervicitis and the causative infectious agent chlamydia.

3. **First-Listed Diagnosis:** **B18.1** Hepatitis, viral, chronic, type B

   Secondary Diagnoses: **K74.60** Cirrhosis, liver;

   F11.21 Addiction, heroin, see Dependence, drug, opioid in remission

   Rationale: The suspected liver failure is not coded because conditions documented as suspected are not coded for outpatient encounters (ICD-10-CM coding guideline IV.H, *Uncertain diagnosis*). In addition, the long-term use of methadone is not coded separately – the Excludes1 note under code Z79.891, *Long term (current) use of opiate analgesic,* indicates that the "use of methadone for treatment of heroin addiction" (F11.2-) is not coded using Z79.891.

5. **First-Listed Diagnosis:** **A46** Erysipelas. Since "acute erysipelas cellulitis" is specified in the scenario, it is also possible to use Index term Cellulitis, erysipelatous *-see* Erysipelas.

   Secondary Diagnoses: None indicated by the documentation provided

   Principal Procedure: Central venous catheter insertion **02HV33Z**

Character	Code	Explanation
Section	0	Medical and Surgical
Body System	2	Heart and Great Vessels
Root Operation	H	Insertion
Body Part	V	Superior Vena Cava
Approach	3	Percutaneous
Device	3	Infusion Device
Qualifier	Z	No Qualifier

INDEX: Insertion of device in, Vena Cava, Superior 02HV

Secondary Procedure(s): None indicated by the documentation provided

Rationale: For the single diagnosis treated during this visit, see the Index entry term erysipelas, or the main term Cellulitis, subterm erysipelatous—*see* Erysipelas.

Insertion of central catheters is based on the end point of catheter placement. In this case, imaging indicated that the catheter tip was located in the superior vena cava, so that is the body part coded.

The group A beta-hemolytic *Streptococcus* is not coded as the causative organism because it was not verified.

7. **First-Listed Diagnosis:**   **A54.01** Urethritis, gonococcal; Cystitis, gonococcal

    Secondary Diagnoses: None indicated by the documentation provided

    Rationale: ICD-10-CM provides a combination code that includes both sites of the infection and the infectious organism.

9. **First-Listed Diagnosis:**   **G14** Syndrome, postpolio

    Secondary Diagnoses: None indicated by the documentation provided

    Rationale: Code B91, *Sequelae of poliomyelitis*, is not used since the specific diagnosis of postpolio syndrome is provided. There is an Excludes1 note present at B91 and G14 to indicate that these two codes may not be assigned together. Postpolio syndrome is a specific condition and is more descriptive of the patient than an unspecified sequela of poliomyelitis. For that reason, postpolio syndrome is coded to G14 instead of B91. The atrophy of the leg muscles is not coded separately as it is a symptom of the postpolio syndrome.

11. **Principal Diagnosis:**   **A41.59** Sepsis, Gram-negative (organism)

    Secondary Diagnoses: **N39.0** Infection, urinary (tract);

    B96.1 Infection, Klebsiella pneumoniae, as cause of disease classified elsewhere;

    E87.1 Hyponatremia;

    E87.6 Hypokalemia;

    C77.3 Metastasis, cancer, to specified site -*see* Neoplasm, secondary, by site. In the Table of Neoplasms, look for subterms lymph, gland (secondary), axilla. C77.3, *Secondary and unspecified malignant neoplasm of axilla and upper limb lymph nodes*, is in the column named Malignant Secondary;

    Z85.3 History, personal malignant neoplasm, breast

    (If information about the surgery [mastectomy, right or left] and acquired absence of breast is available, an additional code could be added, such as Z90.1-, *Acquired absence of breast and nipple*.)

    Principal Procedure: None Indicated by the documentation provided

    Secondary Procedure(s): None indicated by the documentation provided

Rationale: In the Index under the main term of Sepsis, there is no subterm for Klebsiella. However, Klebsiella is a Gram negative organism, so A41.59, *Other Gram-negative sepsis,* is chosen instead of A41.50, *Gram-negative sepsis, unspecified.*

Since the causative organism for the urinary tract infection was identified as Klebsiella pneumoniae, the coder must follow the instructional note under N39.0, *Urinary tract infection, site not specified,* to use an additional code to identify the infectious organism. The coder must use the main term Infection, and subterms Klebsiella pneumoniae NEC, as cause of disease classified elsewhere, to locate the additional code of B96.1, *Klebsiella pneumoniae as the cause of diseases classified elsewhere.*

If the coder uses the main term Infection, and subterm Klebsiella pneumoniae NEC without following the further subterm of *as cause of disease classified elsewhere*, the coder will be incorrectly led to assign A49.8, *Other bacterial infections of unspecified site*. A49.8 does not capture the fact that Klebsiella pneumoniae is the causative organism for the urinary tract infection, so it is not the correct code.

The hyponatremia and hypokalemia are coded as they were treated conditions.

The metastastic cancer of the axillary lymph nodes is coded since the patient underwent evaluation by an oncologist during her hospital stay. The patient's history of primary breast cancer is coded as Z85.3, *Personal history of malignant neoplasm of breast,* since the malignancy at the breast site has already been excised and no further treatment is being directed to that site. As ICD-10-CM coding guideline I.C.2.d, *Primary malignancy previously excised,* states: "When a primary malignancy has been previously excised or eradicated from its site and there is no further treatment directed to that site and there is no evidence of any existing primary malignancy at that site, a code from category Z85, Personal history of malignant neoplasm, should be used to indicate the former site of the malignancy."

13. **First-Listed Diagnosis:**   **B60.13** Keratoconjunctivitis, Acanthamoeba

    Secondary Diagnoses: None indicated by the documentation provided

Rationale: There was a single reason for the office visit that was found to be the keratoconjunctivitis that is coded as the first-listed diagnosis code.

15. **First-Listed Diagnosis:**   **A02.0** Gastroenteritis, due to, food poisoning -*see* Intoxication, foodborne. Intoxication, foodborne, due to, Salmonella, with, (gastro) enteritis

    Secondary Diagnoses: **E86.0** Dehydration

Rationale: The main reason for the emergency department encounter was determined to be the salmonella food poisoning that produced the complication of dehydration. ICD-10-CM has a combination code that identifies salmonella food poisoning with gastroenteritis, so an individual code for the gastroenteritis is not necessary. A secondary code for the dehydration is added to identify the complication of the food poisoning.

17. **Principal Diagnosis:**   **A37.01** Whooping cough due to Bordetella pertussis with pneumonia

    Secondary Diagnoses: None indicated by the documentation provided

    Principal Procedure: None indicated by the documentation provided

    Secondary Procedure(s):   None indicated by the documentation provided

Rationale: The child was in the hospital for a single reason, the diagnosis of whooping cough with complicating pneumonia. ICD-10-CM has a combination code to include both conditions. No other diagnoses were identified during the hospital stay. No procedures were performed.

19. **Principal Diagnosis:**   **A41.4**, Sepsis, Gram-negative, anaerobic

    Secondary Diagnoses: **K61.0** Abscess, perianal

    Principal Procedure: **0D9QXZZ** Incision, abscess -*see* Drainage. Drainage, anus

Character	Code	Explanation
Section	0	Medical and Surgical
Body System	D	Gastrointestinal System
Root Operation	9	Drainage
Body Part	Q	Anus
Approach	X	External
Device	Z	No Device
Qualifier	Z	No Qualifier

INDEX: Incision, abscess -*see* Drainage. Drainage, anus 0D9Q

Secondary Procedure(s): None indicated by the documentation provided

Rationale: *B. fragilis* is a Gram-negative anaerobic bacterium, so the correct principal diagnosis is A41.4, *Sepsis due to anaerobes*. Since the causative organism is already identified by A41.4, no additional code for the *B. fragilis* is needed.

The perianal abscess, which is the localized infection, is coded as a secondary diagnosis. ICD-10-CM coding guideline I.C.1.d.4, *Sepsis and severe sepsis with a localized infection*, states that the systemic infection (the sepsis) is coded first and the localized infection is coded as a secondary diagnosis.

The correct approach value for the incision and drainage of the perianal abscess is X, *External*. According to ICD-10-PCS coding guideline B5.3a: "Procedures performed within an orifice on structures that are visible without the aid of any instrumentation are coded to the approach External." Since the scenario specifies that the perianal abscess is visible just past the anal orifice, the approach to this abscess is External.

Chapter 2

Neoplasms

1. **Principal Diagnosis:** **C34.01** Carcinoma, bronchial or bronchogenic -*see* Neoplasm, lung, malignant. In the Table of Neoplasms: lung, main bronchus, malignant primary, which points to C34.0-. In the Tabular, C34.01 is the correct code for malignant neoplasm of right main bronchus.

   Secondary Diagnoses: **C79.51** Metastasis, metastatic, cancer, to specified site -*see* Neoplasm, secondary, by site. In the Table of Neoplasms: bone, malignant secondary;

   J43.9 Emphysema;

   Z87.891 History, personal, nicotine dependence

   Principal Procedure: Biopsy, *see* Excision with qualifier Diagnostic, Excision, Bronchus, Main, Right **0BB38ZX**

Character	Code	Explanation
Section	0	Medical and Surgical
Body System	B	Respiratory System
Root Operation	B	Excision
Body Part	3	Main Bronchus, Right
Approach	8	Via Natural or Artificial Opening Endoscopic
Device	Z	No Device
Qualifier	X	Diagnostic

INDEX: Excision, Bronchus, Main, Right 0BB3

Secondary Procedure(s): None indicated by the documentation provided

Rationale: The reason for admission was to evaluate the patient's lung disease, which was found to be complicated by the fact that the patient now had lung cancer proven by a bronchoscopic biopsy. Further imaging studies confirmed the presence of metastatic lesions in the bones. The patient's pre-existing conditions that were relevant to this hospital admission were also coded, including the emphysema and the history of smoking. The biopsy is coded in ICD-10-PCS as an excision procedure of the site with the qualifier of X to indicate the excision was a diagnostic procedure. The nuclear medicine bone scan may be coded according to department policy of the types of surgical versus diagnostic procedures to be coded.

3. **Principal Diagnosis:**   **E86.0** Dehydration

   Secondary Diagnoses: **E87.1** Hyponatremia

   C18.7 Carcinoma, intestinal type, specified site – *see* Neoplasm, malignant, by site. In the Table of Neoplasms: colon *-see also* Neoplasm, intestine, large. Intestine, large, colon, sigmoid, malignant primary;

   C78.7 Metastasis, cancer, to specified site *-see* Neoplasm, secondary, by site. In the Table of Neoplasms: liver, malignant, secondary;

   Z51.5 Palliative care;

   Z66 DNR (do not resuscitate)

   Principal Procedure: None indicated by the documentation provided

   Secondary Procedure(s):   None indicated by the documentation provided

   Rationale: The scenario specifies that the focus of the treatment was the dehydration that is due to the malignancy, so E86.0 is the principal diagnosis. As ICD-10-CM coding guideline I.C.2.c.3, *Management of dehydration due to the malignancy,* states: "When the admission/encounter is for management of dehydration due to the malignancy and only the dehydration is being treated (intravenous rehydration), the dehydration is sequenced first, followed by the code(s) for the malignancy."

   The *Use additional* note at E86 instructs the coder to code "any associated disorders of electrolyte and acid-base balance (E87.-)". Therefore, we assign an additional code for the hyponatremia, E87.1.

   The patient chose palliative care and a do-not-resuscitate status prior to being discharged home, so an encounter code for palliative care and a DNR status code are also assigned. No procedures were performed.

5. **First-Listed Diagnosis:**   **C53.9** Carcinoma *-see also* Neoplasm, by site, malignant. In the Table of Neoplasms: cervix, malignant primary

   Secondary Diagnoses: None indicated by the documentation provided

   Principal Procedure: Conization, cervix *see* Excision, Cervix **0UBC8ZX**

Character	Code	Explanation
Section	0	Medical and Surgical
Body System	U	Female Reproductive System
Root Operation	B	Excision
Body Part	C	Cervix
Approach	8	Via Natural or Artificial Opening Endoscopic
Device	Z	No Device
Qualifier	X	Diagnostic

   INDEX: Conization, cervix *see* Excision, Cervix 0UBC

   Secondary Procedure(s):   None indicated by the documentation provided

   Rationale: The patient's diagnosis of cancer of the uterine cervix was confirmed by the procedure. The procedure coded is excision as only part of the cervix was removed. The approach is Via Natural or Artificial Opening Endoscopic" due to the fact that a colposcope was utilized.

7. **First-Listed Diagnosis:**   **C43.39** Melanoma (malignant), skin, forehead

   Secondary Diagnoses: **Z80.8** History, family, malignant neoplasm, specified site NEC;

   Z77.123 Exposure, radiation, naturally occurring NEC

Rationale: Although there was no more malignant tissue found, because the treatment was directed at the site of the melanoma, the code for the malignant melanoma is assigned as the first-listed diagnosis. As ICD-10-CM coding guideline I.C.2.m, *Current malignancy versus personal history of malignancy,* states: "When a primary malignancy has been excised but further treatment, such as an additional surgery for the malignancy…is directed to that site, the primary malignancy code should be used until treatment is completed."

The other conditions or facts relevant to the scenario, namely, the family history of skin cancer and the extensive exposure to radiation from the sun, are coded as additional diagnoses. The outpatient surgical procedure would be coded with CPT procedure codes by the outpatient coders.

9. **First-Listed Diagnosis:** **C79.51** Metastasis, cancer, to specified site -*see* Neoplasm, secondary, by site. In the Tabular: bone, malignant, secondary

   Secondary Diagnoses: **C79.31** Metastasis, cancer, to specified site -*see* Neoplasm, secondary, by site. In the Tabular: brain, malignant secondary;

   C50.912 Cancer, breast -*see also* Neoplasm, breast, malignant C50.91-. In the Tabular: left female breast;

   Z51.5 Palliative care

Rationale: This is not an admission for chemotherapy as the Aredia is used for palliative treatment of bone metastases and not to treat the cancer. The metastatic site of bone cancer is listed first as it is the site where treatment was directed during this encounter. The other metastatic site and the primary site of the malignancy are also coded. The procedure for chemotherapy for an outpatient would be coded with CPT or HCPCS by the outpatient coders.

11. **Principal Diagnosis:** **C18.4** Malignancy -*see also* Neoplasm, malignant, by site. In the Table of Neoplasms: colon -*see also* Neoplasm, intestine, large. Neoplasm, intestine, large, colon, transverse, malignant, primary

    Secondary Diagnoses: **D63.0** Anemia, in, neoplastic disease

    Principal Procedure: Transfusion, Vein, Peripheral, Blood, Red Cells **30233N1**

Character	Code	Explanation
Section	3	Administration
Body System	0	Circulatory
Root Operation	2	Transfusion
Body System/Region	3	Peripheral Vein
Approach	3	Percutaneous
Substance	N	Red Blood Cells
Qualifier	1	Nonautologous

INDEX: Transfusion, Vein, Peripheral, Blood, Red Cells 3023

Secondary Procedure(s): None indicated by the documentation provided

Rationale: The reason for admission was the management of anemia and the anemia was the only condition treated, but ICD-10-CM coding guideline I.C.2.c.1, *Anemia associated with malignancy,* states that "When admission/ encounter is for management of an anemia associated with the malignancy, and the treatment is only for anemia, the appropriate code for the malignancy is sequenced as the principal or first-listed diagnosis followed by the appropriate code for the anemia (such as code D63.0, *Anemia in neoplastic disease*). Also, at code D63.0 in the Tabular there is a note to "*Code first* neoplasm (C00-D49)".

The transfusion code in ICD-10-PCS is found under the main term of Transfusion in the Index. The coder must know the site of the administration (in this scenario, the peripheral vein) and the substance infused (in this scenario, nonautologous red blood cells).

13. **Principal Diagnosis:**   **C71.3** Glioblastoma (multiforme), giant cell, specified site -*see* Neoplasm, malignant, by site. In the Table of Neoplasms: brain, parietal lobe, malignant, primary

    Secondary Diagnoses: **C78.01** Metastasis, cancer, to specified site -*see* Neoplasm, secondary, by site. In the Table of Neoplasms: Neoplasm, lung, malignant, secondary. In the Tabular: right lung;

            F17.210 Dependence, drug, nicotine, cigarettes

            R73.03 Prediabetes

    Principal Procedure: Biopsy, *see* Excision with qualifier Diagnostic. In the Body Part Key, there is an instruction to use Body Part *cerebral hemisphere* for *parietal lobe*. Excision, Cerebral Hemisphere **00B73ZX**

Character	Code	Explanation
Section	0	Medical and Surgical
Body System	0	Central Nervous System and Cranial Nerves
Root Operation	B	Excision
Body Part	7	Cerebral Hemisphere
Approach	3	Percutaneous
Device	Z	No Device
Qualifier	X	Diagnostic

INDEX: Biopsy, *see* Excision with qualifier Diagnostic. In the Body Part Key, there is an instruction to use Body Part *cerebral hemisphere* for *parietal lobe*. Excision, Cerebral Hemisphere **00B7**

Secondary Procedure(s): Biopsy, *see* Excision with qualifier Diagnostic. Excision, Lung, Right **0BBK8ZX**

Character	Code	Explanation
Section	0	Medical and Surgical
Body System	B	Respiratory System
Root Operation	B	Excision
Body Part	K	Lung, Right
Approach	8	Via Natural or Artificial Opening Endoscopic
Device	Z	No Device
Qualifier	X	Diagnostic

INDEX: Biopsy, *see* Excision with qualifier Diagnostic. Excision, Lung, Right 0BBK

Rationale: After study, it was concluded that the patient's symptoms were caused by the glioblastoma. Other studies identified metastases to the right lung. The other conditions addressed during this hospital stay were the nicotine dependence and the prediabetes. Two procedures were performed, both diagnostic procedures. The closed biopsy of the parietal area of the brain was done through a burr hole, which is a Percutaneous (through the skin) approach, with the 7th character of X for Diagnostic. The second procedure was a bronchoscopy with a biopsy of the right lung, which is an Excision with an approach of Via Natural or Artificial Opening Endoscopic, and the 7th character of X for Diagnostic.

15. **First-Listed Diagnosis:**   **C50.912** Cancer *-see also* Neoplasm, by site, malignant. In the Table of Neoplasms: breast, malignant primary. In the Tabular: left female breast

   Secondary Diagnoses: **Z17.0** Status, estrogen receptor, positive;

   Z79.899 Long-term drug therapy, drug, specified NEC;

   Z92.21 History, personal, chemotherapy for neoplastic condition;

   Z92.3 History, personal, radiation therapy

Rationale: The breast cancer is still coded as a currently existing condition, not a history of breast cancer, because the disease is still under treatment with the Herceptin. The positive estrogen receptor status and the patient's history of completed chemotherapy and radiation therapy are relevant secondary diagnoses to be coded.

17. **Principal Diagnosis:**   **C50.211** Carcinoma *-see also* Neoplasm, by site, malignant. In the Table of Neoplasms: breast, upper-inner quadrant, malignant primary. In the Tabular: right female breast

   Secondary Diagnoses: **Z80.3** History, family, malignant neoplasm, breast

   Principal Procedure: Lumpectomy *see* Excision, Breast, Right **0HBT0ZZ**

Character	Code	Explanation
Section	0	Medical and Surgical
Body System	H	Skin and Breast
Root Operation	B	Excision
Body Part	T	Breast, Right
Approach	0	Open
Device	Z	No Device
Qualifier	Z	No Qualifier

INDEX: Lumpectomy *see* Excision, Breast, Right 0HBT

Secondary Procedure(s): None indicated by the documentation provided

Rationale: The patient was admitted for the sole purpose of performing the lumpectomy for the suspected carcinoma of the breast that was confirmed by pathological diagnosis. The family history of breast cancer in this patient is relevant and used as an additional diagnosis code. A lumpectomy is known to be a partial excision of the breast, not a total removal of the breast. Therefore, the ICD-10-PCS definition of excision meets the description of this procedure and is coded. The lumpectomy is a therapeutic procedure to remove the breast tissue, not a diagnostic procedure.

19. **Principal Diagnosis:**   **D09.0** Carcinoma-in-situ *-see also* Neoplasm, in situ, by site. In the Table of Neoplasms: bladder, wall, anterior/lateral, Ca in situ

   Secondary Diagnoses: **E11.9** Diabetes, type 2;

   I10 Hypertension

   Principal Procedure: Fulguration *see* Destruction, Bladder **0T5B8ZZ**

Character	Code	Explanation
Section	0	Medical and Surgical
Body System	T	Urinary System
Root Operation	5	Destruction

Character	Code	Explanation
Body Part	B	Bladder
Approach	8	Via Natural or Artificial Opening Endoscopic
Device	Z	No Device
Qualifier	Z	No Qualifier

INDEX: Fulguration *see* Destruction, Bladder 0T5B

Secondary Procedure: Biopsy, *see* Excision with qualifier Diagnostic, Bladder **0TBB8ZX**

Character	Code	Explanation
Section	0	Medical and Surgical
Body System	T	Urinary system
Root Operation	B	Excision
Body Part	B	Bladder
Approach	8	Via Natural or Artificial Opening Endoscopic
Device	Z	No Device
Qualifier	X	Diagnostic

INDEX: Biopsy, *see* Excision with qualifier Diagnostic, Bladder 0TBB

Rationale: The reason for admission after study and the reason for the procedures was the carcinoma *in situ* of the bladder that is coded as D09.0 regardless of the site treated within the bladder. The patient was also treated for his established type 2 diabetes and hypertension. If documentation in the health record confirmed the patient's diabetes is treated with oral hypoglycemic drugs, code Z79.84 would be assigned. There is no mention of treatment with insulin either. The procedures were performed as a transurethral endoscopic procedure, which would be coded with Approach value 8 for Via Natural or Artificial Opening Endoscopic. The fulguration of the bladder tumor is coded to the root operation of Destruction in ICD-10-PCS. The biopsy of the second site within the bladder is coded to the root operation of Excision with the seventh character using the Diagnostic X character.

21. **Principal Diagnosis:** C76.3 Cancer -*see also* Neoplasm, by site, malignant. In Table of Neoplasms: pelvic, wall

   Secondary Diagnoses: None indicated by the documentation provided

   Principal Procedure: Excision, Retroperitoneum **0WBH0ZZ**

Character	Code	Explanation
Section	0	Medical and Surgical
Body System	W	Anatomical Regions, General
Root Operation	B	Excision
Body Part	H	Retroperitoneum
Approach	0	Open
Device	Z	No Device
Qualifier	Z	No Qualifier

INDEX: Excision, Retroperitoneum 0WBH

Secondary Procedure: Brachytherapy, CivaSheet®, *see* Brachytherapy with qualifier Unidirectional Source. Brachytherapy, Pelvic Region **DW16BB1**

Character	Code	Explanation
Section	D	Radiation Therapy
Body System	W	Anatomical Regions
Modality	1	Brachytherapy
Treatment Site	6	Pelvic Region
Modality Qualifier	B	Low Dose Rate (LDR)
Isotope	B	Palladium 103
Qualifier	1	Unidirectional Source

INDEX: Brachytherapy, CivaSheet®, *see* Brachytherapy with qualifier Unidirectional Source. Brachytherapy, Pelvic Region DW16

Secondary Procedure: Brachytherapy, CivaSheet®, *see* Insertion with device Radioactive Element. Insertion of device in, Retroperitoneum **0WHH01Z**

Character	Code	Explanation
Section	0	Medical and Surgical
Body System	W	Anatomical Regions, General
Root Operation	H	Insertion
Body Part	H	Retroperitoneum
Approach	0	Open
Device	1	Radioactive Element
Qualifier	Z	No Qualifier

INDEX: Brachytherapy, CivaSheet®, *see* Insertion with device Radioactive Element. Insertion of device in, Retroperitoneum 0WHH

Rationale: According to Coding Clinic First Quarter 2019, page 27, pelvic sidewall should be coded using the Body Part *retroperitoneum*. Therefore, the excision of the left pelvic sidewall tumor is coded using root operation Excision and Body Part value H, Retroperitoneum.

ICD-10-PCS guideline D1.a explains that brachytherapy with insertion of a radioactive brachytherapy source left in the body at the end of the procedure is coded with two procedure codes:

1. A brachytherapy code from section D, Radiation Therapy, identifying the treatment site, with the modality Brachytherapy, and the modality qualifier, isotope, and qualifier values appropriate for the case

2. A code from the Medical and Surgical section for the Insertion of the device, using device value Radioactive Element

According to ICD-10-PCS guideline D1.a, two codes are needed because the "Radiation Therapy section code identifies the specific modality and isotope of the brachytherapy," while the "Insertion code identifies the implantation of the brachytherapy source that remains in the body at the end of the procedure."

The CivaSheet® applied to the pelvic sidewall is described in the given scenario as a low dose rate unidirectional brachytherapy device containing palladium 103, so this information is used to choose the correct character values for Modality (Brachytherapy), Treatment Site (Pelvic Region), Modality Qualifier (Low Dose Rate), Isotope (Palladium 103), and Qualifier (Unidirectional Source) to arrive at the brachytherapy code DW16BB1.

To code the insertion of the CivaSheet® device, we follow the Coding Clinic advice referred to above and select Body Part value H, Retroperitoneum for the pelvic sidewall. Although there is a Body Part value in Table 0WH for Pelvic Cavity (value J), we follow the Coding Clinic instruction in this case and choose Retroperitoneum for the Body Part. For Device, value 1, Radioactive Element, should be chosen as that is what the Index instructs.

Chapter 3

Diseases of Blood and Blood-forming Organs and Certain Disorders Involving the Immune Mechanism

1. **Principal Diagnosis:**   **D57.811** Disease, sickle cell Hb-SE, with crisis, with acute chest syndrome

   Secondary Diagnoses: None indicated by the documentation provided

   Principal Procedure: None indicated by the documentation provided

   Secondary Procedure(s):   None indicated by the documentation provided

   Rationale: The patient was admitted with consequences of his known Hb-SE sickle cell disease. ICD-10-CM provides a combination code that includes the type of sickle cell disease as well as the acute chest syndrome due to the sickle cell crisis that prompted the hospital admission in this scenario.

3. **Principal Diagnosis:**   **D50.9** Anemia, iron deficiency

   Secondary Diagnoses: None indicated by the documentation provided

   Principal Procedure: Bone marrow biopsy **07DR3ZX**

Character	Code	Explanation
Section	0	Medical and Surgical
Body System	7	Lymphatic and Hemic Systems
Root Operation	D	Extraction
Body Part	R	Bone Marrow, Iliac
Approach	3	Percutaneous
Device	Z	No Device
Qualifier	X	Diagnostic

INDEX: Extraction, bone marrow, iliac

   Secondary Procedure(s):   None indicated by the documentation provided

   Rationale: The coding in this exercise is limited to the coding of the diagnosis established and the procedure provided by the consultant. The single diagnosis of iron deficiency anemia is coded. The procedure for a bone marrow biopsy is an extraction of bone marrow from the iliac as the root operation is defined in ICD-10-PCS. Biopsy is not coded as an excision because it does not meet the definition of excision in ICD-10-PCS—that is, cutting out a portion of a body part. Aspiration is not the root operation for this case because it does not meet the definition of taking or letting out fluids or gasses from a body part. In this example, the bone marrow is extracted or pulled out of a body part.

5. **Principal Diagnosis:**   **D59.1** Anemia, hemolytic, autoimmune

   Secondary Diagnoses: **M32.9** Lupus, erythematous, systemic

   Principal Procedure: Splenectomy **07TP0ZZ**

Character	Code	Explanation
Section	0	Medical and Surgical
Body System	7	Lymphatic and Hemic Systems
Root Operation	T	Resection
Body Part	P	Spleen
Approach	0	Open
Device	Z	No Device
Qualifier	Z	No Qualifier

INDEX: Splenectomy, see Resection, Spleen

Secondary Procedure(s): None indicated by the documentation provided

Rationale: The patient was admitted to the hospital for surgery (splenectomy) as treatment for the patient's autoimmune hemolytic anemia. The patient's underlying condition of systemic lupus erythematosus was also treated and therefore coded as a secondary diagnosis. The splenectomy, or the removal of the entire spleen, meets the definition of resection in ICD-10-PCS and is coded using the main term in the Index that refers the coder to resection, spleen and table 07TP. No code is assigned for the long term use of prednisone since it had been stopped for several months.

7. **First-Listed Diagnosis:** **K29.40** Gastritis, atrophic (chronic) (without bleeding)

   Secondary Diagnoses: **D51.0** Anemia, pernicious;

   D80.1 Agammaglobulinemia

Rationale: The patient's complaint of chest pain was attributed to her chronic atrophic gastritis that is then the main reason for the outpatient visit and listed as the first-listed diagnosis code. The patient's other medical conditions that were evaluated were also coded as secondary diagnoses.

9. **Principal Diagnosis:** **D66** Hemophilia, A

   Secondary Diagnoses: **M36.2** Arthritis, in hemophilia NEC

   Principal Procedure: Therapeutic plasmapheresis **6A550Z3**

Character	Code	Explanation
Section	6	Extracorporeal or Systemic Therapies
Physiological Systems	A	Physiological Systems
Root Operation	5	Pheresis
Body System	5	Circulatory
Duration	0	Single
Qualifier	Z	No Qualifier
Qualifier	3	Plasma

INDEX: Plasmapheresis, therapeutic

Secondary Procedure(s): None indicated by the documentation provided

Rationale: The reason for admission after study was for the patient's first course of plasmapheresis or extracorporeal immunoadsorption. The condition requiring treatment by plasmapheresis was the patient's hemophilia A condition.

The patient also had arthritis due to the hemophilia, which was evaluated during the hospital stay. The procedure performed is coded using the main term of plasmapheresis, which was a single treatment during this hospital stay.

11. **Principal Diagnosis:**   **L89.153** Ulcer, pressure, sacral, stage 3

    Secondary Diagnoses: **L89.212** Ulcer, pressure, hip, stage 2 (6th character of 2 for right hip);

    R15.9 Incontinence, feces;

    D62 Anemia, posthemorrhagic, acute;

    E11.9 Diabetes, type 2;

    I10 Hypertension;

    M47.26 Osteoarthritis, spine, see Spondylosis with radiculopathy (back pain), lumbar region

    G89.29, Pain, chronic, specified NEC (back)

    Principal Procedure: Diverting colostomy **0D1M0Z4**

Character	Code	Explanation
Section	0	Medical and Surgical
Body System	D	Gastrointestinal System
Root Operation	1	Bypass
Body Part	M	Descending Colon
Approach	0	Open
Device	Z	No Device
Qualifier	4	Cutaneous

INDEX: Colostomy, see Bypass, gastrointestinal system

Secondary Procedure: Blood transfusion, red cells **30233N1**

Character	Code	Explanation
Section	3	Administration
Physiological System	0	Circulatory
Root Operation	2	Transfusion
Body Part	3	Peripheral Vein
Approach	3	Percutaneous
Substance	N	Red Blood Cells
Qualifier	1	Nonautologous

INDEX: Transfusion, vein, peripheral, blood, red cells

Rationale: The principal diagnosis assigned to this case could be debated as either the anemia or the pressure ulcers and could be different in another patient with a similar scenario. In this scenario it was thought that the pressure ulcers were the reason the patient was admitted to the hospital. The ulcers were bleeding, causing the anemia and complicated by the fecal incontinence, which could not be controlled, that was further damaging her skin and pressure ulcers. For this reason, the colostomy was done to eliminate the fecal incontinence and prevent further damage to the skin and the pressure ulcers, which would hopefully heal and no longer bleed, eliminating the anemia. The patient's other conditions were evaluated and treated during the hospital stay, so all were coded as secondary diagnoses. If the documentation in the record identified the type of medication used to treat the diabetes, a code for insulin use or oral hypoglycemic drugs would be assigned. The colostomy meets the definition of bypass in ICD-10-PCS to alter the route of a tubular body part, the descending colon. The approach was Open and the end point of the colostomy was the skin or cutaneous tissue identified in the 7th character for a qualifier. A transfusion was also completed and coded as a secondary procedure using the main term transfusion through a peripheral vein. Whether or not transfusions are coded in the inpatient setting will be determined by facility-specific guidelines.

13. **First-Listed Diagnosis:**   **N18.6** Disease, renal, end stage

    Secondary Diagnoses: **D63.1** Anemia, in, end-stage renal disease;

                                    Z99.2 Dependence, on, renal dialysis

Rationale: In this scenario, it appears the main reason for the outpatient visit was to receive treatment for the anemia due to the ESRD. However, there is a Tabular instruction note under code D63.1 to code first the underlying chronic kidney disease. For this reason, the N18.6 code for ESRD is assigned as the first-listed code and the anemia and dependence on dialysis are coded as secondary diagnoses.

15. **Principal Diagnosis:**   **R55** Syncope

    Secondary Diagnoses: **D56.1** Thalassemia, beta, major

    Principal Procedure: Blood transfusion, red cells **30233N1**

Character	Code	Explanation
Section	3	Administration
Physiological System	0	Circulatory
Root Operation	2	Transfusion
Body Part	3	Peripheral Vein
Approach	3	Percutaneous
Substance	N	Red Blood Cells
Qualifier	1	Nonautologous

INDEX: Transfusion, vein, peripheral, blood, red cells

Secondary Procedure(s): None indicated by the documentation provided

Rationale: The cause for the syncope could not be determined and was not thought to be caused by the thalassemia and, therefore, the symptom code of syncope is listed as the principal diagnosis. The secondary diagnosis of thalassemia is listed as a diagnosis code. The patient's other symptoms (splenomegaly, fatigue, and reduced appetite) are classic symptoms of the thalassemia and therefore not coded. The procedure of the transfusion of the packed red blood cells is coded under the root operation of administration. Coding of transfusions will be based on facility-specific coding guidelines.

17. **Principal Diagnosis:**   **D50.8** Anemia, nutritional, with poor iron absorption

    Secondary Diagnoses: **H25.9** Cataract, senile

    Principal Procedure: None indicated by the documentation provided

    Secondary Procedure(s): None indicated by the documentation provided

Rationale: The reason for the clinic visit was to investigate his abnormal hematocrit that proved to be nutritional anemia with poor iron absorption. The physician documented the senile cataract as a current condition.

Chapter 4

Endocrine, Nutritional, and Metabolic Diseases

1. **Principal Diagnosis:**   **E10.65** Diabetes mellitus, type 1, with, hyperglycemia

   Secondary Diagnoses: **E10.3299** Diabetes mellitus, type 1 with retinopathy, nonproliferative, mild

   Principal Procedure: None indicated by the documentation provided

   Secondary Procedure(s):   None indicated by the documentation provided

   Rationale: The patient was admitted with diabetes that was found after study to be uncontrolled. Diabetes found to be out of control is coded to diabetes by type with hyperglycemia. There is an Index entry for diabetes, out of control, code to Diabetes, by type, with hyperglycemia. The patient also has retinopathy due to her diabetes that is found under Index term diabetes, type 1, with retinopathy, nonproliferative, mild. Although not addressed in the guideline, code Z79.4, long term (current) use of insulin, is not assigned with codes from E10 for type 1 diabetes mellitus. Instead the classification provides a use additional code note to identify any insulin use in all the diabetes categories with the exception of E10 for type 1 diabetes mellitus. The Z79.4 code would not be assigned with type 1 cases because insulin is required or expected to be used with type 1 diabetic patients.

3. **Principal Diagnosis:**   **T85.614A** Complication, insulin pump, mechanical breakdown, initial encounter

   Secondary Diagnoses: **T38.3X6A** Table of Drugs and Chemicals, insulin, underdosing, initial encounter;
   E10.10 Diabetes, type 1, with, ketoacidosis

   Principal Procedure: None indicated by the documentation provided

   Secondary Procedure(s):   None indicated by the documentation provided

   Rationale: The reason for admission after study was the fact the insulin pump had a mechanical breakdown that is coded as a complication of the device. This was the initial encounter for treatment so the 7th character of A is used. The fact the insulin pump was not working produced the ketoacidosis because not enough insulin was being administered. This produced a clinical scenario of underdosing of the insulin. The underdosing of insulin code is found in the Table of Drugs and Chemical under "insulin" with the code chosen from the underdosing column. Seventh character of "A" is used as this is the initial encounter for the care related to the underdosing. The patient had diabetic ketoacidosis as a result and this was coded as a secondary code.

5. **First-Listed Diagnosis:**   **E21.0** Hyperparathyroidism, primary

   Secondary Diagnoses: **D35.1** Adenoma, see Neoplasm, benign by site—Neoplasm, parathyroid, benign

   Rationale: The reason for the visit was evaluation of the abnormal test results that were determined to be caused by the primary hyperparathyroidism. The patient is also known to have the parathyroid adenoma that was addressed with the discussion about surgery.

7. **Principal Diagnosis:**   **E10.65** Diabetes mellitus, type 1, with, hyperglycemia

   Secondary Diagnoses: None indicated by the documentation provided

   Principal Procedure: Insertion of device (insulin pump) subcutaneous abdominal tissue **0JH80VZ**

Character	Code	Explanation
Section	0	Medical and Surgical
Body System	J	Subcutaneous Tissue and Fascia
Root Operation	H	Insertion

Body Part	8	Subcutaneous Tissue and Fascia, Abdomen
Approach	0	Open
Device	V	Infusion Device, Pump
Qualifier	Z	No Qualifier

INDEX: Insertion of device in, subcutaneous tissue and fascia, abdomen

Secondary Procedure: Injection of insulin **3E013VG**

Character	Code	Explanation
Section	3	Administration
Physiological systems	E	Physiological Systems and Anatomical Regions
Root Operation	0	Introduction
Body System/Region	1	Subcutaneous Tissue
Approach	3	Percutaneous
Substance	V	Hormone
Qualifier	G	Insulin

INDEX: Introduction of substance in or on subcutaneous tissue (hormone) insulin

Rationale: The only reason for admission after study was to insert an insulin pump to help take care of the patient's uncontrolled, hyperglycemic, type 1 diabetes. The uncontrolled status is coded to diabetes with hyperglycemia. There were no other complications documented for this encounter. The placement of the insulin pump meets the definition of insertion of a device in ICD-10-PCS. The device is inserted into the subcutaneous tissue of the abdomen or trunk. The injection of insulin is coded in this example as performed as part of the insertion of the insulin pump. The assignment of this procedure code may or may not be coded according to facility-specific guidelines.

9. **Principal Diagnosis:** **E66.01** Obesity, morbid

   Secondary Diagnoses: **I10** Hypertension;

   E11.44 Diabetes, type 2, with, amyotrophy;

   E78.5 Dyslipidemia;

   Z96.653 Presence, knee joint implant (bilateral);

   Z68.43 Body mass index adult 50–59

   Principal Procedure: Gastric banding **0DV64CZ**

Character	Code	Explanation
Section	0	Medical and Surgical
Body System	D	Gastrointestinal System
Root Operation	V	Restriction
Body Part	6	Stomach
Approach	4	Percutaneous Endoscopic

Device	C	Extraluminal Device
Qualifier	Z	No Qualifier

INDEX: Banding, see Restriction, stomach; insertion of port is part of procedure

Secondary Procedure(s): None indicated by the documentation provided

Rationale: The patient's reason for admission after study was the morbid obesity to be treated with the gastric banding procedure. The patient's multiple other conditions were evaluated or treated during the hospital stay and coded as secondary diagnoses. In ICD-10-PCS, the gastric banding procedure meets the definition of restriction of the body part of stomach. The banding is done with an extraluminal device placed internally on the outside of the stomach organ. This procedure was done laparoscopically, so the approach is listed as percutaneous endoscopic.

11. **Principal Diagnosis:**   **E89.1** Postprocedural hypoinsulinemia

    Secondary Diagnoses: **E13.9** Diabetes, secondary or Diabetes, postpancreatectomy, see Diabetes, specified type NEC;

    Z90.411 Absence, pancreas, acquired, partial;

    Z79.4 Long term use of drug, insulin

    Principal Procedure: None indicated by the documentation provided

    Secondary Procedure(s):   None indicated by the documentation provided

    Rationale: The patient's type of diabetes is a "secondary" type as the result of his partial pancreatectomy. The guidelines concerning secondary diabetes mellitus due to pancreatectomy state the hypoinsulinemia is listed first followed by the diabetes code (Guideline I.C.4.a.6.b.i). Other conditions are coded as secondary diagnosis including the absence of part of the pancreas and the long term use of insulin.

13. **Principal Diagnosis:**   **E11.11** Diabetes, type 2, with, ketoacidosis, with coma

    Secondary Diagnoses: **E11.21** Diabetes, type 2, with, nephropathy;

    E11.3419 Diabetes, type 2, with, retinopathy, nonproliferative, severe, with macular edema;

    N39.0 Infection, urinary tract;

    B96.20 Infection, Escherichia coli (E. Coli), as cause of disease classified elsewhere;

    Z87.440 History, personal, urinary tract infection;

    F10.229 Dependence, alcohol, with, intoxication;

    Z91.19 Noncompliance, with, medical treatment

    Principal Procedure: None indicated by the documentation provided

    Secondary Procedure(s):   None indicated by the documentation provided

    Rationale: While the patient had several complications of her diabetes mellitus, the reason for admission after study for this hospital stay was the diabetic ketoacidosis as documented by the physician. Multiple diabetes codes can be used to identify the various organ systems affected. The alcohol dependence was coded with intoxication as evidenced by the positive blood alcohol level.

15. **Principal Diagnosis:**   **E76.1** Mucopolysaccharidosis, type II; Syndrome, Hunter's

    Secondary Diagnoses: None indicated by the documentation provided

    Principal Procedure: None indicated by the documentation provided

    Secondary Procedure(s):   None indicated by the documentation provided

Rationale: The single diagnosis coded, the principal diagnosis, is E76.1 for Mucopolysaccharidosis which is the main term that can be used in the Index. The main term of syndrome, Hunter's may also be used. The symptoms described are known to be due to the condition identified and therefore not coded separately.

17. **Principal Diagnosis:**   **E11.52** Diabetes, type 2, gangrene

    Secondary Diagnoses: **E11.3599** Diabetes, type 2, retinopathy, proliferative

    Principal Procedure: None indicated by the documentation provided

    Secondary Procedure(s):   None indicated by the documentation provided

Rationale: ICD-10-CM provides combination codes for the diabetes with gangrene and the diabetes with proliferative retinopathy with no required additional codes. The combination code includes both conditions in one code. The diabetic gangrene code is listed first as it is the focus of attention on the day of the visit.

19. **Principal Diagnosis:**   **K95.09** Complication, gastric band procedure

    Secondary Diagnoses: **E66.9** Obesity;

                                       Z68.41 BMI, body mass index, 40.0-44.9;

                                         E86.0 Dehydration

    Principal Procedure: Laparoscopic removal of gastric band (includes removal of attached port) **0DP64CZ**

Character	Code	Explanation
Section	0	Medical and Surgical
Body System	D	Gastrointestinal System
Root Operation	P	Removal
Body Part	6	Stomach
Approach	4	Percutaneous Endoscopic
Device	C	Extraluminal Device
Qualifier	Z	No Qualifier

INDEX: Removal of device from, Stomach, 0DP6

    Secondary Procedure(s):   None indicated by the documentation provided

Rationale: The reason for admission after study was found to be the complication of the gastric band. The obesity is coded as it is noted as a current diagnosis for the patient and is the reason why the patient has a gastric band. The dehydration is also coded since it was treated during this admission. The laparoscopic removal of the gastric band (which includes the removal of the attached port) is coded as Removal of an Extraluminal Device from the Stomach via a Percutaneous Endoscopic approach.

Chapter 5

Mental, Behavioral, and Neurodevelopmental Disorders

1. **Principal Diagnosis:**   **F10.231** Dependence, alcohol with withdrawal delirium

    Secondary Diagnoses: **F10.251** Dependence, alcohol with alcohol-induced psychotic disorder with hallucinations;

                                           F17.210 Dependence, nicotine, cigarettes

Principal Procedure: None indicated by the documentation provided

Secondary Procedure(s): None indicated by the documentation provided

Rationale: The physician stated the reason for admission was the impending delirium tremens, so listed as the principal diagnosis. Alcohol dependence and nicotine dependence (smoking cigarettes) were also evaluated and treated, so they are included as secondary diagnoses.

3. **Principal Diagnosis:**   **F14.20** Disorder, cocaine use, moderate

   Secondary Diagnoses: None indicated by the documentation provided

   Principal Procedure: Detoxification Services **HZ2ZZZZ**

Character	Code	Explanation
Section	H	Substance Abuse Treatment
Body System	Z	None
Root Type	2	Detoxification Services
Type Qualifier	Z	None
Qualifier	Z	None
Qualifier	Z	None
Qualifier	Z	None

INDEX: Detoxification Services, for substance abuse

Secondary Procedure: Narcosynthesis **GZGZZZZ**

Character	Code	Explanation
Section	G	Mental Health
Body System	Z	None
Root Type	G	Narcosynthesis
Type Qualifier	Z	None
Qualifier	Z	None
Qualifier	Z	None
Qualifier	Z	None

INDEX: Narcosynthesis

Rationale: The principal diagnosis of cocaine use disorder (dependence) was assigned due to the reason for admission being the need for drug detoxification. No secondary diagnoses were present. The procedures of detoxification and narcosynthesis were coded with the detoxification as principal because it was most closely tied to the reason for admission.

5. **Principal Diagnosis:**   **F41.0** Disorder, panic

   Secondary Diagnoses: **R07.89** Pain, chest, non-cardiac

   Principal Procedure: None indicated by documentation provided

Secondary Procedure(s): None indicated by documentation provided

Rationale: The reason for admission after study was the panic disorder so listed as principal diagnosis. The secondary diagnosis of non-cardiac chest pain was listed by the physician, which is coded even though it has resolved.

7. **Principal Diagnosis:**   **F11.23** Dependence, drug, opioid with withdrawal

   Secondary Diagnoses: None indicated by the documentation provided

   Principal Procedure: Drug detoxification **HZ2ZZZZ**

Character	Code	Explanation
Section	H	Substance Abuse Treatment
Body System	Z	None
Root Type	2	Detoxification Services
Type Qualifier	Z	None
Qualifier	Z	None
Qualifier	Z	None
Qualifier	Z	None

INDEX: Detoxification Services, for substance abuse

Secondary Procedure: Individual substance abuse counseling, motivational **HZ37ZZZ**

Character	Code	Explanation
Section	H	Substance Abuse Treatment
Body System	Z	None
Root Type	3	Individual Counseling
Type Qualifier	7	Motivational Enhancement
Qualifier	Z	None
Qualifier	Z	None
Qualifier	Z	None

INDEX: Substance Abuse Treatment, individual, motivational

Secondary Procedure: Group substance abuse counseling, motivational **HZ47ZZZ**

Character	Code	Explanation
Section	H	Substance Abuse Treatment
Body System	Z	None
Root Type	4	Group Counseling
Type Qualifier	7	Motivational Enhancement

Qualifier	Z	None
Qualifier	Z	None
Qualifier	Z	None

INDEX: Substance Abuse Treatment, group, motivational

Rationale: The ICD-10-CM combination code for the drug dependence and withdrawal is listed as the principal diagnosis and the reason for admission after study. Three procedures are performed with the detoxification procedure most closely described as related to the principal diagnosis.

9. **First-Listed Diagnosis:** **F20.0** Schizophrenia, paranoid

   Secondary Diagnoses: **T43.3X6A** Table of Drugs and Chemicals, Perphenazine, underdosing;

   Z91.120 Underdosing, intentional, due to financial hardship

Rationale: This is an example of a patient with a condition that worsens or exacerbates due to the patient not taking the prescribed medication to manage the condition. The first listed diagnosis is the condition that worsens. Additional diagnoses are used to identify the drug that was underdosed from the Table of Drugs and Chemicals and the reason related to the underdosing by the patient, due to financial hardship.

11. **Principal Diagnosis:** **F33.2** Disorder, depressive, recurrent, current episode, severe

    Secondary Diagnoses: **S13.4XXA** Sprain, cervical, initial encounter;

    J18.9 Pneumonia;

    G89.4 Syndrome, chronic pain;

    S39.012S Sequela, injury-code to injury with seventh character S; strain, back

    F11.20 Dependence, drug, methadone, see Dependence, drug opioid;

    X83.8XXA Index to External causes, suicide, hanging;

    Y92.015 Index to External causes, place of occurrence, residence, house, garage

    Principal Procedure: None indicated by the documentation provided

    Secondary Procedure(s): None indicated by the documentation provided

Rationale: The reason for his admission to the psychiatric unit was the recurrent depressive disorder. This episode was severe. The secondary diagnoses that were treated included the cervical sprain, chronic pain syndrome, drug dependence. (Note: the patient is taking methadone so he is still dependent on opioids.) The external cause codes for the hanging suicide attempt and the place of occurrence identified are also coded as the two facts known about the external cause of the event.

13. **First-Listed Diagnosis:** **F20.81** Disorder, Schizophreniform disorder

    Secondary Diagnoses: **F91.2** Disorder, Conduct, socialized type;

    F90.1 Disorder, Attention-deficit hyperactivity, hyperactive type;

    F81.9 Disability, learning;

    F63.1 Pyromania;

    Z81.8 History, Family mental disorders

Rationale: In addition to the diagnoses listed by the physician at the end of the scenario, the patient is also described with the diagnosis of pyromania and having a history of family mental illness/disorders.

15. **Principal Diagnosis:** **F43.12** Disorder, post-traumatic stress, chronic

    Secondary Diagnoses: **R45.851** Ideation, suicidal

    Principal Procedures: Individual supportive individual psychotherapy **GZ56ZZZ**

Character	Code	Explanation
Section	G	Mental Health Services
Body System	Z	None
Root Type	5	Individual Psychotherapy
Type Qualifier	6	Supportive
Qualifier	Z	None
Qualifier	Z	None
Qualifier	Z	None

INDEX: Psychotherapy, individual, mental health services, supportive

Secondary Procedure(s): Individual cognitive-behavioral psychotherapy **GZ58ZZZ**

Character	Code	Explanation
Section	G	Mental Health Services
Body System	Z	None
Root Type	5	Individual Psychotherapy
Type Qualifier	8	Cognitive Behavioral
Qualifier	Z	None
Qualifier	Z	None
Qualifier	Z	None

INDEX: Psychotherapy, individual, mental health services, cognitive-behavioral

Rationale: The scenario describes a patient with both post-traumatic stress disorder (PTSD) and suicide ideation that were treated during the hospital stay. The PTSD appears to be the reason for admission after study and, therefore, the principal diagnosis with the additional diagnosis coded for the suicide ideation.

The two psychotherapy services provided were also coded and either one could probably be listed as principal.

17. **Principal Diagnosis:** **F33.9** Disorder, depressive, major, recurrent

    Secondary Diagnoses: **F41.9** Disorder, anxiety;

    F45.0 Disorder, somatization

    Principal Procedure: Medication management **GZ3ZZZZ**

Character	Code	Explanation
Section	G	Mental Health Services
Body System	Z	None

Root Type	3	Medication management
Type Qualifier	Z	None
Qualifier	Z	None
Qualifier	Z	None
Qualifier	Z	None

INDEX: Medication Management

Secondary Procedure(s): None indicated by the documentation provided

Rationale: The patient was admitted because she was not responding to outpatient therapy for her known major depression that was described as recurrent. The physician added the secondary diagnoses of anxiety disorder and somatization disorder, which were coded. The physician described the procedure performed as medication management. All the diagnoses were accessed in the Alphabetic Index under the main term of "disorder."

Chapter 6

Diseases of the Nervous System

1. **First-Listed Diagnosis:** G30.1 Disease, Alzheimer's, late onset, with behavioral disturbance

   Secondary Diagnoses: F02.81 Disease, Alzheimer's, late onset, with behavioral disturbances;

   Z91.83 Wandering in diseases classified elsewhere

   Rationale: The main reason the patient was brought to the physician's office was for management of her symptoms caused by the Alzheimer's dementia. Coding notes require the coder to code first the Alzheimer's disease followed by codes for the manifestation of the disease. Under code F02.81, there is a note to "Use additional code, if applicable, to identify wandering in dementia in conditions classified elsewhere (Z91.83))." Therefore, we assign Z91.83 for the wandering due to the dementia.

3. **Principal Diagnosis:** G20 Disease, Parkinson's

   Secondary Diagnoses: L02.212 Abscess, cutaneous, see Abscess, by site, back

   Principal Procedure: Drainage, subcutaneous tissue and fascia, back **0J970ZZ**

Character	Code	Explanation
Section	0	Medical and Surgical
Body System	J	Subcutaneous Tissue and Fascia
Root Operation	9	Drainage
Body Part	7	Subcutaneous Tissue and Fascia, Back
Approach	0	Open
Device	Z	No Device
Qualifier	Z	No Qualifier

INDEX: Incision, abscess, see Drainage, subcutaneous tissue and fascia, back

Secondary Procedure(s): None indicated by the documentation provided

Rationale: The reason for admission after study was the patient's Parkinsonism, but a secondary condition (abscess) was surgically treated. The other symptoms described in the scenario (rigidity, loss of speech, and loss of ambulation) are not coded as these are integral conditions to the Parkinsonism disease. The incision and drainage procedure performed is coded to the root operation of drainage as it is the objective of the procedure.

5. | **Principal Diagnosis:** | **A41.9** Sepsis |
    | --- | --- |
    | **Secondary Diagnoses:** | **R65.21** Sepsis, severe, with septic shock; |
    | | **N17.9** Failure, renal, acute; |
    | | **K72.00** Failure, hepatic acute; |
    | | **G31.83** Lewy body dementia; Dementia, Lewy body |
    | | **F02.80** Dementia without behavioral disturbance; |
    | | **J69.0** Pneumonia, aspiration, due to food; |
    | | **R13.10** Difficulty, swallowing, see Dysphagia; |
    | | **L89.153** Ulcer, pressure, sacrum, stage III; |
    | | **Z74.01** Status, bed, confinement; |
    | | **Z66** DNR |
    | | **Z51.5**, Palliative care |
    | **Principal Procedure:** | None indicated by the documentation provided |
    | **Secondary Procedure(s):** | None indicated by the documentation provided |

Rationale: The diagnosis of severe sepsis and shock requires codes for the blood stream infection (sepsis) severe sepsis status with shock (specifically the organ failure, renal and hepatic). In addition, the patient's dementia, dysphagia, pressure ulcer, bed confinement status, and DNR status were also managed and, therefore, coded for this hospital stay. The dementia code is added because of the use additional code note that appears under category G31, other degenerative diseases of the nervous system, not elsewhere classified. The family elected hospice care with no further aggressive care. No procedures were performed.

7. | **First-Listed Diagnosis:** | **G51.0** Palsy, Bell's or Palsy, facial |
    | --- | --- |
    | **Secondary Diagnoses:** | **E11.9** Diabetes, type 2; |
    | | **Z79.84** Long-term drug therapy, oral hypoglycemic drugs (glipizide) |
    | | **F17.210** Dependence, drug, nicotine, cigarettes |

Rationale: The primary reason the patient was in the physician's office was to diagnosis the condition that was causing the symptoms she was experiencing, that is, Bell's Palsy. Her other conditions were also evaluated and therefore coded and reported.

9. | **Principal Diagnosis:** | **G45.9** Attack, transient ischemic |
    | --- | --- |
    | **Secondary Diagnoses:** | **I69.354** Sequela, infarction, cerebral, hemiplegia, left nondominant; |
    | | **I10** Hypertension, essential; |
    | | **E11.22** Diabetes, type 2, with chronic kidney disease; |
    | | **N18.2** Disease, kidney, chronic, stage 2 |
    | **Principal Procedure:** | None indicated by the documentation provided |
    | **Secondary Procedure(s):** | None indicated by the documentation provided |

Rationale: The patient was admitted with diagnosis of a possible stroke, but it was determined after study the patient had suffered a transient ischemic attack (TIA). The symptoms the patient was experiencing on admission are not coded separately when present with a TIA. However, the residuals of the original stroke are coded. The patient's other medical conditions were also evaluated and treated during the hospital stay and, therefore, are coded. If there was documentation in the health record on what type of medication was used to treat the diabetes (insulin or oral hypoglycemic medications), an additional code could be assigned. According to the coding guideline I.C.9.a.2 for hypertensive chronic kidney disease the "CKD should not be coded as hypertensive if the physician has specified a different cause." For this reason, the hypertension is coded as I10 and not coded to I12. The type 2 diabetes is coded "with chronic kidney disease" as the scenario describes the CKD as due to the diabetes and not the hypertension.

11. **Principal Diagnosis:**   **G90.01** Syndrome, carotid, sinus

    Secondary Diagnoses: None indicated by the documentation provided

    Principal Procedure: Insertion of dual chamber cardiac pacemaker generator **0JH606Z**

Character	Code	Explanation
Section	0	Medical and Surgical
Body System	J	Subcutaneous Tissue and Fascia
Root Operation	H	Insertion
Body Part	6	Subcutaneous Tissue and Fascia, Chest
Approach	0	Open
Device	6	Pacemaker Dual Chamber
Qualifier	Z	No Qualifier

INDEX: Pacemaker, Dual Chamber, Chest

Secondary Procedure: Insertion of pacemaker lead into right atrium **02H63JZ**

Character	Code	Explanation
Section	0	Medical and Surgical
Body System	2	Heart and Great Vessels
Root Operation	H	Insertion
Body Part	6	Atrium, Right
Approach	3	Percutaneous
Device	J	Cardiac Lead, Pacemaker
Qualifier	Z	No Qualifier

INDEX: Insertion of device in, Atrium, right

Secondary Procedure: Insertion of lead into right ventricle **02HK3JZ**

Character	Code	Explanation
Section	0	Medical and Surgical
Body System	2	Heart and Great Vessels

Root Operation	H	Insertion
Body Part	K	Ventricle, Right
Approach	3	Percutaneous
Device	J	Cardiac Lead, Pacemaker
Qualifier	Z	No Qualifier

INDEX: Insertion of device in, Ventricle, right

Rationale: That patient was admitted to the hospital for a singular reason, the carotid sinus syndrome. The procedure performed involved the insertion of three devices, the cardiac pacemaker generator into the subcutaneous tissue of the chest and the insertion of two pacemaker leads, one into the right atrium and one into the right ventricle.

13. **Principal Diagnosis:**   **R42** Vertigo

   Secondary Diagnoses: **R51** Headache

   R11.0 Nausea

   R20.8 Loss, sense of, touch

   G65.2 Polyneuropathy, in, toxic agent NEC, sequelae

   Principal Procedure: None indicated by the documentation provided

   Secondary Procedure(s): None indicated by the documentation provided

   Rationale: This patient's scenario does not describe a current episode of herbicide toxicity. Instead, the patient is experiencing conditions as a result of the toxicity. For this reason, the coder should assign the sequelae or the conditions present as a result of the herbicide toxicity. Under category G65 is an instruction in the Tabular List to code first the condition resulting from the polyneuropathy, any of which could be the first listed code. There were no procedures performed to be coded.

15. **Principal Diagnosis:**   **G00.1** Meningitis, bacterial, pneumococcal

   Secondary Diagnoses: **J13** Pneumonia, Streptococcus pneumoniae

   H66.003 Otitis, media, suppurative, acute, bilateral

   Principal Procedure: Diagnostic lumbar puncture **009U3ZX**

Character	Code	Explanation
Section	0	Medical and Surgical
Body System	0	Central Nervous System and Cranial Nerves
Root Operation	9	Drainage
Body Part	U	Spinal Canal
Approach	3	Percutaneous
Device	Z	No Device
Qualifier	X	Diagnostic

INDEX: Drainage, spinal canal

Secondary Procedure(s): None indicated by the documentation provided

Rationale: The patient's symptoms at the time of admission were caused by the bacterial meningitis that is coded as the principal diagnosis. The patient was also diagnosed and treated for pneumonia and otitis media during the admission, which were therefore coded as secondary diagnoses. One procedure was performed, a diagnostic spinal puncture.

17. **Principal Diagnosis:**   **G61.0** Syndrome, Guillain-Barre or Guillain-Barre Disease or Syndrome

Secondary Diagnoses: None indicated by the documentation provided

Principal Procedure: Plasmapheresis **6A550Z3**

Character	Code	Explanation
Section	6	Extracorporeal Therapies
Body System	A	Physiological Systems
Root Operation	5	Pheresis
Body Part	5	Circulatory
Approach	0	Single
Device	Z	No Qualifier
Qualifier	3	Plasma

INDEX: Plasmapheresis

Secondary Procedure: Diagnostic lumbar puncture **009U3ZX**

Character	Code	Explanation
Section	0	Medical and Surgical
Body System	0	Central Nervous System
Root Operation	9	Drainage
Body Part	U	Spinal Canal
Approach	3	Percutaneous
Device	Z	No Device
Qualifier	X	Diagnostic

INDEX: Puncture, see Drainage, spinal canal

Rationale: The patient's symptoms and history of a viral infection along with the physical examination and diagnostic studies led both physicians to conclude the patient was having an initial attack of Guillain-Barre Syndrome. The coding of this condition is straight forward using the main terms of "syndrome" or "Guillain-Barre." Two procedures were performed. The therapeutic procedure of plasmapheresis was listed first with the diagnostic procedure listed second. The ICD-10-PCS Index includes the complete code for the plasmapheresis. The code for the spinal tap may first be located under the main term of "puncture" that states see drainage. The coder must recognize that the procedure is a puncture of the spinal canal, not the spinal cord. The qualifier of X is used because the spinal tap/puncture is a diagnostic procedure to establish a diagnosis.

19. **Principal Diagnosis:**   **G83.4** Syndrome, cauda equina

    Secondary Diagnoses: **M48.062** Stenosis, spinal, lumbar region, with neurogenic claudication

    Principal Procedure: L5 laminectomy **00NY0ZZ**

Character	Code	Explanation
Section	0	Medical and Surgical
Body System	0	Central Nervous System and Cranial Nerves
Root Operation	N	Release
Body Part	Y	Lumbar Spinal Cord
Approach	0	Open
Device	Z	No Device
Qualifier	Z	No Qualifier

INDEX: Laminectomy, *see* Release, Central Nervous System and Cranial Nerves

Secondary Procedure(s):   None indicated by the documentation provided

Rationale: Cauda equina syndrome is the medical emergency that caused the patient to be admitted to the hospital for surgery, so it is the principal diagnosis. The patient's longstanding lumbar spinal stenosis with neurogenic claudication is coded as a secondary diagnosis. The laminectomy of L5 is coded as a Release since its goal is to decompress the spinal cord.

Chapter 7

Diseases of the Eye and Adnexa

1. **First-Listed Diagnosis:**   **H40.10X1** Glaucoma, open angle (bilateral), mild

   Secondary Diagnoses: None indicated by the documentation provided

   Rationale: Per ICD-10-CM coding guideline I.C.7.a.2, when a patient has bilateral glaucoma, and both eyes are documented as being the same type and stage, and ICD-10-CM does not provide a code for bilateral glaucoma (i.e., H40.10), the coding professional should report only one code for the type of glaucoma with the appropriate seventh character for the stage (i.e., 1 = mild).

3. **First-Listed Diagnosis:**   **H11.052** Pterygium, peripheral, progressive, left eye

   Secondary Diagnoses: None indicated by the documentation provided

   Rationale: The symptom the patient described to the physician as the reason for the visit was diagnosed as pterygium and was the first-listed diagnosis.

5. **First-Listed Diagnosis:**   **E11.3392** Diabetes, type 2 with retinopathy, nonproliferative, moderate without macular edema, left eye

   Z79.84 Long-term drug therapy, oral hypoglycemic

   Secondary Diagnoses: None indicated by the documentation provided

   Rationale: ICD-10-CM contains combination codes for diabetes including the type of diabetes, the body system affected, and the specific condition related to the diabetes.

7. **Principal Diagnosis:**   **H16.072** Ulcer, cornea, perforated, left

   Secondary Diagnoses: **Z94.7** Transplant (status), cornea;

   Q90.9 Syndrome, Down

   Principal Procedure: Keratoplasty, see Replacement, cornea, left **08R93KZ**

Character	Code	Explanation
Section	0	Medical and Surgical
Body System	8	Eye
Root Operation	R	Replacement
Body Part	9	Cornea, Left
Approach	3	Percutaneous
Device	K	Nonautologous Tissue Substitute
Qualifier	Z	No Qualifier

INDEX: Keratoplasty, see Replacement, cornea, left **08R93KZ**

Secondary Procedure: Removal of previous corneal tissue (device), eye left **08P13KZ**

Character	Code	Explanation
Section	0	Medical and Surgical
Body System	8	Eye
Root Operation	P	Removal
Body Part	1	Eye, Left
Approach	3	Percutaneous
Device	K	Nonautologous Tissue Substitute
Qualifier	Z	No Qualifier

INDEX: Removal of device, eye, left

Rationale: The reason for admission after study, the principal diagnosis, is the corneal ulcer. The surgical procedure is a replacement of the cornea for the second time. The cornea is replaced with donor material, not repaired or supplemented according to PCS definitions of those procedures. The other conditions present are coded as secondary diagnoses. A corneal transplant is a replacement procedure where a body part is replaced by a device, in this case, a tissue substitute. A removal procedure is coded for taking out the device (corneal tissue) used in a previous replacement procedure before the second corneal replacement can be performed. This is a second corneal transplant, so the first corneal tissue "device" has to be removed. If this had been a first-time corneal transplant, the natural cornea would not be coded as removed because that is integral to the replacement. But, according to ICD-10-PCS coding guideline B6.1c, procedures performed on a device only and not on a body part are specified in the root operations Change, Irrigation, Removal and Revision, and are coded to the procedure performed. This case was a removal and replacement of the corneal tissue. The removal of the corneal tissue is coded to "eye" instead of "cornea" because the ICD-10-PCS table, 08P, does not include the body part of "cornea" but does include body part for "eye" as the removal procedure tables in ICD-10-PCS are often less specific for the body parts involved when a device is removed.

9. **First-Listed Diagnosis:**   **H25.11** Cataract, nuclear, sclerosis, see Cataract, senile nuclear, right

   Secondary Diagnoses: **H40.2213** Glaucoma, angle closure, chronic, right, severe stage

   Rationale: The reason for the office visit was to consider what could be done to correct his eye conditions, specifically the cataract and glaucoma. Since both conditions were addressed, either could be listed as the first-listed diagnosis code.

11. **Ophthalmic Diagnosis:**   **H44.011** Panophthalmitis

    Principal Procedure: Sclerotomy **08943ZX**

Character	Code	Explanation
Section	0	Medical and Surgical
Body System	8	Eye
Root Operation	9	Drainage
Body Part	4	Vitreous, Right
Approach	3	Percutaneous
Device	Z	No Device
Qualifier	X	Diagnostic

INDEX: Sclerotomy, see Drainage, eye, vitreous

Secondary Procedure: Injection of antibiotic, eye **3E0C329**

Character	Code	Explanation
Section	3	Administration
Physiological System	E	Physiological Systems and Anatomical Regions
Root Operation	0	Introduction
Body System/Region	C	Eye
Approach	3	Percutaneous
Substance	2	Anti-infective
Qualifier	9	Other Anti-infective

INDEX: Introduction of substance into eye, anti-infective

Rationale: Only the ophthalmic diagnosis code was coded in this example in a patient with other unknown conditions, so the principal diagnosis code could not be identified. The ophthalmic procedures performed include the drainage of the vitreous and an injection or introduction of substance into the eye, that is, anti-infective agents. The "Diagnostic" qualifier was chosen for the sclerotomy based on the fact that there was pus in the eye and the fluid was sent for culture. However, if there is any doubt as to whether the procedure is therapeutic or diagnostic, the coder should query the physician.

13. **First-Listed Diagnosis:** **H40.31X2** Glaucoma secondary to trauma, moderate stage, right

Secondary Diagnoses: **T65.91XS** Table of Drugs and Chemicals, Chemical substance NEC, accidental, sequela

T26.91XS Burn, chemical, see Corrosion by site, eye, sequela

Rationale: This is an example of the sequela of an eye injury, so the current condition (glaucoma) is listed first with identification of the original injury with the injury code using the seventh character of S for sequela. A code first note with code T26.91XS indicates the need to identify the chemical and intent with a code from T51-T65. The ICD-10-CM first listed diagnosis code included two facts—the glaucoma is due to the original trauma and is present in the moderate stage.

15. **First-Listed Diagnosis:** **H44.511** Glaucoma, absolute, right

Secondary Diagnoses: **H57.11** Pain, ocular, right eye

D66 Hemophilia, A

Principal Procedure: Evisceration **08R00JZ**

Character	Code	Explanation
Section	0	Medical and Surgical
Body System	8	Eye
Root Operation	R	Replacement
Body Part	0	Eye, Right
Approach	0	Open
Device	J	Synthetic Substitute
Qualifier	Z	No Qualifier

INDEX: Evisceration, Eyeball with prosthetic implant *see* Replacement, Eye 08R

Rationale: The eye pain may be identified as the main reason for the clinic visit but the cause of the pain is known to be the absolute glaucoma. Because the ocular pain is not always present with the glaucoma, the pain code should be used to further explain the conditions evaluated during the clinic visit and used in making the decision to perform the upcoming surgery. The procedure "Evisceration" gives coders a different root operation option if an ocular implant is used, so select "Replacement" over "Resection".

17. **First-Listed Diagnosis:** **H43.12** Hemorrhage, vitreous, left

Secondary Diagnoses: **H33.42** Detachment, retina, traction, left;

I10 Hypertension;

R94.31 Abnormal, electrocardiogram;

I09.9 Rheumatic, heart, see Disease, heart, rheumatic

Rationale: The main reason the patient came to the ophthalmologist's office was to check on the status of her left eye vitreous hemorrhage; therefore, it is coded as the first diagnosis. The retinal detachment coded as an additional diagnosis. The medical conditions acknowledged by the ophthalmologist that required further evaluation by the primary care physician were also coded as secondary diagnoses.

Chapter 8

Diseases of the Ear and Mastoid Process

1. **First-Listed Diagnosis:**   **H90.41** Loss, hearing, see also Deafness, sensorineural, unilateral (right ear)

   Secondary Diagnoses: **W42.9XXA** Index to External Causes, Main term, Noise, initial

   Rationale: The main reason for the clinic visit is the hearing loss on the right side, identified as sensorineural type. There was no hearing loss identified on left side. The external cause code is optional as there is no national requirement for reporting external causes of injuries or conditions.

3. **First-Listed Diagnosis:**   **H81.13** Vertigo, benign paroxysmal (positional)

   Secondary Diagnoses: None indicated by the documentation provided.

   Rationale: The patient was seen for one condition that had been evaluated by diagnostic testing, the vertigo, as stated by the physician. In ICD-10-CM the fifth character of "3" is used to describe a bilateral condition.

5. **First-Listed Diagnosis:**   **H72.02** Perforation, tympanic (membrane), central, left ear

   Secondary Diagnoses: None indicated by the documentation provided

   Rationale: The patient had a single reason for coming to the emergency department, which was found to have been caused by a perforation of his left tympanic membrane. The ICD-10-CM diagnosis code includes the laterality of left ear.

7. **First-Listed Diagnosis:**   **H60.42** Cholesteatoma, external ear, left

   Secondary Diagnoses: **H66.92** Otitis, media, chronic, left

                           Q87.410 Syndrome, Marfan's, with, cardiovascular manifestations, aortic dilation

   Primary Procedure: Mastoidectomy **0NB60ZZ**

Character	Code	Explanation
Section	0	Medical and Surgical
Body System	N	Head and Facial Bones
Root Operation	B	Excision
Body Part	6	Temporal Bone, Left
Approach	0	Open
Device	Z	No Device
Qualifier	Z	No Qualifier

INDEX: Mastoid process *use* Temporal Bone, Left, Excision, Bone, Temporal, Left 0NB6

Secondary Procedure: Insertion of TORP **09RA0JZ**

Character	Code	Explanation
Section	0	Medical and Surgical
Body System	9	Ear, Nose, Sinus
Root Operation	R	Replacement
Body Part	A	Auditory Ossicle, Left

Approach	0	Open
Device	J	Synthetic Substitute
Qualifier	Z	No Qualifier

INDEX: Replacement, Auditory Ossicle, Left (TORP=Total Ossicular Replacement Prosthesis)

Rationale: The left side conditions of the cholesteatoma and otitis media can be identified with the laterality included in the ICD-10-CM diagnosis codes. The Marfan's syndrome with the aortic dilation cardiovascular condition should also be coded. The mastoidectomy is an excision procedure of the mastoid process; coders must follow the instruction to code to excision of temporal bone. The TORP is a replacement of the ossicles that have been damaged with a synthetic device.

9. **First-Listed Diagnosis:** **H66.005** Otitis, media, suppurative, acute, recurrent, left

   Secondary Diagnoses: None indicated by the documentation provided

   Rationale: The emergency department physician identifies the reason for the patient's symptoms to be the acute otitis media that is coded as the single reason for the emergency department visit. The ICD-10CM diagnosis codes allow for the laterality to be identified with the code as occurring on the left side.

11. **First-Listed Diagnosis:** **H60.21** Otitis, externa, malignant, right

    Secondary Diagnoses: **E11.65** Diabetes, type 2, with, hyperglycemia

    Rationale: The main reason for the office visit was to re-examine the patient's symptoms related to his ear disease and provide further management. The patient's uncontrolled diabetes mellitus was also addressed as important in the patient's overall condition. The possible osteomyelitis is not coded because of the coding guideline that states in the outpatient setting an uncertain diagnosis is not coded as if it existed. ICD-10-CM allows for the laterality to be identified with the otitis codes. The patient's uncontrolled diabetes is identified with the code for the type of diabetes present with hyperglycemia. If the type of medication (insulin or oral hypoglycemic medications) was identified in the record that was used to treat the diabetes, an additional code from Z79 category would be assigned.

13. **First-Listed Diagnosis:** **H81.03** Meniere's Disease, bilateral

    Secondary Diagnoses: None indicated by the documentation provided

    Rationale: The patient in this example was seen in her physician's office for a known problem, Meniere's disease. The patient was treated for the condition. ICD-10-CM diagnosis codes for Meniere's disease allow for the laterality to be identified, but in this example, the physician described the condition as bilateral.

15. **First-Listed Diagnosis:** **H81.23** Neuronitis, vestibular, bilateral

    Secondary Diagnoses: None indicated by the documentation provided

    Rationale: This scenario describes a follow up visit in the consultant's office after an emergency department visit. The consultant identified the cause of the patient's symptoms as bilateral vestibular neuronitis, which can be coded in ICD-10-CM with the bilateral nature of the disease identified.

17. **First-Listed Diagnosis:** **H61.012** Perichondritis, ear, acute, left

    Secondary Diagnoses: **B96.5** Pseudomonas, aeruginosa, as cause of disease classified elsewhere or Infection, bacterial, as cause of disease classified elsewhere, Pseudomonas

    Rationale: The physician concluded the patient had acute perichondritis of the left external ear (pinna) based on the patient's history of ear cartilage piercing and the physical appearance of the area as well as the culture results. Culture results specified organism responsible for condition.

Chapter 9

Diseases of the Circulatory System

1. **Principal Diagnosis:**   **I21.19** Infarction, myocardium, ST elevation, inferior

   Secondary Diagnoses: **I25.10** Arteriosclerosis, coronary;

   I25.83 Arteriosclerosis, coronary, due to lipid rich plaque;

   I48.19 Fibrillation, atrial, persistent

   Principal Procedure: Combined right and left heart catheterization **4A023N8**

Character	Code	Explanation
Section	4	Measurement and Monitoring
Body System	A	Physiological Systems
Root Operation	0	Measurement
Body System	2	Cardiac
Approach	3	Percutaneous
Function/Device	N	Sampling and Pressure
Qualifier	8	Bilateral (Right and Left Heart)

INDEX: Catheterization, heart, see Measurement, cardiac

Secondary Procedure: Combined right and left heart angiocardiography **B2161ZZ**

Character	Code	Explanation
Section	B	Imaging
Body System	2	Heart
Root Type	1	Fluoroscopy
Body Part	6	Heart, Right and Left
Contrast	1	Low Osmolar
Qualifier	Z	None
Qualifier	Z	None

INDEX: Angiocardiography, Combined right and left heart *see* Fluoroscopy, heart, Right and Left

Secondary Procedure: Multiple Vessel Coronary arteriography **B2111ZZ**

Character	Code	Explanation
Section	B	Imaging
Body System	2	Heart
Root Type	1	Fluoroscopy
Body Part	1	Coronary Arteries, Multiple

Contrast	1	Low Osmolar
Qualifier	Z	None
Qualifier	Z	None

INDEX: Arteriography, see Fluoroscopy, heart

Rationale: The statement in this scenario is the chest pain was determined to be the result of an inferior wall myocardial infarction, and he was treated for it. The code I21.19 is the principal diagnosis code. The coronary artery disease was found to be present in the coronary angiography. A "code first coronary atherosclerosis" note is present at code I25.83 so code I25.10 is listed before the I25.83 code. The statement of persistent atrial fibrillation was coded with I48.19. Three cardiac diagnostic procedures were performed as typically is done with the radiology modality of fluoroscopy: left and right heart catheterization is a measurement of cardiac function, specifying sampling and pressure measurements. Both the left and right sides of the heart were examined with the angiocardiography using low osmolar contrast material. Multiple coronary arteries were examined (arteriography) by fluoroscopy to arrive at the diagnosis of coronary artery disease, again with low osmolar contrast.

3. **First-Listed Diagnosis:** **I69.351** Hemiplegia, following, cerebrovascular disease, cerebral infarction

   Secondary Diagnoses: **I69.321** Dysphasia, following, cerebrovascular disease, cerebral infarction;

   I10 Hypertension;

   I48.91 Fibrillation, atrial

Rationale: The patient has two sequela conditions or neurologic deficits as a result of having a cerebral infarction six months ago. It appears she was being evaluated for both conditions, so either one of the I69 category codes could be listed first. She was also treated for hypertension and atrial fibrillation that are coded as additional diagnoses.

5. **First-Listed Diagnosis:** **I46.9** Arrest, cardiac

   Secondary Diagnoses: **I11.9** Hypertension, heart (disease);

   Y93.H1 External cause code—Activity, shoveling, snow;

   Y92.014 Place of occurrence, residence, house, single family, driveway

   Y99.8 External cause status, specified NEC;

   Principal Procedure: Cardioversion **5A2204Z**

Character	Code	Explanation
Section	5	Extracorporeal or Systemic Assistance and Performance
Body System	A	Physiological Systems
Root Operation	2	Restoration
Body System	2	Cardiac
Duration	0	Single
Qualifier	4	Rhythm
Qualifier	Z	No Qualifier

INDEX: Cardioversion

Secondary Procedure(s): Cardiopulmonary resuscitation **5A12012**

Character	Code	Explanation
Section	5	Extracorporeal or Systemic Assistance and Performance
Body System	A	Physiological Systems
Root Operation	1	Performance
Body System	2	Cardiac
Duration	0	Single
Qualifier	1	Output
Qualifier	2	Manual

INDEX: Resuscitation, External chest compression

Rationale: This case is an outpatient visit in the emergency department. The physician describes the myocardial infarction as "probable." Probable conditions are not coded for outpatient cases. See Coding Guideline IV.H. For these reasons, the cardiac arrest is listed as the first diagnosis. The known hypertensive heart disease is also coded. The family said the patient had an enlarged heart, but it was not coded because it is not stated as a diagnosis by the physician. The external cause codes are not required by a national standard but may be coded according to state regulations or internal hospital coding policies.

7. **Principal Diagnosis:** **I25.10** Atherosclerosis, coronary artery

   Secondary Diagnoses: **I24.9** Syndrome, coronary, acute

   Principal Procedure: PTCA of one site **02703DZ**

Character	Code	Explanation
Section	0	Medical and Surgical
Body System	2	Heart and Great Vessels
Root Operation	7	Dilation
Body Part	0	Coronary Artery, One Artery
Approach	3	Percutaneous
Device	D	Intraluminal Device
Qualifier	Z	No Qualifier

INDEX: PTCA, see dilation, heart and great vessels

Secondary Procedure: Cardiac catheterization, left **4A023N7**

Character	Code	Explanation
Section	4	Measurement and Monitoring
Body System	A	Physiological Systems

Root Operation	0	Measurement
Body Part	2	Cardiac
Approach	3	Percutaneous
Function/Device	N	Sampling and Pressure
Qualifier	7	Left Heart

INDEX: Catheterization, heart, see Measurement, cardiac

Secondary Procedure: Coronary arteriogram **B2111ZZ**

Character	Code	Explanation
Section	B	Imaging
Body System	2	Heart
Root Operation	1	Fluoroscopy
Body Part	1	Coronary Arteries Multiple
Contrast	1	Low Osmolar
Qualifier	Z	None
Qualifier	Z	None

INDEX: Arteriography, see Fluoroscopy, Heart

Secondary Procedure: Infusion of platelet inhibitor **3E033PZ**

Character	Code	Explanation
Section	3	Administration
Physiological System	E	Physiological Systems and Anatomical Regions
Root Operation	0	Introduction
Body System	3	Peripheral Vein
Approach	3	Percutaneous
Substance	P	Platelet Inhibitor
Qualifier	Z	No Qualifier

INDEX: Infusion, see Introduction of substance in or on

Rationale: The patient's reason for admission was the acute coronary syndrome but after study it was determined to be due to arteriosclerotic coronary artery disease. For this reason, code I25.10 is listed as principal with an additional code for the acute coronary syndrome, I24.9. Four procedures were performed: dilation of the coronary artery with insertion of a stent (PTCA), the diagnostic cardiac catheterization to measure intracardiac pressures and to take samples, imaging of the coronary arteries with fluoroscopy (arteriogram), and infusion of the Integrilin or the platelet inhibitor. The PTCA with the insertion of the coronary stent is the therapeutic procedure related to the principal diagnosis and therefore listed as the principal procedure.

9. **Principal Diagnosis:**   **I82.431** Thrombosis, vein, popliteal

    Secondary Diagnoses: **I50.9** Failure, heart, congestive

    Principal Procedure: Intravascular ultrasound, popliteal vein **B54BZZ3**

Character	Code	Explanation
Section	B	Imaging
Body System	5	Veins
Root Type	4	Ultrasonography
Body Part	B	Lower Extremity Veins, Right
Contrast	Z	None
Qualifier	Z	None
Qualifier	3	Intravascular

INDEX: Ultrasonography, vein, lower extremity, right, intravascular

Secondary Procedure(s): None indicated by the documentation provided

Rationale: The diagnostic ultrasound study located the presence of a thrombus in the right popliteal vein that explained the symptoms the patient was experiencing and; therefore, it is coded as the principal diagnosis. The patient's heart failure was also coded. The only procedure performed was the imaging study of an intravascular ultrasound, which may or may not be coded according to hospital procedure coding guidelines.

11. **Principal Diagnosis:**   **I11.0**, Hypertension, heart, with heart failure

    Secondary Diagnoses: **I50.42** Failure, heart, systolic combined with diastolic, chronic;

    J96.10 Failure, respiratory, chronic;

    Z99.81 Dependence, oxygen;

    S52.502A Fracture, traumatic, radius, lower end, initial encounter;

    N39.0 Infection, urinary;

    Z87.440 History, personal, urinary (tract) infection;

    Z51.5 Palliative care;

    W18.11 XA External cause, fall, from toilet, initial encounter;

    Y92.013 External cause, place of occurrence, residence, house, single family, bedroom;

    Y99.8 External cause status, specified

    Principal Procedure: Application wrist splint **2W3DX1Z**

Character	Code	Explanation
Section	2	Placement
Anatomical Regions	W	Anatomical Regions
Root Operation	3	Immobilization
Body Region	D	Lower Arm Left

Approach	X	External
Device	1	Splint
Qualifier	Z	No Qualifier

INDEX: Splinting, musculoskeletal, see Immobilization, anatomical regions

Secondary Procedure: None indicated by the documentation provided

Rationale: The patient was admitted for treatment of her congestive heart failure, specifically the chronic combined systolic with diastolic type. Code I50.42 includes all of these descriptions. Another code for "congestive" heart failure (I50.9) is not necessary because the code I50.42 description includes congestive in (parentheses) as part of that code. The hypertensive heart disease has a "Use additional code" note for the heart failure and therefore indicates the hypertensive code is sequenced first. All other stated medical conditions present are coded including the fact that palliative care was accepted. The external cause codes are not required by a national standard but may be coded according to state regulations or internal hospital coding policies.

13. **Principal Diagnosis:** **I11.0** Hypertension, with heart failure

    Secondary Diagnoses: **I50.32** Failure, heart, diastolic (congestive);

    E11.40 Diabetes, type 2, with neuropathy

Rationale: The main reason the physician went to the nursing home to see the patient was to evaluate the patient's difficulty breathing and fatigue. The physician diagnosed the patient as having chronic congestive diastolic heart failure, which is combined into one code when heart failure is present with hypertension. The classification presumes a relationship unless the physician indicates they are not related. In this case, the principal diagnosis or the first code would be I11.0. The patient's diabetes with neuropathy is also coded with a combination code in ICD-10-CM. Hypertension was also evaluated and coded. If the documentation in the health record indicated what type of medication was used to treat the diabetes (insulin or oral hypoglycemic medication), an additional code from category Z79 would be used.

15. **Principal Diagnosis:** **I21.09** Infarct, myocardium, ST elevation, anterior

    Secondary Diagnoses: **I25.10** Disease, artery, coronary

    Principal Procedure: PTCA of 2 sites with intraluminal stents **02713EZ**

Character	Code	Explanation
Section	0	Medical and Surgical
Body System	2	Heart and Great Vessels
Root Operation	7	Dilation
Body Part	1	Coronary Artery, Two Arteries
Approach	3	Percutaneous
Device	E	Intraluminal Device, two stents
Qualifier	Z	No Qualifier

INDEX: PTCA, see Dilation, heart and great vessels

Secondary Procedure: PTCA of 1 site **02703ZZ**

Character	Code	Explanation
Section	0	Medical and Surgical
Body System	2	Heart and Great Vessels
Root Operation	7	Dilation
Body Part	0	Coronary Artery, One Artery
Approach	3	Percutaneous
Device	Z	No Device
Qualifier	Z	No Qualifier

INDEX: PTCA, see Dilation, heart and great vessels

Rationale: The patient's reason for transfer and reason for admission after study at Hospital B was the STEMI that continued to be treated and evaluated. The diagnosis of coronary artery disease was established upon the completion of the cardiac studies at Hospital A and continued to be the reason for the further study and treatment at Hospital B. For the procedures, a total of three vessels were treated with PTCA or angioplasty. Of the three vessels angioplastied, two stents were inserted into two coronary arteries. This requires two procedure codes: dilation of two coronary artery sites with two intraluminal devices inserted and dilation of one coronary artery site that did not have a device inserted.

17. **Principal Diagnosis:** **I08.3** Stenosis, aortic (valve), rheumatic, with mitral valve disease, with tricuspid valve disease

    Secondary Diagnoses: **I13.2**, Hypertensive cardiorenal with stage 5 chronic kidney disease or end-stage renal disease

    I50.32 Failure, heart, diastolic, chronic (congestive);

    N18.6 Disease, renal, End stage;

    Z99.2 Dependence on renal dialysis;

    D63.1 Anemia in chronic kidney disease;

    E78.5 Hyperlipidemia, unspecified;

    Z86.19 History, Personal, hepatitis C

    Principal Procedure: Replacement of aortic valve with porcine graft **02RF08Z**

Character	Code	Explanation
Section	0	Medical and Surgical
Body System	2	Heart and Great Vessels
Root Operation	R	Replacement
Body Part	F	Aortic Valve
Approach	0	Open
Device	8	Zooplastic Tissue (Porcine)
Qualifier	Z	No Qualifier

INDEX: Replacement, valve, aortic

Secondary Procedure: Supplement mitral valve with annuloplasty ring **02UG0JZ**

Character	Code	Explanation
Section	0	Medical and Surgical
Body System	2	Heart and Great Vessels
Root Operation	U	Supplement
Body Part	G	Mitral Valve
Approach	0	Open
Device	J	Synthetic Substitute
Qualifier	Z	No Qualifier

INDEX: Annuloplasty ring is supplementing the function of the mitral valve. Annuloplasty, see Supplement, heart and great vessels.

Secondary Procedure: Cardiopulmonary Bypass **5A1221Z**

Character	Code	Explanation
Section	5	Extracorporeal Assistance and Performance
Physiological Systems	A	Physiological Systems
Root Operation	1	Performance
Body System	2	Cardiac
Duration	2	Continuous
Function	1	Output
Qualifier	Z	No Qualifier

INDEX: Bypass, cardiopulmonary

Rationale: Multiple heart valve disease specified as rheumatic or unspecified are assigned as rheumatic disorders. There are several ways to locate the I08 code in the Alphabetic Index, for example, under insufficiency or stenosis. The important fact is to find the combined code for the multiple valves involved. The anemia code is a manifestation code and must be sequence after the code for the underlying disease, the chronic kidney disease. The procedure performed was the replacement of the aortic valve with a porcine valve, which is from an animal or referred to as zooplastic tissue in ICD-10-PCS. Another term, bioprosthesis valve means it is a porcine valve. Operative reports may also refer to this type of valve as a bioprosthesis. Replacement involves removing the natural valve as integral to the procedure. The mitral valve was repaired with an annuloplasty ring, which is a supplement type procedure in ICD-10-PCS as it supports the structure of the mitral valve. The tricuspid valve was examined, but not repaired in this case.

19. **Principal Diagnosis:**   I25.110 Disease, artery, coronary, with angina pectoris, see Arteriosclerosis, coronary. Arteriosclerosis, coronary, native vessel, with angina pectoris, unstable

    Secondary Diagnoses: F17.210 Dependence, nicotine, cigarettes

    Principal Procedure: Aortocoronary bypass, three sites **021209W**

Character	Code	Explanation
Section	0	Medical and Surgical
Body System	2	Heart and Great Vessels
Root Operation	1	Bypass
Body Part	2	Coronary Artery, Three Arteries
Approach	0	Open
Device	9	Autologous Venous Tissue
Qualifier	W	Aorta

INDEX: Bypass, artery, coronary, three sites

Secondary Procedure: Excision of left greater saphenous vein **06BQ0ZZ**

Character	Code	Explanation
Section	0	Medical and Surgical
Body System	6	Lower Veins
Root Operation	B	Excision
Body Part	Q	Greater Saphenous Veins Left
Approach	0	Open
Device	Z	No Device
Qualifier	Z	No Qualifier

INDEX: Excision, vein, greater saphenous, left

Secondary Procedure: Cardiopulmonary Bypass **5A1221Z**

Character	Code	Explanation
Section	5	Extracorporeal Assistance and Performance
Physiological Systems	A	Physiological Systems
Root Operation	1	Performance
Body System	2	Cardiac
Duration	2	Continuous
Function	1	Output
Qualifier	Z	No Qualifier

INDEX: Bypass, cardiopulmonary

Rationale: ICD-10-CM provides a combination code for coronary artery disease when present with angina pectoris. The Alphabetic Index entry of disease, artery, coronary, with angina pectoris, leads the coder to see Arteriosclerosis, coronary. The complete entry is arteriosclerosis, coronary, native vessel, with angina pectoris, unstable. The only other diagnosis given for this patient was her nicotine dependence that was coded. Three procedures are coded with ICD-10-PCS including the aortocoronary bypass with excision of the greater saphenous veins for the grafting and the cardiopulmonary bypass used during the surgery.

21. **First-Listed Diagnosis:**   I69.320 Sequelae, stroke NOS, aphasia

    Secondary Diagnoses: I69.392 Sequelae, stroke NOS, facial weakness

Rationale: The aphasia due to the past stroke appears to be the main reason for the visit and is listed as the first diagnosis code. The aphasia is a neurologic deficit or sequelae of the previous stroke. The facial weakness is also coded as sequelae of the stroke. Another Index entry is not helpful to code this scenario because the main term of "aphasia" with entry for "following, cerebrovascular disease" does not have a subterm for "stroke."

23. **Principal (Nursing Home) Diagnosis:**   I69.398 Sequelae, stroke, specified effect; Use additional code to identify sequelae present

    Secondary Diagnoses: G40.909 Disorder, seizure

Rationale: The patient's seizure disorder was stated as caused by the stroke that occurred ten months ago and is considered a "sequela" of the stroke. Using the Alphabetic Index main term of sequelae, stroke with the listing of neurological deficits under that entry is the most efficient way to code the condition in ICD-10-CM. However, in this scenario, there is no entry for "seizure disorder," but it is a specified condition, and there is an entry for specified effect NEC. Under code I69.398, there is a note to "use additional code" to identify the sequelae. A secondary code is assigned for G40.909 to identify the seizure disorder as the specified effect.

25. **Principal Diagnosis:**   I49.5 Syndrome, sick sinus

    Secondary Diagnoses: I50.9 Failure, heart

    Principal Procedure: Insertion, dual chamber pacemaker generator **0JH606Z**

Character	Code	Explanation
Section	0	Medical and Surgical
Body System	J	Subcutaneous Tissue and Fascia
Root Operation	H	Insertion
Body Part	6	Subcutaneous Tissue and Fascia, Chest
Approach	0	Open
Device	6	Pacemaker, Dual Chamber
Qualifier	Z	No Qualifier

INDEX: Insertion of device in, subcutaneous tissue and fascia, chest

    Secondary Procedure: Insertion, pacemaker lead into right atrium **02H63JZ**

Character	Code	Explanation
Section	0	Medical and Surgical
Body System	2	Heart and Great Vessels
Root Operation	H	Insertion
Body Part	6	Atrium, Right

Approach	3	Percutaneous
Device	J	Cardiac Lead, Pacemaker
Qualifier	Z	No Qualifier

INDEX: Insertion of device in, atrium right

Secondary Procedure: Insertion, pacemaker lead into right ventricle **02HK3JZ**

Character	Code	Explanation
Section	0	Medical and Surgical
Body System	2	Heart and Great Vessels
Root Operation	H	Insertion
Body Part	K	Ventricle, Right
Approach	3	Percutaneous
Device	J	Cardiac Lead, Pacemaker
Qualifier	Z	No Qualifier

INDEX: Insertion of device in, ventricle right

Rationale: The reason for admission after study and the principal diagnosis is the sick sinus syndrome, found easily in the Alphabetic Index to Diseases under the main term of syndrome. The patient's congestive heart failure is also treated and coded as a secondary diagnosis. The procedure performed is the insertion of a dual-chamber pacemaker that is coded in ICD-10-PCS as three procedures. The root operation for all three procedures is "Insertion of device in" subcutaneous tissue and fascia (body part value 6, pacemaker dual chamber, device 6), right atrium (body part value 6, device cardiac lead pacemaker J), and right ventricle (body part value K, device cardiac lead pacemaker J). The approach for placing the pacemaker generator in the chest subcutaneous tissue is open. The insertion of the leads into the heart was done by percutaneous approach by puncturing into the subclavian vein for inserting the leads. There is no qualifier (7th character) required for any of the three procedures.

Chapter 10

Diseases of the Respiratory System

1. **Principal Diagnosis:** **J44.1** Disease, lung, obstructive, with acute exacerbation

   Secondary Diagnoses: **Z87.891** History, personal, nicotine dependence

   Principal Procedure: None indicated by the documentation provided

   Secondary Procedure(s): None indicated by the documentation provided

   Rationale: The patient was admitted with symptoms of acute respiratory insufficiency that were determined to be an acute exacerbation of the chronic obstructive lung disease. The respiratory insufficiency is a symptom of and integral to COPD and not coded separately. The history of smoking was addressed and coded as a secondary diagnosis.

3. **First-Listed Diagnosis:** **J45.909** Asthma, childhood

   Secondary Diagnoses: None indicated by the documentation provided

Rationale: The reason for the office visit was to treat the patient for his childhood asthma. The allergic rhinitis is not coded separately—the Tabular List includes a note under category J45 Asthma. The Index also includes the entry for rhinitis, allergic, with asthma for code J45.909.

5. **Principal Diagnosis:**   **J18.9** Pneumonia

   Secondary Diagnoses: **D61.810** Pancytopenia, antineoplastic, chemotherapy induced;

        T45.1X5A Table of Drugs and chemical, antineoplastic, adverse effect;

        C90.00 Myeloma (multiple);

   Principal Procedure: Blood transfusion **30233N1**

Character	Code	Explanation
Section	3	Administration
Body System	0	Circulatory
Root Operation	2	Transfusion
Body Part	3	Peripheral Vein
Approach	3	Percutaneous
Substance	N	Red Blood Cells
Qualifier	1	Nonautologous

INDEX: Transfusion, vein, peripheral, blood, red cells

Secondary Procedure(s): None indicated by the documentation provided

Rationale: The reason for admission after study, and therefore the principal diagnosis, was the patient's pneumonia. The patient's other conditions, the multiple myeloma, pancytopenia, and the anxiety were also coded. The pancytopenia is an adverse effect of the chemotherapy. In order to identify the drug involved, the coder would access the Table of Drugs and Chemicals for the substance of antineoplastic agent or chemotherapy and select the code for adverse effect from the column for adverse. The code would require a 7th character of A for the initial encounter for care for the pancytopenia. The blood transfusion of packed red blood cells would be coded as a procedure. The patient was recommended to have an evaluation for his anxiety (F41.9), but the psychiatric consultation was refused by the patient. If there is any doubt as to whether to code anxiety as a diagnosis, the physician should be asked to clarify the patient's diagnosis.

7. **First-Listed Diagnosis:**   **J02.0** Pharyngitis, streptococcal

   Secondary Diagnoses: **H66.003** Otitis, media, suppurative acute

   Rationale: Because this is an outpatient visit, the "possible" early tonsillar abscess is not coded as confirmed. Instead, the conditions known for certain are the diagnosis codes reported for the outpatient visit, including the streptococcal pharyngitis, are listed first because the patient was complaining of a sore throat and the otitis media was also diagnosed and treated.

9. **First-Listed Diagnosis:**   **J01.10** Sinusitis, frontal, acute

   Secondary Diagnoses: **J01.00** Sinusitis, maxillary, acute

   Rationale: The reason for the office visit was the patient's acute sinusitis that explained the signs and symptoms the patient was experiencing. ICD-10-CM has separate codes for acute frontal and acute maxillary sinusitis. Either code could be listed as the first diagnosis code. In this scenario the codes were assigned for the conditions in sequence of how the physician documented the two conditions.

11. **Principal Diagnosis:**   **R09.1** Pleurisy

    Secondary Diagnoses: **M32.14** Lupus, erythematosus, systemic with organ involvement, renal (nephritis);

    E86.0 Dehydration;

    R19.7 Diarrhea;

    E87.1 Hyponatremia;

    E87.6 Hypokalemia;

    R79.89 Azotemia

    Principal Procedure: None indicated by the documentation provided

    Secondary Procedure(s):   None indicated by the documentation provided

    Rationale: The patient was admitted to the hospital because of respiratory symptoms that were determined to be pleurisy. For this reason, pleurisy was listed as the principal diagnosis code. It was not certain that the pleurisy was related to her lupus. However, she was known to have nephritis due to her lupus and it was treated, as were other conditions including dehydration, diarrhea, hyponatremia, hypokalemia, and azotemia.

13. **Principal Diagnosis:**   **J12.9** Pneumonia, viral

    Secondary Diagnoses: **E86.0** Dehydration

    Principal Procedure: None indicated by the documentation provided

    Secondary Procedure(s):   None indicated by the documentation provided

    Rationale: The physician's conclusion in the discharge summary was that the patient had "pneumonia, possibly viral origin, complicated by dehydration." For this reason, the viral pneumonia is coded as principal diagnosis because "possible" diagnoses are coded as if confirmed for an inpatient. The additional code for dehydration was added.

15. **Principal Diagnosis:**   **C34.12** Neoplasm, lung, upper lobe

    Secondary Diagnoses: **J91.0** Effusion, pleural, malignant

    Principal Procedure: Thoracentesis for drainage **0W9B3ZZ**

Character	Code	Explanation
Section	0	Medical and Surgical
Body System	W	Anatomical regions, general
Root Operation	9	Drainage
Body Part	B	Pleural cavity, left
Approach	3	Percutaneous
Device	Z	No Qualifier
Qualifier	Z	No Qualifier

INDEX: Thoracentesis or Drainage, pleural cavity

Secondary Procedure: Talc pleurodesis **3E0L3GC**

Character	Code	Explanation
Section	3	Administration
Body System	E	Physiological Systems and Anatomical Regions

Root Operation	0	Introduction
Body Part	L	Pleural Cavity
Approach	3	Percutaneous
Substance	G	Other Therapeutic Substance
Qualifier	C	Other Substance

INDEX: Pleurodesis, Chemical injection *see* Introduction, of substance in or on, Pleural Cavity 3E0L

Secondary Procedure(s): Thoracoscopy **0BJQ4ZZ**

Character	Code	Explanation
Section	0	Medical and Surgical
Body System	B	Respiratory System
Root Operation	J	Inspection
Body Part	Q	Pleura
Approach	4	Percutaneous Endoscopic
Device	Z	No Device
Qualifier	Z	No Qualifier

INDEX: Inspection, Pleura

Rationale: The reason for admission for this patient was the malignant pleural effusion due to his lung cancer. There is an instruction note under code J91.0 to "code first the underlying neoplasm." For this reason, the malignant neoplasm of the lung was coded as principal diagnosis. A therapeutic thoracentesis was performed to remove fluid, and this objective meets the definition of drainage performed in the pleural cavity. There is no indication that a drainage tube was left in place after the thoracentesis so no qualifier is used for device for this procedure code. The video-assisted talc pleurodesis requires two codes: one for the pleurodesis, which is the introduction of the talc used to prevent fluid accumulation, and the other code to capture the thoracoscopy portion which cannot be done with the approach for pleurodesis. In this case, the thoracoscopy is coded to inspection of the pleural cavity via the percutaneous endoscopic method.

17. **Principal Diagnosis:**   **J69.0** Pneumonia, aspiration

    Secondary Diagnoses: **J96.00** Failure, respiratory, acute;

    J44.9 Bronchitis, chronic, obstructive

    Principal Procedure: Intermittent positive pressure breathing **5A09458**

Character	Code	Explanation
Section	5	Extracorporeal Assistance & Performance
Physiological Systems	A	Physiological Systems
Root Operation	0	Assistance
Body Part	9	Respiratory

Duration	4	24-96 Consecutive Hours
Function	5	Ventilation
Qualifier	8	Intermittent Positive Airway Pressure

INDEX: Intermittent positive airway pressure, 24–96 hours

Secondary Procedure(s): None indicated by the documentation provided

Rationale: The patient was admitted with symptoms of three conditions (chronic lung disease, aspiration pneumonia, and respiratory failure) all present on admission, and any could have been the reason after study for the admission to the hospital. In order to determine the correct principal diagnosis, a physician query is appropriate in this scenario. The physician stated the aspiration pneumonia was the patient's principal diagnosis because it was one of the main reasons for the admission and required the greatest intensity of care and use of resources. The other two conditions were then coded as secondary diagnoses. The patient's respiratory procedure was intermittent positive pressure airway breathing and coded using that title in the ICD-10-PCS Index that led to the appropriate table for the code identification. What was aspirated by the patient and caused the aspiration pneumonia is not stated in the question and may not have been known. Most types of aspiration—that is, food, gastric secretions, mild, vomit—would code to J69.0. If a specific substance, such as oils or solids, were documented as the substance aspirated, the pneumonia code would change to J69.1 or J69.8.

19. **Diagnosis for the operative procedure:**   **J96.21** Failure, respiratory, acute on chronic, with, hypoxia

    Secondary Diagnoses: **J43.1** Emphysema, panlobular;

                                           J15.6 Pneumonia, gram-negative;

                                           Z99.11 Dependence, on, respirator or ventilator

    Principal Procedure: Tracheostomy **0B110F4**

Character	Code	Explanation
Section	0	Medical and Surgical
Body System	B	Respiratory System
Root Operation	1	Bypass
Body Part	1	Trachea
Approach	0	Open
Device	F	Tracheostomy Device
Qualifier	4	Cutaneous

INDEX: Tracheostomy, see Bypass, respiratory system (trachea)

Secondary Procedure(s): None indicated by the documentation provided

Rationale: The instruction for this exercise was to code the reason for the procedure as the first diagnosis so the acute on chronic respiratory failure with hypoxia was coded first. The patient's underlying conditions of panlobular emphysema, gram-negative pneumonia, and dependence on the respirator were also coded. The tracheostomy is a bypass procedure according to the definitions of the root operations in ICD-10-PCS. The device that remains in the patient after the procedure is the tracheostomy device that is identified in the 6th character for device. The 7th character of "cutaneous" is used with the tracheostomy. A bypass procedure in ICD-10-PCS is coded by identifying the body part bypassed "from" (trachea) and the body part bypassed "to" which would be the skin of the neck or the value 4 for cutaneous.

21. **Principal Diagnosis:**   **J90** Effusion, pleural

    Secondary Diagnoses: None indicated by the documentation provided.

    Principal Procedure: Infusion of tissue plasminogen activator (tPA) into pleural cavity **3E0L3GC**

Character	Code	Explanation
Section	3	Administration
Body System	E	Physiological Systems and Anatomical Regions
Root Operation	0	Introduction
Body Part	L	Pleural Cavity
Approach	3	Percutaneous
Device	G	Other Therapeutic Substance
Qualifier	C	Other Substance

INDEX: Introduction of substance in or on, Pleural Cavity 3E0L

Secondary Procedure(s):   None indicated by the documentation provided

Rationale: The patient was admitted for treatment of her pleural effusion, so J90 is the principal diagnosis. The empyema has already been treated and the infection has resolved, so it is no longer coded as a current condition. The tPA is infused into the patient's pleural cavity via a catheter, so the procedure is coded as an introduction of other therapeutic substance into the pleural cavity via a percutaneous approach.

Chapter 11

Diseases of the Digestive System

1. **Principal Diagnosis:**   **K80.10** Calculus, gallbladder, with cholecystitis, chronic

   Secondary Diagnoses: **Z53.31** Procedure, converted, laparoscopic to open

   Principal Procedure: Open cholecystectomy **0FT40ZZ**

Character	Code	Explanation
Section	0	Medical and Surgical
Body System	F	Hepatobiliary System and Pancreas
Root Operation	T	Resection
Body Part	4	Gallbladder
Approach	0	Open
Device	Z	No Device
Qualifier	Z	No Qualifier

INDEX: Cholecystectomy, see Resection, gallbladder

Secondary Procedure: Laparoscopy attempt **0FJ44ZZ**

Character	Code	Explanation
Section	0	Medical and Surgical
Body System	F	Hepatobiliary System and Pancreas
Root Operation	J	Inspection
Body Part	4	Gallbladder
Approach	4	Percutaneous Endoscopic
Device	Z	No Device
Qualifier	Z	No Qualifier

INDEX: Laparoscopy, see Inspection

Rationale: There is one reason for admission and, therefore, it is the principal diagnosis. The conversion of the laparoscopic to an open procedure is also coded. ICD-10-PCS guideline B3.2.d states during the same operative episode multiple procedures are coded if the intended root operation is attempted using one approach, but is converted to a different approach. For example, laparoscopic converted to open cholecystectomy is coded as an open resection and the laparoscopic attempt is coded as a percutaneous endoscopic inspection.

3. **Principal Diagnosis:** **K40.90** Hernia, inguinal

    Secondary Diagnoses: **Z53.09** Canceled procedure, because of contraindication;

    R07.2 Pain, chest, precordial;

    I10 Hypertension;

    J44.9 Disease, lung, obstructive

    Principal Procedure: None indicated by the documentation provided

    Secondary Procedure(s): None indicated by the documentation provided

    Rationale: The reason for admission after study was the inguinal hernia and listed as the principal diagnosis even though the surgery was canceled. The reason for the canceled surgery (chest pain) and the other conditions treated (hypertension and COPD) were coded as secondary diagnoses as conditions evaluated or treated. The canceled procedure because of contraindication is coded to explain why the surgery was not performed.

5. **Principal Diagnosis:** **K52.9** Gastroenteritis

    Secondary Diagnoses: **E86.0** Dehydration;

    J18.9 Pneumonia;

    K44.9 Hernia, hiatal;

    K21.0 Esophagitis, reflux

    Principal Procedure: None indicated by the documentation provided

    Secondary Procedure(s): None indicated by the documentation provided

    Rationale: When asked the physician stated the main reason for the hospital stay was the gastroenteritis, so it is coded as the principal diagnosis. The other conditions that were present, evaluated, and treated during the hospital stay were coded as secondary diagnoses.

7. **Principal Diagnosis:**   **I86.4** Varix, gastric

   Secondary Diagnoses: **K92.0** Hematemesis;

   K70.30 Cirrhosis, alcoholic;

   K70.10 Hepatitis, alcoholic

   I85.00 Varix, esophagus;

   F10.20 Alcoholism;

   Principal Procedure: Transjugular intrahepatic portosystemic (venous) shunt (TIPS) **06183J4**

Character	Code	Explanation
Section	0	Medical and Surgical
Body System	6	Lower Veins
Root Operation	1	Bypass
Body Part	8	Portal Vein
Approach	3	Percutaneous
Device	J	Synthetic Substitute
Qualifier	4	Hepatic Vein

INDEX: Shunt creation, see Bypass vein portal (between portal and hepatic veins)

Secondary Procedure(s): None indicated by the documentation provided

Rationale: The upper GI bleeding was found after study to be due to a gastric varix that was then coded as the principal diagnosis. The other findings of the study and the patient's known diseases were coded as secondary diagnoses with sequencing guidance I85.10 followed. The procedure performed, known as TIPS, is the creation of a shunt between the portal and hepatic veins, which meets the definition in ICD-10PCS as a bypass, the rerouting of the contents of a tubular body part with the body part identify the part bypassed "from" and the qualifier as the part bypassed "to."

9. **Principal Diagnosis:**   **K85.90** Pancreatitis, acute

   Secondary Diagnoses: **K86.1** Pancreatitis, chronic;

   F10.229 Alcoholic, intoxication, with dependence

   Principal Procedure: None indicated by the documentation provided

   Secondary Procedure(s): None indicated by the documentation provided

Rationale: When a patient has both the acute and chronic forms of the same disease (pancreatitis) and there are individual codes to identify each condition, the acute diagnosis code is selected as the principal diagnosis with the chronic condition coded as a secondary diagnosis. In this scenario, the acute pancreatitis is the principal diagnosis and the secondary diagnoses are the chronic pancreatitis and the chronic alcoholism. If the physician had indicated the pancreatitis was alcohol induced there would be a more specific code for the pancreatitis. The neurologist evaluated the patient for a "seizure disorder," but none was found, and no medications were prescribed for it, so it was not coded.

11. **Principal Diagnosis:**   **K55.029** Gangrene, intestine see also Infarct, intestine, small

    Secondary Diagnoses: **K55.049** Infarction, intestine, large;

    J96.00 Failure, respiratory, acute;

    A41.51 Sepsis, Escherichia coli;

    R65.20 Sepsis, severe;

I10 Hypertension;

E03.9 Hypothyroidism;

Z51.5 Palliative Care

Principal Procedure: Exploratory laparotomy **0WJG0ZZ**

Character	Code	Explanation
Section	0	Medical and Surgical
Body System	W	Anatomical Regions, General
Root Operation	J	Inspection
Body Part	G	Peritoneal Cavity
Approach	0	Open
Device	Z	No Device
Qualifier	Z	No Qualifier

INDEX: Laparotomy, exploratory, see Inspection, peritoneal cavity

Secondary Procedure: Mechanical ventilation **5A1945Z**

Character	Code	Explanation
Section	5	Extracorporeal Assistance and Performance
Physiological system	A	Physiological Systems
Root Operation	1	Performance
Body System	9	Respiratory
Duration	4	24-96 Consecutive Hours
Function	5	Ventilation
Qualifier	Z	No Qualifier

INDEX: Mechanical ventilation, see Performance, respiratory

Secondary Procedure(s): Endotracheal intubation **0BH17EZ**

Character	Code	Explanation
Section	0	Medical and Surgical
Physiological System	B	Respiratory System
Root Operation	H	Insertion
Body Part	1	Trachea
Duration	7	Via natural or artificial opening
Function	E	Intraluminal device, endotracheal airway
Qualifier	Z	No Qualifier

INDEX: Intubation, airway – see Insertion of device in, Trachea 0BH1-

Rationale: The patient was admitted to the hospital for abdominal pain, nausea, and vomiting and was found, after study including surgery, to have gangrene or an infarction of the small and large intestine. The small intestine infarction was selected as the principal diagnosis. The other diagnoses listed as the physician's final diagnoses were coded as secondary diagnoses. The exploratory laparotomy procedure that did not involve any other procedure such as a resection or excision was coded as Inspection in ICD10-PCS because that met the definition of manually and visually exploring a body part. The mechanical ventilation was coded as extracorporeal performance for the 24 hours it was performed. The endotracheal intubation procedure is also coded.

13. **First-Listed Diagnosis:**   **K21.9** Reflux, gastroesophageal

    Secondary Diagnoses: **K44.9** Hernia, hiatal;

                                       K26.7 Ulcer, duodenum, chronic

                                       R19.5 Abnormal, stool

Rationale: The diagnoses are coded in the sequence as listed by the physician as reasonable explanations for the patient's symptoms and complaints. The diagnosis of R19.5, abnormal stool, was added because it was a complaint of the patient that was evaluated with a recommendation to discontinue the Pepto-Bismol medication. The procedures are coded with CPT and HCPCS coding systems for outpatient visits.

15. **Principal Diagnosis:**   **K70.30** Disease, liver, alcoholic, cirrhosis

    Secondary Diagnoses: **I85.11** Varix, esophageal, in cirrhosis of liver, bleeding;

                                       F10.239 Dependence, alcohol, with withdrawal;

                                       D69.6 Thrombocytopenia

    Principal Procedure: EGD **0DJ08ZZ**

Character	Code	Explanation
Section	0	Medical and Surgical
Body System	D	Gastrointestinal System
Root Operation	J	Inspection
Body Part	0	Upper Intestinal Tract
Approach	8	Via Natural and Artificial Endoscopic
Device	Z	No Device
Qualifier	Z	No Qualifier

INDEX: EGD (esophagogastroduodenoscopy)

Secondary Procedure: Detoxification **HZ2ZZZZ**

Character	Code	Explanation
Section	H	Substance Abuse Treatment
Body System	Z	None
Root Type	2	Detoxification
Type qualifier	Z	None
Qualifier	Z	None

Character	Code	Explanation
Qualifier	Z	None
Qualifier	Z	None

INDEX: Detoxification services for substance abuse

Rationale: The patient was admitted for GI bleeding that was found to be due to bleeding esophageal varices in alcoholic liver cirrhosis, so the cirrhosis coded as the principal diagnosis. The patient's underlying medical conditions of bleeding esophageal varices, alcohol dependence with withdrawal, and thrombocytopenia were coded as secondary diagnoses. The principal procedure was the EGD with no other procedures performed through the scope that was done to evaluate the bleeding source. The management of the withdrawal symptoms was coded with the procedure of detoxification.

17. **Principal Diagnosis:**   **K40.91** Hernia, inguinal, unilateral, recurrent

    Secondary Diagnoses: None indicated by the documentation provided

    Principal Procedure: Right inguinal hernia repair **0YQ50ZZ**

Character	Code	Explanation
Section	0	Medical and Surgical
Body System	Y	Anatomical Regions, Lower Extremities
Root Operation	Q	Repair
Body Part	5	Inguinal Region Right
Approach	0	Open
Device	Z	No Device
Qualifier	Z	No Qualifier

INDEX: Herniorrhaphy, see Repair, anatomical regions, lower extremities

Secondary Procedure(s): None indicated by the documentation provided

Rationale: The single reason for the hospital admission was the recurrent inguinal hernia, so it was listed as the principal diagnosis. The surgery performed was an inguinal herniorrhaphy. In the ICD-10-PCS Index, the term herniorrhaphy states "with synthetic substitute, see Supplement" or "see Repair, anatomical regions, general or lower extremities." Because there was no synthetic material used to repair the inguinal hernia in this scenario, such as mesh, the correct root operation would be repair. On the ICD-10-PCS table 0WQ, there is no body part for inguinal area. The coder should refer to the table 0YQ that does include the inguinal region. This was an open procedure performed through an incision.

19. **Principal Diagnosis:**   **K56.50** Obstruction, intestine, with adhesions

    Secondary Diagnoses: **E03.9** Hypothyroidism;

                            I10 Hypertension;

                            E78.5 Hyperlipidemia;

                            F43.0 Reaction, stress, acute

Principal Procedure: Lysis/release of small intestine **0DN80ZZ**

Character	Code	Explanation
Section	0	Medical and Surgical
Body System	D	Gastrointestinal System
Root Operation	N	Release
Body Part	8	Small intestine
Approach	0	Open
Device	Z	No device
Qualifier	Z	No Qualifier

INDEX: Lysis, see Release, intestine, small

Secondary Procedure: Placement of Seprafilm adhesion barrier **3E0M05Z**

Character	Code	Explanation
Section	3	Administration
Physiological system	E	Physiological system and anatomical regions
Root Operation	0	Introduction
Body system/region	M	Peritoneal cavity
Approach	0	Open
Substance	5	Adhesion barrier
Qualifier	Z	No Qualifier

INDEX: Introduction of substance in or on, peritoneal cavity, adhesion barrier

Rationale: The patient was admitted to the hospital with signs and symptoms of gastrointestinal disease with dilated loops of the small bowel trapped between the abdominal wall and intestines. During surgery it was determined the patient had a small bowel obstruction due to adhesions that were lysed. The principal diagnosis is the small bowel obstruction with adhesions. All the patient's other medical conditions that were evaluated and treated were coded as secondary diagnoses. The elevated blood pressure reading was not assigned a code as it was stated this was thought to be due to the stress reaction the patient was having concerning her condition and impending surgery. In ICD-10-PCS the main term of lysis for an operative procedure directs the coder to the term of release of the body part being released. The application of the adhesion barrier to reduce further adhesions from forming is coded to the root operation of introduction. If the coder had used the main term of application, it would have directed the coder to the main term of introduction of substance in or on and the coder would pick the anatomic site where the substance was introduced.

21. **Principal Diagnosis:**   **K26.0** Ulcer, duodenum, acute with hemorrhage

   Secondary Diagnoses: **K44.9** Hernia, hiatal

   Principal Procedure: Cauterization bleeding points in duodenum **0D598ZZ**

Character	Code	Explanation
Section	0	Medical and Surgical
Body System	D	Gastrointestinal System
Root Operation	5	Destruction
Body Part	9	Duodenum
Approach	8	Via Natural or Artificial Opening Endoscopic
Device	Z	No Device
Qualifier	Z	No Qualifier

INDEX: Cauterization, see Destruction, duodenum

Secondary Procedure(s): None indicated by the documentation provided

Rationale: The patient was admitted to the hospital because of vomiting blood. After study with the performance of an EGD and cauterization of bleeding points in the duodenum, the diagnosis of acute hemorrhaging duodenal ulcer was made, and this was listed as the principal diagnosis. A secondary diagnosis of hiatal hernia was also assigned based on the findings of the EGD procedure. The endoscopic procedure included cauterization of the bleeding points within the duodenum. In ICD-10-PCS the main term of cauterization leads the coder to the root operation Destruction to identify the body part involved. No other procedures were performed.

23. **Principal Diagnosis:**   **T18.128A** Foreign body, esophagus, causing, injury NEC, food, initial encounter
    Secondary Diagnoses: None indicated by the documentation provided
    Principal Procedure: EGD with removal of foreign body from lower esophagus **0DC38ZZ**

Character	Code	Explanation
Section	0	Medical and Surgical
Body System	D	Gastrointestinal System
Root Operation	C	Extirpation
Body Part	3	Esophagus, Lower
Approach	8	Via Natural or Artificial Opening Endoscopic
Device	Z	No Device
Qualifier	Z	No Qualifier

INDEX: Extirpation, Esophagus, Lower 0DC3

Secondary Procedure(s): None indicated by the documentation provided

Rationale: The patient was admitted for surgical removal of the food impacted in his esophagus, so the principal diagnosis is T18.128A. According to Coding Clinic First Quarter 2015, pages 23-24: "An esophageal foreign body is any object that does not belong in the esophagus that becomes stuck there, and so it is classified as causing injury in ICD-10-CM." Therefore, the coding path we use in the Index is *Foreign body, esophagus, causing, injury NEC, food.* The removal of the impacted food bolus from the esophagus is an Extirpation. The approach is Via Natural or Artificial Opening Endoscopic since an EGD was used.

Chapter 12

Diseases of the Skin and Subcutaneous Tissue

1. **Principal Diagnosis:**   **L89.313** Ulcer, pressure, stage 3, buttock, right

   Secondary Diagnoses: **L97.411** Ulcer, lower limb, heel, right, skin breakdown only;

   I70.203 Arteriosclerosis, extremities, leg, bilateral

   Principal Procedure: Debridement of hip **0KBN0ZZ**

Character	Code	Explanation
Section	0	Medical and Surgical
Body System	K	Muscle
Root "No	B	Excision
Body Part	N	Hip Muscle, Right
Approach	0	Open
Device	Z	No Device
Qualifier	Z	No Qualifier

INDEX: Debridement, excisional, see Excision, muscle, hip, right

   Secondary Procedure: Debridement foot **0HBMXZZ**

Character	Code	Explanation
Section	0	Medical and Surgical
Body System	H	Skin and Breast
Root Operation	B	Excision
Body Part	M	Skin, Right Foot
Approach	X	External
Device	Z	No Device
Qualifier	Z	No Qualifier

INDEX: Debridement, excisional, see Excision, skin, foot, right

Rationale: The reason for admission after study was the severe decubitus ulcer of the right buttock so it was selected as the principal diagnosis. The chronic ulcer and the atherosclerosis were coded as secondary diagnoses. The pressure ulcer code includes the site, laterality and stage. The non-pressure ulcer code for the condition on the right foot includes the site and laterality with the depth of the wound instead of the stage. Excisional debridement procedures are coded in ICD-10-PCS according to the root operation Excision and the depth of the wound, such as skin or muscle.

3. **First-Listed Diagnosis:**   **L23.2** Dermatitis, contact, allergic, due to cosmetics

   Secondary Diagnoses: **L70.0** Acne, cystic

Rationale: The patient came to the physician's office because of inflammation and irritation on her eyelids and under eyebrows. The physician diagnosed this as contact dermatitis due to cosmetics, so this was listed as the first diagnosis. The physician also evaluated the patient's cystic acne during this visit, and this would be coded as a secondary diagnosis.

5. **Dermatology Diagnosis:**   **L56.5** DSAP;

   Secondary Dermatology Diagnoses: **Z77.123** Contact, radiation, naturally occurring NEC;

        X32.XXXA External Cause Index, exposure, sunlight, initial

   Dermatology Procedure: Biopsy skin right lower arm **0HBDXZX**

Character	Code	Explanation
Section	0	Medical and Surgical
Body System	H	Skin and Breast
Root Operation	B	Excision
Body Part	D	Skin, right lower arm
Approach	X	External
Device	Z	No device
Qualifier	X	Diagnostic

INDEX: Biopsy, see Excision, skin, lower arm, right, with qualifier diagnostic

Secondary Procedure(s): None indicated by the documentation provided

Rationale: The dermatology diagnosis was DSAP that was determined to be the type of lesion present on the patient's skin. A secondary code from the external cause chapter, identifying the cause of the lesions as sun exposure, is optional. If the procedure, skin biopsy, was performed for an inpatient, it would be coded to the root operation of excision with the qualifier of diagnostic.

7. **First-Listed Diagnosis:**   **L23.81** Dermatitis, contact, allergic, dander

   Secondary Diagnoses: None indicated by the documentation provided

Rationale: The single reason for the patient coming to the office for this visit was determined to be contact dermatitis resulting from exposure to animal dander. There is one code for this condition regardless of the sites on which it occurs.

9. **First-Listed Diagnosis:**   **E10.621** Diabetes, type I, with foot ulcer

   Secondary Diagnoses: **L97.415** Ulcer, lower limb, heel, right, with muscle involvement without evidence of necrosis

Rationale: The first-listed code is the diabetes code that includes the foot ulcer. A note appears under code E10.621to use an additional code for the site of the ulcer and muscle involvement, L97.415.

11. **Dermatology Diagnosis:**   **C44.41** Neoplasm, scalp, basal cell carcinoma

   Secondary Dermatology Diagnoses: **L57.0** Keratosis, actinic

   Principal Procedure: Punch biopsy, skin, scalp **0HB0XZX**

Character	Code	Explanation
Section	0	Medical and Surgical
Body System	H	Skin and Breast
Root Operation	B	Excision
Body Part	0	Skin, scalp
Approach	X	External
Device	Z	No device
Qualifier	X	Diagnostic

INDEX: Punch biopsy, see Excision, skin, scalp, with qualifier diagnostic

Secondary Procedure: Excision, skin, scalp **0HB0XZZ**

Character	Code	Explanation
Section	0	Medical and Surgical
Body System	H	Skin and Breast
Root Operation	B	Excision
Body Part	0	Skin, Scalp
Approach	X	External
Device	Z	No Device
Qualifier	Z	No Qualifier

INDEX: Excision, skin, scalp

Rationale: The lesion that was biopsied was a basal cell carcinoma of the skin. The second lesion that was removed was an actinic keratosis. Either condition could have been listed first, with the procedure performed for the first listed condition listed as the first procedure. In ICD-10-PCS, the procedure code for the biopsy requires the use of the X character for the qualifier.

13. **Principal Diagnosis:**   **L03.311** Cellulitis, abdominal wall

  Secondary Diagnoses: **R78.81** Bacteremia;

  B96.5 Infection, bacterial as cause of disease classified elsewhere, pseudomonas, as cause of disease classified elsewhere;

  I87.2 Dermatitis, stasis;

  L03.115 Cellulitis, lower limb, right;

  L03.116 Cellulitis, lower limb, left;

  K70.30 Cirrhosis, alcoholic;

  E88.09 Hypoalbuminemia;

  E66.01 Obesity, morbid

Principal Procedure: None indicated by the documentation provided

Secondary Procedure(s): None indicated by the documentation provided

Rationale: The patient was admitted because of the cellulitis of his abdominal wall which after study still proved to be the principal diagnosis. The physician's stated discharge diagnoses provide the secondary diagnoses to be coded. A second code is needed to report the pseudomonas infection as the bacteremia code does not specify the organism involved. Even though the physician identified the patient as having alcoholic cirrhosis, the physician did not document alcohol abuse or dependence. Therefore, it was not coded. However, the physician could be asked for clarification to decide if it should be coded.

15. **Principal Diagnosis:** L89.156 Ulcer, pressure, coccyx Also – Damage, deep tissue, pressure-induced – see also L89 with final character.6. Also – Pressure, area, skin – see Ulcer, pressure, by site

    Secondary Diagnoses: I50.32 Failure, heart, diastolic, chronic;

    I25.10 Arteriosclerosis, coronary;

    I25.82 Occlusion, coronary, chronic total

    Principal Procedure: Debridement **0QBS0ZZ**

Character	Code	Explanation
Section	0	Medical and Surgical
Body System	Q	Lower Bones
Root Operation	B	Excision
Body Part	S	Coccyx
Approach	0	Open
Device	Z	No Device
Qualifier	Z	No Qualifier

INDEX: Debridement, excisional was done down to the coccyx bone, the body system is lower bones, see Excision, coccyx (Not Excision, bone, coccyx)

Secondary Procedure(s): None indicated by the documentation provided

Rationale: The patient was admitted to the hospital for surgical treatment of her stage 4 sacral pressure ulcer, so it is listed as the principal diagnosis. The physician documents the other medical conditions that were treated during the stay and therefore coded as secondary diagnoses. The debridement procedure is an excision procedure in ICD-10-PCS and the body part involved is the bone involved in the debridement procedure.

17. **First-Listed Diagnosis:** L10.2 Pemphigus, foliaceous

    Secondary Diagnoses: I10 Hypertension (essential)

    Rationale: The reason for the dermatology clinic visit was the recurrence of pemphigus foliaceus. After updating the patient's history and conducting a physical examination, the physician concluded the patient again had pemphigus foliaceus and prescribed medications to treat it. The physician also considered the fact the patient had essential hypertension under treatment. The pemphigus foliaceus was listed as the first-listed diagnosis code as the reason for the visit with a secondary code of hypertension.

Chapter 13

Diseases of the Musculoskeletal System and Connective Tissue

1. **Principal Diagnosis:**   **M51.26** Displacement, intervertebral disc, lumbar

   Secondary Diagnoses: **M47.26** Osteoarthritis, spine, see Spondylosis, Spondylosis, with radiculopathy, lumbar region

   Principal Procedure: Excision of lumbar vertebral disc 0SB20ZZ

Character	Code	Explanation
Section	0	Medical and Surgical
Body System	S	Lower Joints
Root Operation	B	Excision
Body Part	2	Lumbar Vertebral Disc
Approach	0	Open
Device	Z	No Device
Qualifier	Z	No Qualifier

INDEX: Resection, disc, lumbar vertebral

Secondary Procedure(s):   None indicated by the documentation provided

Rationale: In the Alphabetic Index, the main term herniation, nucleus pulposus (vertebrae) led the coder to the main term displacement, lumbar region. The reason for the admission and the surgery is the displacement of the intervertebral disc, so it is listed as the principal diagnosis. The patient also has osteoarthritis, which is an additional code. An intervertebral discectomy involves removing the nucleus pulpous but leaving the annulus fibrosus intact. Therefore, this procedure is considered an excision. The laminotomy is the approach for this procedure and is not coded separately.

3. **First-Listed Diagnosis:**   **M15.9** Arthritis, degenerative, see Osteoarthritis, osteoarthritis, generalized

   Secondary Diagnoses: **M47.817** Arthritis, degenerative, see Osteoarthritis, spine, see Spondylosis, without myelopathy, lumbosacral spine;

                                    I10 Hypertension;

                                      I25.719 Disease, artery, coronary, with angina pectoris, see Arteriosclerosis, coronary, artery, bypass graft, autologous vein, with angina pectoris;

                                      Z95.1 Status, aortocoronary bypass

Rationale: The main reason for the visit is to evaluate the patient's arthritis, which is listed as the first diagnosis. Other medical conditions were also evaluated and treated; therefore, the secondary codes are included. There is an Excludes2 note under section M15–M19 for osteoarthritis of spine M47 so an additional code can be used to describe the osteoarthritis of spine for this patient.

5. **First-Listed Diagnosis:**   **M84.361A** Fracture, traumatic, stress, tibia, right, initial

   Secondary Diagnoses: **M84.362A** Fracture, traumatic, stress, tibia, left, initial;

                                      M84.374A Fracture, traumatic, stress, metatarsus, right foot; initial

                                      S39.012A Strain, low back, initial;

> **X50.3XXA** Index to external cause, overexertion, repetitive movements, initial;
>
> **Y93.02** Index to external cause, activity, running;
>
> **Y99.8** Index to external cause, recreation or sport not for income or while a student

Rationale: Given the fact that the patient has multiple traumatic stress fractures, any of the three codes from M84.36- could be listed as the first code. The other sites of the stress fractures as well as the strain of the low back are listed as secondary diagnosis codes. The use of the external cause codes for injury due to repetitive movements by running for recreation are optional codes as there is no national requirement for external cause reporting.

7. **First-Listed Diagnosis:**   **M24.411** Dislocation, recurrent, shoulder

   Secondary Diagnoses: **M12.511** Arthritis, traumatic, see Arthropathy, traumatic, shoulder;

   X50.0XXA External cause index: Lifting, heavy objects, initial;

   Y92.025 External cause index: Place of occurrence, garage, mobile home

Rationale: The reason the patient came to the ER is the recurrent dislocation of his shoulder. The secondary diagnosis of traumatic arthritis is a co-existing condition that should be listed as a secondary diagnosis.

Practice procedure coding: Closed reduction of shoulder dislocation, **0RSJXZZ**

Character	Code	Explanation
Section	0	Medical and Surgical
Body System	R	Upper joints
Root Operation	S	Reposition
Body Part	J	Shoulder Joint Right
Approach	X	External (closed)
Device	Z	No Device
Qualifier	Z	No Qualifier

INDEX: Reduction, dislocation, see Reposition, joint, shoulder, right

9. **Principal Diagnosis:**   **M23.221** Tear, meniscus, old—see Derangement, knee, meniscus, due to old tear, medial posterior horn

   Secondary Diagnoses: **I11.9** Hypertension, heart (disease)

   Principal Procedure: Meniscectomy or excision knee joint arthroscopic **0SBC4ZZ**

Character	Code	Explanation
Section	0	Medical and Surgical
Body System	S	Lower Joints
Root Operation	B	Excision
Body Part	C	Knee Joint, Right
Approach	4	Percutaneous Endoscopic
Device	Z	No Device
Qualifier	Z	No Qualifier

INDEX: Meniscectomy, knee *see* Excision, Joint, Knee, Right

Secondary Procedure(s): None indicated by the documentation provided

Rationale: The patient was admitted to the hospital for surgical treatment of the old tear of the meniscus in the right knee. The patient's secondary condition of hypertensive heart disease is coded as a secondary diagnosis as it is also a reason the patient was admitted. The partial meniscectomy is coded as an excision in ICD-10-PCS as the total meniscus was not excised. The code includes the arthroscopic approach for the 5th character.

11. **Principal Diagnosis:**   **M54.5** Pain, low back

   Secondary Diagnoses: **C50.911** Neoplasm breast, malignant, primary;

   D75.81 Myelofibrosis, secondary;

   D46.9 Myelodysplastic syndrome;

   T45.1X5S Table of drugs, antineoplastic, adverse effect;

   Z90.11 Absence, breast, right

   Principal Procedure: None indicated by the documentation provided

   Secondary Procedure(s): None indicated by the documentation provided

Rationale: The reason for admission after study was the pain in the low back. Had the pain not been present, there was no reason to admit the patient to the hospital. The patient's underlying conditions were also coded. The code for the drug involved in this patient's care would require the use the 7th character of "S" since this patient was known to have the myelodysplastic syndrome previously as a result of the drug therapy and not discovered during this current episode of care.

13. **Principal Diagnosis:**   **M16.4** Osteoarthritis post-traumatic hip bilateral

   Secondary Diagnoses: None indicated by the documentation provided

   Principal Procedure: Left hip replacement **0SRB039**

Character	Code	Explanation
Section	0	Medical and Surgical
Body System	S	Lower Joints
Root Operation	R	Replacement
Body Part	B	Hip Joint Left
Approach	0	Open
Device	3	Synthetic Substitute, Ceramic
Qualifier	9	Cemented

INDEX: Replacement, joint, hip, left

Secondary Procedure(s): None indicated by the documentation provided

Rationale: There is a single reason for the admission and the surgery, that is, the traumatic arthritis of both the hips. The procedure is a hip replacement using a ceramic cemented device. The removal of the diseased hip joint is integral to the replacement procedure. If required under organization coding policy, a code may be assigned for the hysterectomy status by indexing the term "Status (post)" and choosing hysterectomy leading to code Z90.710.

15. **First-Listed Diagnosis:**   **M62.561** Atrophy, muscle, lower leg, right

   Secondary Diagnoses: **M62.562** Atrophy, muscle, lower leg, left;

   G14, Syndrome, postpolio

Rationale: Either of the muscle atrophy codes (right or left) could be listed first as the bilateral condition was the reason for the clinic visit. Code G14, a more specific neurological condition, has an Excludes1 note for code B91 for sequela of polio so the B91 code is not used.

17. **Diagnosis Codes:**   **M22.42** Chondromalacia, patella, left knee;

    Secondary Diagnoses: **M70.42** Bursitis, knee, prepatellar

    Principal Procedure: Debridement, left knee joint arthroscope **0SBD4ZZ**

Character	Code	Explanation
Section	0	Medical and Surgical
Body System	S	Lower Joints
Root Operation	B	Excision
Body Part	D	Knee Joint Left
Approach	4	Percutaneous Endoscopic
Device	Z	No Device
Qualifier	Z	No Qualifier

INDEX: Debridement, excisional, see Excision, joint, knee, left

Secondary Procedure(s): None indicated by the documentation provided

Rationale: The procedure of arthroscopic debridement of the knee joint was done to treat the chondromalacia of the left patella. A secondary diagnosis of prepatellar bursitis was also established during the procedure. The procedure performed was a debridement of the patella. In ICD-10-PCS, the Alphabetic Index the main term of debridement states "excisional see Excision." Under the main term of excision there is a subterm of patella but more than the patella was debrided so the subterm of joint was used instead.

Chapter 14

Diseases of the Genitourinary System

1. **Principal Diagnosis:**   **N39.0** Infection, urinary (tract)

   Secondary Diagnoses: **B96.4** Infection, bacteria, as cause of disease classified elsewhere, proteus; **I10** Hypertension;

   I25.10 Arteriosclerosis, coronary (artery);

   Z98.61 Status (post) angioplasty, coronary artery;

   J44.9 Disease, lung obstructive;

   Z87.440 History, personal, urinary infection(s)

   Principal Procedure: IV infusion of medication **3E03329**

Character	Code	Explanation
Section	3	Administration
Body System	E	Physiological Systems and Anatomical Regions
Root Operation	0	Introduction

Body Part	3	Peripheral Vein
Approach	3	Percutaneous
Device	2	Anti-infective
Qualifier	9	Other anti-infective

INDEX: Infusion *see* Introduction of substance in or on, Vein, Peripheral, Anti-infective

Secondary Procedure(s): None indicated by the documentation provided

Rationale: The reason for admission after study, the principal diagnosis, is the urinary tract infection with proteus as the cause of the infection. The patient's underlying medical conditions, including the fact the patient has had previous urinary tract infections, were coded as secondary diagnoses. A procedure code was assigned for the IV antibiotic infusion, which may or may not be coded according to facility-specific guidelines.

3. **Principal Diagnosis:**   **N81.12** Cystocele, female, paravaginal

    Secondary Diagnoses: **N39.3** Incontinence, stress;

    E11.9 Diabetes, type 2

    Z79.84, Long-term (current) drug therapy (use of), oral, antidiabetic

    H81.4, Vertigo, central

    Principal Procedure: Colporrhaphy **0UQG0ZZ**

Character	Code	Explanation
Section	0	Medical and Surgical
Body System	U	Female Reproductive System
Root Operation	Q	Repair
Body Part	G	Vagina
Approach	0	Open
Device	Z	No Device
Qualifier	Z	No Qualifier

INDEX: Colporrhaphy, see Repair, vagina

Secondary Procedure(s): None indicated by the documentation provided

Rationale: The patient was admitted to the hospital for surgical treatment of a paravaginal cystocele so this is the principal diagnosis. The cystocele caused urinary incontinence, and the patient was also treated for the diabetes. The surgery colporrhaphy is coded with the root operation of repair in ICD-10-PCS per the direction in the Index and table 0UQ. If documentation in the record identified the type of medication used to treat the type 2 diabetes, an additional code would be assigned for insulin therapy (Z79.4) or oral hypoglycemic medication (Z79.84).

5. **Principal Diagnosis:**   **N10** Pyelonephritis, acute

    Secondary Diagnoses: **N17.9** Failure, renal, acute;

    I10 Hypertension;

    Z87.442 History, personal, calculi, renal

    Principal Procedure: Hemodialysis performed, 4 hours **5A1D70Z**

Character	Code	Explanation
Section	5	Extracorporeal assistance and performance
Body System	A	Physiological systems
Root Operation	1	Performance
Body System	D	Urinary
Duration	7	Intermittent, Less than 6 Hours Per Day
Function	0	Filtration
Qualifier	Z	No Qualifier

INDEX: Hemodialysis *see* Performance, Urinary, Intermittent, less than 6 hours per day

Secondary Procedure(s): IV infusion of antibiotics **3E03329**

Character	Code	Explanation
Section	3	Administration
Body System	E	Physiological Systems and Anatomical Regions
Root Operation	0	Introduction
Body Part	3	Peripheral Vein
Approach	3	Percutaneous
Device	2	Anti-infective
Qualifier	9	Other anti-infective

INDEX: Infusion *see* Introduction of substance in or on, Vein, Peripheral, Anti-infective

Rationale: The reason for admission after study was the acute pyelonephritis complicated by acute renal failure. The acute pyelonephritis was the principal diagnosis and the acute renal failure was the secondary diagnosis. The patient was also known to have hypertension and a history of renal calculi that were coded as secondary diagnoses. The intermittent hemodialysis was performed for 4 hour sessions during the hospital stay so the duration was intermittent less than 6 hours per day. The coding of the infusion will be based on facility-specific coding guidelines, shown here for practice purposes.

7. **Principal Diagnosis:**   **N80.0** Endometriosis, uterus

    Secondary Diagnoses: **N80.1** Endometriosis, ovary;

                                N80.2 Endometriosis, fallopian tube;

                                N80.3 Endometriosis, peritoneal;

                                D06.9 Neoplasm, cervix, carcinoma in situ

    Principal Procedure: Vaginal Hysterectomy **0UT97ZZ**

Character	Code	Explanation
Section	0	Medical and Surgical
Body System	U	Female Reproductive System

Character	Code	Explanation
Root Operation	T	Resection
Body Part	9	Uterus
Approach	7	Via Natural or Artificial Opening
Device	Z	No Device
Qualifier	Z	No Qualifier

INDEX: Hysterectomy, see Resection, uterus

Secondary Procedure: Removal of the uterine cervix **0UTC7ZZ**

Character	Code	Explanation
Section	0	Medical and Surgical
Body System	U	Female Reproductive System
Root Operation	T	Resection
Body Part	C	Cervix
Approach	7	Via Natural or Artificial Opening
Device	Z	No Device
Qualifier	Z	No Qualifier

INDEX: Laparoscopy, see Inspection

Secondary Procedure: Bilateral salpingectomy **0UT77ZZ**

Character	Code	Explanation
Section	0	Medical and Surgical
Body System	U	Female Reproductive system
Root Operation	T	Resection
Body Part	7	Fallopian Tubes, Bilateral
Approach	7	Via Natural or Artificial Opening
Device	Z	No Device
Qualifier	Z	No Qualifier

INDEX: Salpingectomy, see Resection, female reproductive system

Secondary Procedure: Bilateral oophorectomy **0UT27ZZ**

Character	Code	Explanation
Section	0	Medical and Surgical
Body System	U	Female Reproductive system
Root Operation	T	Resection

Body Part	2	Ovaries, bilateral
Approach	7	Via natural or artificial opening
Device	Z	No device
Qualifier	Z	No qualifier

INDEX: Oophorectomy, see Resection, female reproductive system

Rationale: The patient was admitted for a scheduled hysterectomy and bilateral salpingo-oophorectomy. Even though the endometriosis was present in several anatomic locations, the principal diagnosis of endometriosis of the uterus was selected over the other sites. The principal procedure was selected to be the hysterectomy. All of the other sites affected, as well as the pathological diagnosis of the carcinoma in situ of the cervix, were coded as secondary procedures. The removal of the entire uterus, fallopian tubes, ovaries, and cervix were coded to the root operation of resection in ICD-10-PCS.

9. **First-Listed Diagnosis:**   **N20.0** Calculus, kidney

    Secondary Diagnoses: None indicated by the documentation provided

Rationale: As an outpatient visit for a diagnostic test that has a report written by a physician, the coder is able to use the diagnosis provided by the radiologist in the IVP report. The bilateral nephrolithiasis is coded as the first-listed and only diagnosis code. The renal colic is not coded as it is a symptom of the calculus in the kidney.

11. **Principal Diagnosis:**   **N39.0** Infection, urinary (tract)

    Secondary Diagnoses: **E86.0** Dehydration;

      C67.5 Neoplasm, bladder, neck, malignant, primary;

      I25.10 Disease, artery, coronary, see Arteriosclerosis, coronary

      Z95.1 Status, aortocoronary bypass;

      Z93.6 Status, nephrostomy;

      E11.9 Diabetes, type 2;

      Z79.84, Long-term (current) drug therapy (use of), oral, antidiabetic

      E78.00 Hypercholesterolemia

    Principal Procedure: None indicated by the documentation provided

    Secondary Procedure(s):   None indicated by the documentation provided

Rationale: It is stated the reason for admission was the urinary tract infection so the code for it is listed as a principal diagnosis. The fact the patient also has dehydration and cancer of the bladder are significant conditions to code. In addition, the patient's medical conditions are also coded as secondary diagnoses.

13. **Principal Diagnosis:**   **N17.9** Failure, renal, acute

    Secondary Diagnoses: **E86.0** Dehydration

    Principal Procedure: None indicated by the documentation provided

    Secondary Procedure(s):   None indicated by the documentation provided

Rationale: This could be a scenario where there is a coder debate as to whether the acute renal failure or the dehydration was the principal diagnosis. The question is, what brought the patient into the hospital? If she just had dehydration, could that have been treated as an outpatient? The physician's conclusion that the patient had "acute renal failure due to dehydration" appears to say the reason for admission was the acute renal failure, which is then the principal diagnosis.

15. **First-Listed Diagnosis:**   **N93.8** Bleeding, uterus, dysfunctional

      Secondary Diagnoses: **Z30.2** Encounter (for), sterilization

      Practice Procedure Coding: Diagnostic D& C **0UDB7ZX**

Character	Code	Explanation
Section	0	Medical and Surgical
Body System	U	Female Reproductive System
Root Operation	D	Extraction
Body Part	B	Endometrium
Approach	7	Via Natural or Artificial Opening
Device	Z	No Device
Qualifier	X	Diagnostic

INDEX: Curettage, see excision, see Extraction. Uterine curettage is extraction

      Practice Procedure Coding: Laparoscopic bilateral tubal ligation (occlusion) with Falope ring application **0UL74CZ**

Character	Code	Explanation
Section	0	Medical and Surgical
Body System	U	Female Reproductive System
Root Operation	L	Occlusion
Body Part	7	Fallopian Tubes, Bilateral
Approach	4	Percutaneous endoscopic
Device	C	Extraluminal Device (Falope ring)
Qualifier	Z	No Qualifier

INDEX: Ligation, see Occlusion, Fallopian Tubes bilateral, 0UL7. A Falope ring is applied to the outside of the Fallopian tube or extraluminal type.

Rationale: This is an outpatient visit and, normally, the two procedures performed would be coded with CPT/HCPCS codes but were coded for this exercise as ICD-10-PCS coding practice. Each condition had a procedure performed for it. For that reason, either condition could be listed as the first diagnosis.

17. **Principal Diagnosis:**   **N39.0** Infection, urinary tract

      Secondary Diagnoses: **N41.0** Prostatitis, acute;

                                    N41.1 Prostatitis, chronic;

                                    N40.0 Hypertrophy, prostate, see Enlarged prostate, without lower urinary tract symptoms (LUTS);

                                    I48.20 Fibrillation, atrial, chronic;

                                    Z79.01 Long term drug therapy (current) anticoagulants

                                    Z87.440 History, personal, urinary (tract) infections

Principal Procedure: None indicated by the documentation provided

Secondary Procedure(s):   None indicated by the documentation provided

Rationale: Based on the answer to the physician query, that the diagnosis was urinary tract infection and not sepsis, the code for urinary tract infection was listed as the principal diagnosis code. The related conditions, the prostatitis and enlarged prostate, were included as additional diagnoses. The diagnosis code for enlarged prostate without lower urinary tract symptoms was selected because no incomplete bladder emptying, nocturia, or any of the other conditions listed under code N40.1 were documented. The patient's atrial fibrillation and treatment on anticoagulants were addressed during the hospital stay and were, therefore, coded as secondary diagnoses. Any diagnosis qualified as "possible" for an inpatient is coded as if it was confirmed.

Chapter 15

Pregnancy, Childbirth, and the Puerperium

1. **First-Listed Diagnosis:**   **O99.810** Pregnancy, complicated by, abnormal glucose tolerance

   Secondary Diagnoses: **O09.512** Pregnancy, supervision of, elderly mother, primigravida, second trimester (22 weeks)

   Z3A.22 Pregnancy, weeks of gestation, 22 weeks

   Rationale: Rule out conditions cannot be coded for outpatient visits. What appeared to be known about the patient was that she had abnormal glucose tolerance screening, and that is the reason for this laboratory test. At the beginning of ICD-10-CM Chapter 15, Pregnancy, Childbirth and the Puerperium, there is an instruction note "Use additional code from category Z3A, weeks of gestation, to identify the specific week of gestation, if known."

3. **Principal Diagnosis:**   **O33.9** Delivery, cesarean, cephalopelvic disproportion

   Secondary Diagnoses: **O34.211** Delivery, cesarean, previous cesarean delivery, low;

   Z3A.39 Pregnancy, weeks of gestation, 39 weeks;

   Z37.0 Outcome of delivery, single, liveborn

   Principal Procedure: Repeat low Cesarean delivery **10D00Z1**

Character	Code	Explanation
Section	1	Obstetrics
Body System	0	Pregnancy
Root Operation	D	Extraction
Body Part	0	Products of Conception
Approach	0	Open
Device	Z	No Device
Qualifier	1	Low

INDEX: Caesarean section, see Extraction, products of conception; Delivery, cesarean – see Extraction, products of conception

Secondary Procedure(s):   None indicated by the documentation provided

Rationale: The patient had a previous cesarean delivery for cephalopelvic disproportion. The cesarean delivery was performed again for this second pregnancy because the patient had the same cephalopelvic disproportion. At the beginning of ICD-10-CM Chapter 15, Pregnancy, Childbirth and the Puerperium, there is an instruction note "Use additional code from category Z3A, weeks of gestation, to identify the specific week of gestation, if known." The outcome of delivery code is assigned for every patient who has a delivery. The Index entry for cesarean section refers the coder in ICD-10-PCS to locate the main term of extraction, products of conception for the cesarean delivery code.

5. **Principal Diagnosis:**   **O80** Delivery, normal

    Secondary Diagnoses: **Z3A.40** Pregnancy, weeks of gestation, 40 weeks;

                                  Z37.0 Outcome of delivery, single liveborn

    Principal Procedure: Manually assisted delivery **10E0XZZ**

Character	Code	Explanation
Section	1	Obstetrics
Body System	0	Pregnancy
Root Operation	E	Delivery
Body Part	0	Products of Conception
Approach	X	External
Device	Z	No Device
Qualifier	Z	No Qualifier

INDEX: Delivery, manually assisted

    Secondary Procedure: Artificial rupture of membranes **10907ZC**

Character	Code	Explanation
Section	1	Obstetrics
Body System	0	Pregnancy
Root Operation	9	Drainage
Body Part	0	Products of Conception
Approach	7	Via Natural or Artificial Opening
Device	Z	No Device
Qualifier	C	Amniotic Fluid, Therapeutic

INDEX: Induction of labor, artificial rupture of membranes, see Drainage, products of conception, amniotic fluid, therapeutic (The term rupture does not apply here)

Rationale: This patient had a normal full-term pregnancy with a completely normal delivery. The artificial rupture of membranes can be coded with a diagnosis code of normal delivery O80. The vaginal delivery (manually assisted) is assigned as the principal procedure code. The artificial rupture of membranes is a drainage procedure by the definition of drainage in ICD-10-PCS and the body part being drained is the amniotic fluid from the uterus, which is part of the products of conception. At the beginning of ICD-10-CM Chapter 15, Pregnancy, Childbirth and the Puerperium, there is an instruction note "Use additional code from category Z3A, weeks of gestation, to identify the specific week of gestation, if known."

7. **First-Listed Diagnosis:**   **O91.12** Abscess, breast, puerperal, see Mastitis, obstetric, purulent, associated with puerperium

   Secondary Diagnoses: None indicated by the documentation provided

   Rationale: The reason for the office visit is found to be the postpartum purulent breast abscess, and that is the only diagnosis code required as the first-listed diagnosis.

9. **Principal Diagnosis:**   **O07.1** Abortion, attempted, complicated by, hemorrhage

   Secondary Diagnoses: **O99.019** Pregnancy, complicated by anemia; (weeks not known)

   D62 Anemia, blood loss, acute

   Principal Procedure: Dilatation and curettage following abortion **10D17ZZ**

Character	Code	Explanation
Section	1	Obstetrics
Body System	0	Pregnancy
Root Operation	D	Extraction
Body Part	1	Products of Conception Retained
Approach	7	Via Natural or Artificial Opening
Device	Z	No Device
Qualifier	Z	No Qualifier

INDEX: Curettage – see Extraction. Extraction, products of conception, retained

Secondary Procedure(s): None indicated by the documentation provided

Rationale: The reason for admission after study was found to be retained products of conception following an elective abortion during a previous healthcare encounter. The vaginal bleeding is occurring because the elective abortion was not completed. The complication of the abortion code is listed as principal diagnosis. The patient was also diagnosed and treated for anemia associated with the pregnancy, and this is coded as a secondary diagnosis. The weeks of pregnancy code is not assigned here because the codes are not applicable for pregnancies with abortive outcomes, according to ICD-10-CM Chapter 15 coding guidelines. The ICD-10-PCS root operation of extraction is used to describe the dilatation and curettage following the abortion to remove the retained products of conception from the uterus. Refer to ICD-10-PCS coding guideline C.2 for procedures following delivery or abortion.

11. **Principal Diagnosis:**   **O44.33** Pregnancy, complicated by, placenta previa, partial with hemorrhage third trimester

    Secondary Diagnoses: **O30.043** Pregnancy, twin, dichorionic/diamniotic, third trimester;

    O60.14X1 Pregnancy, complicated by, preterm labor, third trimester, 34 weeks;

    O60.14X2 Pregnancy, complicated by, preterm labor, third trimester, 34 weeks;

    O99.013 Pregnancy, complicated by, anemia, third trimester;

    D62 Anemia, blood loss, acute;

    Z3A.34 Pregnancy, weeks of gestation, 34 weeks;

    Z37.2 Outcome of delivery, twins, both liveborn

    Principal Procedure: Cesarean delivery **10D00Z1**

Character	Code	Explanation
Section	1	Obstetrics
Body System	0	Pregnancy
Root Operation	D	Extraction
Body Part	0	Products of Conception
Approach	0	Open
Device	Z	No Device
Qualifier	1	Low

INDEX: Cesarean section, see Extraction, products of conception

Secondary Procedure(s): None indicated by the documentation provided

Rationale: The reason for the admission and the cesarean delivery was the patient's pregnancy complicated by partial placenta previa. The vaginal bleeding is a symptom of the placenta previa and not coded separately. The patient is also diagnosed with acute blood loss anemia that is coded as complicating the pregnancy. Some of these pregnancy chapter codes require the use of the character to identify the trimester of pregnancy. In this scenario, it is the third trimester of pregnancy. At the beginning of ICD-10-CM Chapter 15, Pregnancy, Childbirth and the Puerperium, there is an instruction note to "Use additional code from category Z3A, weeks of gestation, to identify the specific week of gestation, if known." On admission, the patient had completed 34 weeks of gestation (guideline I.C.21.c.11). The Index entry for cesarean section refers the coder in ICD-10-PCS to locate the main term of extraction, products of conception for the cesarean delivery code. The outcome of delivery code is assigned for every patient who has a delivery.

13. **Principal Diagnosis:** **O76** Delivery, complicated by, fetal, heart rate irregularity

    Secondary Diagnoses: **O99.013** Pregnancy, complicated by, anemia;

    D50.9 Anemia, iron deficiency;

    Z3A.38 Pregnancy, weeks of gestation, 38 weeks;

    Z37.0 Outcome of delivery, single, liveborn

    Principal Procedure: Cesarean delivery **10D00Z1**

Character	Code	Explanation
Section	1	Obstetrics
Body System	0	Pregnancy
Root Operation	D	Extraction
Body Part	0	Products of Conception
Approach	0	Open
Device	Z	No Device
Qualifier	1	Low

INDEX: Cesarean section, extraction, products of conception

Secondary Procedure: Artificial rupture of membranes **10907ZC**

Character	Code	Explanation
Section	1	Obstetrics
Body System	0	Pregnancy
Root Operation	9	Drainage
Body Part	0	Products of Conception
Approach	7	Via Natural or Artificial Opening
Device	Z	No Device
Qualifier	C	Amniotic Fluid, Therapeutic

INDEX: Induction of labor, artificial rupture of membranes, see Drainage, pregnancy, 109; AROM (artificial rupture of membranes) 10907ZC

Secondary Procedure: Fetal monitoring **4A1HXCZ**

Character	Code	Explanation
Section	4	Measurement and Monitoring
Physiologic system	A	Physiological System
Root Operation	1	Monitoring
Body Part	H	Products of Conception, Cardiac
Approach	X	External
Function/device	C	Rate
Qualifier	Z	No Qualifier

Index: Monitoring, products of conception, cardiac rate

Rationale: The patient was in labor on admission but was found to have fetal distress with fetal heart rate decelerations, and the management of the patient was changed to performance of a cesarean delivery for her. Based on the fetal decelerations leading to distress, code O76 was chosen as the principal diagnosis. However, O77.8 (fetal stress) or O36.8330 (Pregnancy, complicated by fetal, heart rate or rhythm) may alternatively be selected as the principal diagnosis. A physician query may be necessary to help with the appropriate principal diagnosis code selection. The patient also had microcytic anemia related to her pregnancy, which was treated. The principal procedure was the cesarean delivery. The Index entry for cesarean section refers the coder in ICD-10-PCS to locate the main term of extraction, products of conception for the cesarean delivery code. Two other procedures were performed, including the rupture of membranes (drainage as the root operation in ICD-10-PCS) and the fetal heart rate monitoring (which may or may not be coded depending on facility-specific coding guidelines). At the beginning of ICD-10-CM Chapter 15, Pregnancy, Childbirth and the Puerperium, there is an instruction note "Use additional code from category Z3A, weeks of gestation, to identify the specific week of gestation, if known." The outcome of delivery code is assigned for every patient who has a delivery.

15. **Principal Diagnosis:**   **O44.13** Delivery, cesarean for, placenta previa, complete, with hemorrhage, third trimester

    Secondary Diagnoses: **O32.8XX0** Delivery, cesarean for, breech presentation, incomplete (double footling);

    O13.3 Hypertension, gestational;

    O34.211 Delivery, cesarean, previous, cesarean delivery, low transverse scar;

    O41.1230 Pregnancy, complicated by, chorioamnionitis;

    Z3A.32 Pregnancy, weeks of gestation, 32 weeks;

    Z37.0 Outcome of delivery, single, liveborn

    Principal Procedure: Cesarean delivery **10D00Z1**

Character	Code	Explanation
Section	1	Obstetrics
Body System	0	Pregnancy
Root Operation	D	Extraction
Body Part	0	Products of Conception
Approach	0	Open
Device	Z	No Device
Qualifier	1	Low

INDEX: Cesarean section, extraction, products of conception

Secondary Procedure(s):   None indicated by the documentation provided

Rationale: The patient has multiple conditions treated during this pregnancy. The patient needed to be admitted and have the cesarean delivery because of the vaginal bleeding that was occurring due to the total placenta previa that was known to be present. The other conditions treated and evaluated were the breech presentation of the infant, the fact the patient had a previous cesarean delivery, gestational hypertension, and the presence of amnionitis found on pathological exam of the placenta. A code for preterm labor is not assigned as the patient did not go into labor. At the beginning of ICD-10-CM Chapter 15, Pregnancy, Childbirth and the Puerperium, there is an instruction note "Use additional code from category Z3A, weeks of gestation, to identify the specific week of gestation, if known." The Index entry for cesarean section refers the coder in ICD-10-PCS to locate the main term of extraction, products of conception for the cesarean delivery code. The outcome of delivery code is assigned for every patient who has a delivery.

17. **Principal Diagnosis:**   **O00.102** Pregnancy, ectopic, tubal, without intrauterine pregnancy

    Secondary Diagnoses: None indicated by the documentation provided

    Principal Procedure: Resection, fallopian tube, left **0UT60ZZ**

Character	Code	Explanation
Section	0	Medical and Surgical
Body System	U	Female Reproductive System
Root Operation	T	Resection
Body Part	6	Fallopian Tube, Left
Approach	0	Open

Character	Code	Explanation
Device	Z	No Device
Qualifier	Z	No Qualifier

INDEX: Resection, fallopian tube, left

Secondary Procedure: Diagnostic D&C (no products of conception) **0UDB7ZX**

Character	Code	Explanation
Section	0	Medical and Surgical
Body system	U	Female Reproductive System
Root Operation	D	Extraction
Body Part	B	Endometrium
Approach	7	Via Natural or Artificial Opening
Device	Z	No Device
Qualifier	X	Diagnostic

INDEX: Curettage, see Extraction, endometrium

Secondary Procedure: Removal of contents of fallopian tube, salpingectomy with products of conception (Need OB chapter code as patient is pregnant) **10T20ZZ**

Character	Code	Explanation
Section	1	Obstetrics
Body system	0	Pregnancy
Root Operation	T	Resection
Body Part	2	Products of Conception, Ectopic
Approach	0	Open
Device	Z	No Device
Qualifier	Z	No Qualifier

INDEX: Resection, products of conception, ectopic

Rationale: After study, it was determined the patient had an ectopic pregnancy in the left fallopian tube, so it was chosen as the principal diagnosis. There was no documentation of a pregnancy also present in the uterus. The estimated eight weeks of pregnancy would not be assigned as a secondary diagnosis code. As the coding guidelines for Chapter 21 stated, category Z3A codes should not be used for pregnancies with abortive outcomes, categories O00–O08. The patient had three procedures. The definitive procedure related to the principal diagnosis is the removal of the entire left fallopian tube that would be coded with the root operation of resection in ICD-10-PCS. It was an open procedure for the approach. Prior to deciding the fallopian tube had to be removed, the surgeon removed the contents of the fallopian, the ectopic pregnancy products of conception. Therefore, the body part is the products of conception that were removed in their entirety, so the root operation of resection is used again. The first procedure performed was a diagnostic procedure, a dilatation and curettage, to determine if there was an intrauterine pregnancy or possibly an incomplete abortion or a missed abortion. There were no villi in the uterus; therefore, there was no pregnancy in the uterus. The D&C is identified as an "extraction" in ICD-10-PCS and is coded as a diagnostic with the 7th character of X as it was not treating the ectopic pregnancy.

Chapter 16

Certain Conditions Originating in the Perinatal Period

1. **Principal Diagnosis:**   **P07.03** Low, birth weight, extreme, with weight of 750–999 grams

   Secondary Diagnoses: **P07.32** Premature, newborn, less than 37 completed weeks, see Preterm infant, newborn, gestational age, 29 completed weeks;

   P22.0 Syndrome, respiratory, distress, newborn

   Principal Procedure: Continuous positive airway pressure, 24-96 consecutive hours ventilation

Character	Code	Explanation
Section	5	Extracorporeal or Systemic Assistance and Performance
Body System	A	Physiological Systems
Root Operation	0	Assistance
Body System	9	Respiratory
Duration	4	24-96 consecutive hours
Function	5	Ventilation
Qualifier	7	Continuous positive airway pressure

INDEX: Continuous positive airway pressure, 24-96 consecutive hours ventilation, 5A09457

Secondary Procedure(s): None indicated by the documentation provided

Rationale: The reason for the transfer to the university hospital is the infant's prematurity. See the note located under Category P07 Disorders of newborn related to short gestation and low birth weight, not elsewhere classified: when both birth weight and gestational age of the newborn are available, both should be coded with birth weight sequenced before gestational age. In addition, a code for the neonatal respiratory distress syndrome is coded.

3. **First-Listed Diagnosis:**   **Z00.111** Newborn, examination, 8 to 28 days old

   Secondary Diagnoses: **P38.9** Omphalitis without hemorrhage

Rationale: The purpose of the visit was for the well-baby exam. The use additional code for any identified abnormal findings appears under code Z00.11 so the omphalitis is also coded and reported.

5. **Principal Diagnosis:**   **P29.30,** Hypertension, pulmonary, of newborn

   Secondary Diagnoses: **P84** Hypoxemia, newborn

   Principal Procedure: ECMO, see performance, circulatory **5A1522G**

Character	Code	Explanation
Section	5	Extracorporeal Assistance and Performance
Physiological System	A	Physiological Systems
Root Operation	1	Performance
Body System	5	Circulatory
Duration	2	Continuous

Function	2	Oxygenation
Qualifier	G	Membrane, peripheral veno-arterial

INDEX: ECMO, see Performance circulatory 5A15

Secondary Procedure: Ultrasound, heart **B24DYZZ**

Character	Code	Explanation
Section	B	Imaging
Body System	2	Heart
Root Type	4	Ultrasonography
Body Part	D	Pediatric Heart
Contrast	Y	Other Contrast
Qualifier	Z	None
Qualifier	Z	None

INDEX: Echocardiogram, see Ultrasonography, heart pediatric B24

Rationale: The infant was transferred to the hospital and found to have pulmonary hypertension in a newborn as the reason after study for the hospital admission. The hypoxemia was also treated and not integral to the pulmonary hypertension. The ECMO procedure was the principal therapeutic procedure performed. The ultrasound of the heart may or may not be required to be coded based on the coding guidelines of the hospital as it is a diagnostic imaging procedure.

7. **Principal Diagnosis:**   **P96.1** Withdrawal state, newborn infant of dependent mother

    Secondary Diagnoses: **P05.18** Small-for-dates with weight of 2400 grams

    Principal Procedure: None indicated by the documentation provided

    Secondary Procedure(s):   None indicated by the documentation provided

Rationale: The infant was transferred to the university hospital as an infant of an addicted mother and found to be suffering withdrawal and this was the principal diagnosis. The physician also described the infant as "small for dates." There is no code assigned for the weeks of gestation for this full-term infant. The procedure of weaning the infant from the narcotics does not have a code.

9. **First-Listed Diagnosis:**   **P04.41** Crack baby

    Secondary Diagnoses: **P22.1** Tachypnea, of newborn (transitory) (idiopathic)

Rationale: The infant was brought to the pediatric clinic for evaluation of her status as a "crack baby," so this should be the first-listed diagnosis code. The physician also diagnosed the infant as having transitory tachypnea.

11. **Principal Diagnosis:**   **Z38.01** Newborn, born in hospital, by cesarean

    Secondary Diagnoses: **P05.07** Light-for-dates with weight of 1920 grams;

    P07.35 Preterm infant, newborn gestational age, 32 completed weeks;

    Z05.1 Observation, newborn (for) suspected condition, ruled out, infectious

Principal Procedure: None indicated by the documentation provided

Secondary Procedure(s):   None indicated by the documentation provided

Rationale: The principal diagnosis for an infant born in the hospital during a current admission should be the Z38 category code describing the infant's status and type of delivery. This infant was premature and also described as "light for dates." Both of these conditions were added as secondary diagnoses. The gestational age of the infant and the fact the infant was suspected of acquiring an infectious disease from the mother, but found not to have an infection, was also coded as secondary diagnoses.

13. **First Listed Diagnosis:**   **Z00.110** Newborn, examination, under 8 days old

    Secondary Diagnoses: **P39.1** Conjunctivitis, chlamydial, neonatal

Rationale: The 7-day old infant was brought to the physician's office for her first post-discharge examination and, therefore, this is the first-listed diagnosis. The findings of the exam are coded and reported as a secondary diagnosis.

15. **Principal Diagnosis:**   **P07.16** Low, birth weight, with weight of, 1600 grams

    Secondary Diagnoses: **P07.36** Preterm infant, newborn, gestational age, 33 completed weeks;

        Q76.0 Spina Bifida, occulta

    Principal Procedures: None indicated by the documentation provided

    Secondary Procedure(s):   None indicated by the documentation provided

Rationale: The reason the infant was transferred to the university hospital because of his prematurity and respiratory difficulties. No diagnosis was made to explain the suspected respiratory condition. Additional diagnosis codes were assigned to reflect the infant's gestational age and the spina bifida occulta. No procedures were performed.

17. **Principal Diagnosis:**   **Z38.01** Newborn, born in hospital, by cesarean

    Secondary Diagnoses: **P22.1** Tachypnea, newborn (transitory)

    Principal Procedure: Oxygen therapy (introduction) **3E0F7GC**

Character	Code	Explanation
Section	3	Administration
Physiological System	E	Physiological Systems and Anatomical Regions
Root Operation	0	Introduction
Body System/Region	F	Respiratory Tract
Approach	7	Via Natural or Artificial Opening
Substance	G	Other Therapeutic Substance
Qualifier	C	Other Substance

INDEX: Introduction of substance in or on, respiratory tract, 3E0F

Secondary Procedure(s):   None indicated by the documentation provided

Rationale: The infant was born during the current hospital stay by cesarean delivery and weighed 3150 grams after a 38-week gestation. The principal diagnosis is the Z38.01 code to indicate the birth. The pediatrician also described the infant as having transient tachypnea that is coded with a secondary diagnosis of P22.1. The ICD-10-PCS code for the supplemental oxygen is coded as an introduction of a therapeutic substance into the respiratory tract. The approach is via the natural opening (nose). The coding of oxygen therapy may or may not be coded based on hospital coding policies as it not a surgical procedure that is required to be coded.

Chapter 17

Congenital Malformations, Deformations, and Chromosomal Abnormalities

1. **Principal Diagnosis:** **H90.6** Loss, hearing, see also Deafness, mixed, conductive and sensorineural, bilateral
   Secondary Diagnoses: **Q16.5** anomaly, ear, inner
   Principal Procedure: Insertion of cochlear prosthesis, right **09HD05Z**

Character	Code	Explanation
Section	0	Medical and Surgical
Body System	9	Ear, Nose, Sinus
Root Operation	H	Insertion
Body Part	D	Inner Ear, Right
Approach	0	Open
Device	5	Hearing Device, Single Channel Cochlear Prosthesis
Qualifier	Z	No Qualifier

INDEX: Cochlear implant, single channel, use hearing device, single channel cochlear prosthesis, right

Secondary Procedure: Insertion of cochlear prosthesis, left **09HE05Z**

Character	Code	Explanation
Section	0	Medical and Surgical
Body System	9	Ear, Nose, Sinus
Root Operation	H	Insertion
Body Part	E	Inner Ear, Left
Approach	0	Open
Device	5	Hearing Device, Single Channel Cochlear Prosthesis
Qualifier	Z	No Qualifier

INDEX: Cochlear implant, single channel, use hearing device, single channel cochlear prosthesis, left

Rationale: The principal diagnosis, reason for admission after study, was bilateral hearing loss. The underlying congenital anomaly of the inner ear was also assigned as a secondary diagnosis. A bilateral cochlear implant procedure was performed. Two procedure codes are assigned, one for the right ear and one for the left ear.

3. **Principal Diagnosis:** **Q25.1** Coarctation, aorta
   Secondary Diagnoses: None indicated by the documentation provided
   Principal Diagnosis: Excision of the thoracic aorta **02BW0ZZ**

Character	Code	Explanation
Section	0	Medical and Surgical
Body System	2	Heart and Great Vessels
Root Operation	B	Excision
Body Part	W	Thoracic, Aorta, Descending
Approach	0	Open
Device	Z	No Device
Qualifier	Z	No Qualifier

INDEX: Excision, aorta, thoracic, descending 02BW

Secondary Procedure: Cardiopulmonary bypass **5A1221Z**

Character	Code	Explanation
Section	5	Extracorporeal Assistance and Performance
Physiological System	A	Physiological Systems
Root Operation	1	Performance
Body System	2	Cardiac
Duration	2	Continuous
Function	1	Output
Qualifier	Z	No Qualifier

INDEX: Bypass, cardiopulmonary 5A1221Z

Rationale: The reason for admission (transfer) for this infant was the congenital condition, coarctation of the aorta, that was surgically repaired. An excision of the thoracic aorta was performed with an end-to-end anastomosis. Procedure steps necessary to reach the operative site and close the operative site, including any anastomosis of a tubular body part, are not coded separately. The use of the pump oxygenator or cardiopulmonary bypass is coded as an additional procedure.

5. **Principal Diagnosis:**   **Q22.1** Stenosis, pulmonary valve, congenital

   Secondary Diagnoses: **Q25.6** Stenosis, pulmonary artery (congenital);

   Z98.890 History, personal, surgery, NEC;

   Z87.74 History, personal, congenital malformation, circulatory system

   Principal Procedure: Replacement of the pulmonary valve **02RH0KZ**

Character	Code	Explanation
Section	0	Medical and Surgical
Body System	2	Heart and Great Vessels
Root Operation	R	Replacement

Body Part	H	Pulmonary Valve
Approach	0	Open
Device	K	Nonautologous Tissue Substitute
Qualifier	Z	No Qualifier

INDEX: Replacement, valve, pulmonary 02RH

Secondary Procedure: Repair of the pulmonary artery, left **02QR0ZZ**

Character	Code	Explanation
Section	0	Medical and Surgical
Body System	2	Heart and Great Vessels
Root Operation	Q	Repair
Body Part	R	Pulmonary Artery, Left
Approach	0	Open
Device	Z	No Device
Qualifier	Z	No Qualifier

INDEX: Arterioplasty, see Repair, artery, pulmonary

Secondary Procedure: Repair of the pulmonary artery, right **02QQ0ZZ**

Character	Code	Explanation
Section	0	Medical and Surgical
Body System	2	Heart and Great Vessels
Root Operation	Q	Repair
Body Part	Q	Pulmonary Artery, Right
Approach	0	Open
Device	Z	No Device
Qualifier	Z	No Qualifier

INDEX: Arterioplasty, see Repair, artery, pulmonary

Secondary Procedure: Cardiopulmonary bypass **5A1221Z**

Character	Code	Explanation
Section	5	Extracorporeal Assistance and Performance
Physiological System	A	Physiological Systems
Root Operation	1	Performance
Body System	2	Cardiac

Duration	2	Continuous
Function	1	Output
Qualifier	Z	No Qualifier

INDEX: Bypass, cardiopulmonary

Secondary Procedure: Ultrasound of the heart, intraoperative, pediatric **B24DZZ4**

Character	Code	Explanation
Section	B	Imaging
Body System	2	Heart
Root Type	4	Ultrasonography
Body Part	D	Pediatric Heart
Contrast	Z	None
Qualifier	Z	None
Qualifier	4	Transesophageal

INDEX: Echocardiogram, see Ultrasonography, heart, B24 (pediatric heart)

Rationale: The reason for admission after study was to repair the child's congenital heart defects that had previously been repaired, but this was a planned next procedure. The principal diagnosis was identified by the physician as the pulmonary valve stenosis and secondary conditions of stenosis of the pulmonary artery. The other conditions produced by the congenital defect of right ventricular outflow obstruction and pulmonary insufficiency are symptoms of the underlying congenital condition and are not coded separately. The personal history of cardiac surgery and personal history of congenital malformation of the circulatory system are relevant to the patient's current admission and are therefore coded as secondary diagnoses. The principal procedure is to replace the pulmonary value with a homograft, a nonautologous tissue graft. The bilateral repair of the pulmonary arteries is reported with two codes because each is a separate body part in ICD-10-PCS. The ICD-10-PCS root operation of "repair" is used for the arterioplasty as the type of reconstruction of the artery and is not included in other ICD-10-PCS root operations definitions. The cardiopulmonary bypass and intraoperative echocardiogram are also coded as secondary procedures relevant to the overall surgery.

7. **First-Listed Diagnosis:**   **Q37.8** Cleft, lip, bilateral, with cleft palate

   Secondary Diagnoses: **R63.3** Difficult, feeding;

   Z98.890 Status, postsurgical (postprocedural)

Rationale: The reason for the clinic visit was to evaluate the child's complete bilateral cleft lip and palate deformity that was coded as the first-listed diagnosis. The child's feeding difficulties as a result of the congenital deformity as well as the fact that the child had previous surgery for the condition were relevant to the current clinic visit and coded as secondary diagnoses.

9. **First-Listed Diagnosis:**   **Q13.4** Embryotoxon

   Secondary Diagnoses: **Q91.7** Trisomy 13

Rationale: The infant was seen in the ophthalmologist's office for an eye examination and the physician made the diagnosis of an embryotoxon or a congenital corneal malformation. There was no evidence of a retinoblastoma.

The child was previous diagnoses with Trisomy 13, which is relevant to the current examination, so it was coded as a secondary diagnosis.

11. **First-Listed Diagnosis:**   **Q30.0** Atresia, choanal

   Secondary Diagnoses: None indicated by the documentation provided

   Rationale: The reason for the visit to the physician's office was to evaluate the symptoms the infant was demonstrating after feeding. Examination by the physician and the CT scan concluded with the diagnosis of choanal atresia left side being made, so it was listed as the first diagnosis for this outpatient visit.

13. **First-Listed Diagnosis:**   **Q51.3** Bicornate uterus

   Secondary Diagnoses: None indicated by the documentation provided

   Rationale: The reason for the visit to the physician's office was to review the findings of a recent ultrasound examination. Based on the imaging study, the physician concluded the patient had a congenital condition of a partial bicornuate uterus. The physician orders another radiology study for a possible kidney abnormality, but this was not proven and suspected conditions are not coded on the outpatient records.

15. **First-Listed Diagnosis:**   **Q54.0** Hypospadias, balanic

   Secondary Diagnoses: None indicated by the documentation provided

   Rationale: The reason for the physician office visit was to re-evaluate the established hypospadias. That is the only option for the first-listed diagnosis code for this visit. There were no other diagnoses established.

17. **First-Listed Diagnosis:**   **Q75.0** Craniosynostosis

   Secondary Diagnoses: None indicated by the documentation provided

   Rationale: The coding of this congenital condition is straightforward using the main term of craniosynostosis. The child's misshaped head and deviated nose were symptoms of the congenital condition and are not coded separately.

Chapter 18

Symptoms, Signs, and Abnormal Clinical and Laboratory Findings, Not Elsewhere Classified

1. **Principal Diagnosis (for colonoscopy services):**   **R19.4** Change, bowel habits

   Secondary Diagnoses: **Z80.0** History, family, malignant neoplasm, gastrointestinal tract

   Principal Procedure (for colonoscopy services):   Colonoscopy with biopsy of descending colon **0DBM8ZX**

Character	Code	Explanation
Section	0	Medical and Surgical
Body System	D	Gastrointestinal System
Root Operation	B	Excision
Body Part	M	Descending colon
Approach	8	Via Natural or Artificial Opening Endoscopic

Device	Z	No Device
Qualifier	X	Diagnostic

INDEX: Biopsy, see excision with qualifier diagnostic. Excision, colon, descending

Secondary Procedure(s): None indicated by the documentation provided

Rationale: Coding the diagnoses and procedure performed for the colonoscopy and biopsy services provided to an inpatient was the purpose of this exercise. The reason for the colonoscopy was change in bowel habits in a patient with a family history of colon cancer. No abnormal findings were identified during the exam so the main reason for the colonoscopy was the change in bowel habits. The possible colonic polyps were not found and therefore not coded. The family history of colon cancer is another reason for the colonoscopy, so this fact is also coded.

3. **Principal Diagnosis:**   **R91.8** Mass, lung

   Secondary Diagnoses: **R05** Cough;

   R07.89 Pressure, chest

   R00.1 Bradycardia;

   Z53.09 Procedure not done because of contraindication

   Principal Procedure: Bronchoscopy **0BJ08ZZ**

Character	Code	Explanation
Section	0	Medical and Surgical
Body System	B	Respiratory System
Root Operation	J	Inspection
Body Part	0	Tracheobronchial Tree
Approach	8	Via Natural or Artificial Opening Endoscopic
Device	Z	No Device
Qualifier	Z	No Qualifier

INDEX: Bronchoscopy

Secondary Procedure(s): None indicated by the documentation provided

Rationale: The reason for admission, even though the diagnostic study could not be completed, was to evaluate the etiology of the lung mass. The patient's other symptoms of cough and chest pressure would be secondary diagnosis codes. During the bronchoscopy when a biopsy was planned, the patient developed bradycardia so it would also be listed as a secondary diagnosis as the reason the biopsy procedure was canceled. The Z53.09 code is added to indicate that a planned procedure was canceled. The only procedure performed was the bronchoscopy, considered to be an inspection procedure in ICD10-PCS when no other procedure is performed through the bronchoscope.

5. **First-Listed Diagnosis:**   **R20.0** Numbness

   Secondary Diagnoses: **R26.2** Difficulty in walking;

   R27.9 Lack of coordination;

   R25.1 Tremor

Rationale: While the neurologist considered the patient's condition to be "consistent with multiple sclerosis" the patient's physician was not 100% certain and was sending the patient for further evaluation and study. Because this is an outpatient visit and that qualified diagnoses such as possible or probable are not coded for outpatients, the patient's symptoms were coded as the diagnoses for the office visit. Any of the diagnoses could be listed first. The author chose to list the diagnoses in the sequence listed by the physician in the documentation.

7. **First-Listed Diagnosis:**   **R87.810** Human papillomavirus (HPV), DNA test positive, high risk, cervix

    Secondary Diagnoses: None listed by the documentation provided

Rationale: The main reason for the follow-up visit was to review the results of a recent abnormal Pap smear that produced the diagnosis of DNA positive for cervical high-risk human papillomavirus (HPV). A secondary diagnosis for genital warts (A63.0) was not included as a secondary diagnosis because of the Excludes1 note that includes code A63.0 with code R87.810.

9. **First-Listed Diagnosis:**   **R51** Headache

    Secondary Diagnoses: **R50.9** Fever;

    R11.2 Nausea with vomiting;

    R29.1 Meningismus

Rationale: This is an outpatient visit, so any diagnosis stated as a "rule out" condition is not coded as if it were confirmed. Instead the reasons for the visit are the conditions known to be present. Any of the symptoms could have been listed as the first-listed diagnosis but the author chose the diagnosis of headache as it was the first symptom identified in the documentation. The physician added the diagnosis of meningismus at the conclusion of the visit, so it was also coded.

11. **Principal Diagnosis:**   **R13.10** Dysphagia

    Secondary Diagnoses: **F41.9** Anxiety disorder;

    E86.0 Dehydration

    Principal Procedure: EGD **0DJ08ZZ**

Character	Code	Explanation
Section	0	Medical and Surgical
Body System	D	Gastrointestinal System
Root Operation	J	Inspection
Body Part	0	Upper Intestinal Tract
Approach	8	Via Natural or Artificial Opening Endoscopic
Device	Z	No Device
Qualifier	Z	No Qualifier

INDEX: EGD (Esophagogastroduodenoscopy)

Secondary Procedure(s): None indicated by the documentation provided

Rationale: The reason for admission after study was the dysphagia even though no cause for the dysphagia was found during the examinations. This symptom was coded as the principal diagnosis. The other diagnoses documented by the physician for anxiety and dehydration were coded as second diagnoses.

13. **First-Listed Diagnosis:**   **R94.39** Findings, abnormal, stress test

    Secondary Diagnoses: **R03.0** Elevation, blood pressure reading

Rationale: The reason the patient was seen in the cardiologist's office was to "diagnose and treat possible cardiac disease" because the patient had a previous abnormal stress test. Based on the repeated blood pressure readings taken in the office the physician included in his impression at the conclusion of the visit that the patient had elevated blood pressure readings and rule out hypertension. Because this was an outpatient visit, the rule out diagnosis of hypertension is not coded.

15. **First-Listed Diagnosis:** **R10.83** Colic

    Secondary Diagnoses: None indicated by the documentation provided

Rationale: The clearly stated reason for the office visit for this infant is colic. It appears much of the visit included advising and counseling the parents on how to soothe the infant, but these are not diagnoses to be coded and instead reflect the work of the physician in the professional fee evaluation and management procedure code for the office visit.

17. **First-Listed Diagnosis:** **N40.1** Enlarged, prostate, with lower urinary tract symptoms

    Secondary Diagnoses: **R35.1** Nocturia;

    R39.16 Straining, on urination;

    R35.0 Frequency, micturition;

    I10 Hypertension (essential);

    E78.5 Hyperlipidemia

Rationale: The patient presents to the physicians with symptoms of an enlarged prostate and the diagnosis was confirmed after the physical examination. In ICD-10-CM under the code N40.1, there is a note to use additional codes for associated symptoms. For that reason, symptom codes for nocturia, straining, and frequency were added. Usually the integral symptoms of a disease are not coded when the cause of the symptoms are known. However, the direction in the ICD-10-CM code book to use additional code for associated symptoms over-rules the practice of not assigning the symptom codes. Additional codes were assigned for the hypertension and hyperlipidemia because the conditions were evaluated and prescription management continued.

Chapter 19A

Injuries, Effects of Foreign Body, Burns and Corrosions, and Frostbite

*Note: List all applicable codes **excluding** the External Cause codes*

1. **First-Listed Diagnosis:** **T21.31XA** Burn, chest wall, third degree, chest, initial encounter

   Secondary Diagnoses: **T22.232A** Burn, above elbow, left, second degree, initial encounter;

   T22.231A Burn, above elbow, right, second degree initial encounter;

   T31.20 Burn, extent, 20–29% with 0–9% third degree burns

Rationale: The most severe burn, the third degree burn of the chest, is listed first. The second degree burn, and the extent of burn codes are listed as additional diagnoses.

3. **Principal Diagnosis:** **S72.402A** Fracture, traumatic, femur, lower end, initial encounter

   Secondary Diagnoses: **S92.112A** Fracture, traumatic, talus, - See fracture, tarsal, talus, neck, initial encounter

   Principal Procedure: Open reduction, internal fixation fracture left femur **0QSC04Z**

Character	Code	Explanation
Section	0	Medical and Surgical
Body System	Q	Lower Bones
Root Operation	S	Reposition
Body Part	C	Lower Femur, Left
Approach	0	Open
Device	4	Internal Fixation Device
Qualifier	Z	No Qualifier

INDEX: Reduction, fracture, see Reposition, femur, lower left

Secondary Procedure: Open reduction, internal fixation fracture talus **0QSM04Z**

Character	Code	Explanation
Section	0	Medical and Surgical
Body System	Q	Lower Bones
Root Operation	S	Reposition
Body Part	M	Tarsal, Left
Approach	0	Open
Device	4	Internal Fixation Device
Qualifier	Z	No Qualifier

INDEX: Reduction, fracture, see Reposition, tarsal,

Rationale: The most severe injury is coded first so the principal diagnosis is the fracture of the lower femur. The second fracture is listed as the secondary code. The principal procedure most closely related to the principal diagnosis is the open reduction of the femur fracture. A second procedure code is added for the open reduction of the talus.

5. **Principal Diagnosis:**   S06.9X2A Injury, head, with loss of consciousness initial encounter

   Secondary Diagnoses: S01.411A Laceration, cheek, right, initial encounter;

   S01.81XA Laceration, forehead and jaw (specified site of head), initial encounter;

   S01.511A Laceration, lip, initial encounter;

   S60.511A Abrasion, hand, right, initial encounter;

   S60.512A Abrasion, hand, left, initial encounter;

   S30.1XXA Contusion, abdominal wall, initial encounter;

   S80.01XA Contusion, knee, right, initial encounter,

   S80.02XA Contusion, knee, left, initial encounter;

   S80.11XA Contusion, lower leg, right, initial encounter;

   S80.12XA Contusion, lower leg, left, initial encounter

   Principal Procedure: Repair of skin, face, **0HQ1XZZ**

Character	Code	Explanation
Section	0	Medical and Surgical
Body System	H	Skin and Breast
Root Operation	Q	Repair
Body Part	1	Skin, Face
Approach	X	External
Device	Z	No Device
Qualifier	Z	No Qualifier

INDEX: Suture, laceration repair, see Repair, skin, face

Secondary Procedure: Repair laceration of upper lip **0CQ0XZZ**

Character	Code	Explanation
Section	0	Medical and Surgical
Body System	C	Mouth and Throat
Root Operation	Q	Repair
Body Part	0	Upper Lip
Approach	X	External
Device	Z	No Device
Qualifier	Z	No Qualifier

INDEX: Suture, laceration repair, see Repair, lip

Rationale: The most severe injury is coded as the principal diagnosis, which appears to be the head injury with loss of consciousness for this patient. The patient also had multiple lacerations that are coded individually per site. The patient had other injuries, including abrasions and contusions on different body sites that are coded individually per site. Lesser injuries that occur at the same site as a more severe injury are not coded separately, but in this scenario, there are multiple sites on the body with different injuries. For the procedures, each body part that is repaired is coded separately. There were multiple lacerations on the face, the forehead and the cheek, that were individual repaired, but all these sites are on the "face" which is the body part character 4 so reported once per ICD-10-PCS guideline B3.2a. The coding of the MRI of the brain would be determined by hospital procedure coding guidelines.

7. **Principal Diagnosis:**   **S97.82XA** Crush, foot, left, initial encounter
    Secondary Diagnoses: **S92.312B** Fracture, traumatic, metatarsal, first, initial encounter
    Principal Procedure: Fasciotomy, left foot **0J8R0ZZ**

Character	Code	Explanation
Section	0	Medical and Surgical
Body System	J	Skin and Breast
Root Operation	8	Division

Body Part	R	Subcutaneous Tissue and Fascia, Left Foot
Approach	0	Open
Device	Z	No Device
Qualifier	Z	No Qualifier

INDEX: Fasciotomy, see Division, subcutaneous tissue and fascia

Secondary Procedure: Open reduction, internal fixation fracture first metatarsal **0QSP04Z**

Character	Code	Explanation
Section	0	Medical and Surgical
Body System	Q	Lower Bones
Root Operation	S	Reposition
Body Part	P	Metatarsal, Left
Approach	0	Open
Device	4	Internal Fixation Device
Qualifier	Z	No Qualifier

INDEX: Reduction, fracture, see Reposition, metatarsal

Rationale: The most severe injury for the principal diagnosis appears to be the crushing injury to the foot but there could probably be a coder debate on that so the physician should designate the most severe injury. There is an instructional note at category S97 to code all associated injuries, so a secondary code was added, S92.312B, for the fracture of the first metatarsal. The surgical repair included the fasciotomy and the open reduction and internal fixation. Depending on which of the diagnoses was selected by the physician as principal, the matching surgical repair (fasciotomy versus reduction) should be selected as the principal procedure.

9. **Principal Diagnosis:**   S32.022A Fracture, traumatic, vertebra, lumbar, second, burst, unstable, initial encounter

Secondary Diagnoses: S32.032A Fracture, traumatic, vertebra, lumbar, third, burst, unstable, initial encounter

Principal Procedure: Open reduction vertebral fracture, lumbar **0QS00ZZ**

Character	Code	Explanation
Section	0	Medical and Surgical
Body System	Q	Lower Bones
Root Operation	S	Reposition
Body Part	0	Lumbar Vertebra
Approach	0	Open
Device	Z	No Device
Qualifier	Z	No Qualifier

INDEX: Reduction, fracture, see Reposition, vertebra, lumbar

Secondary Procedure: Fusion of Lumbar vertebrae with device **0SG00AJ**

Character	Code	Explanation
Section	0	Medical and Surgical
Body System	S	Lower Joints
Root Operation	G	Fusion
Body Part	0	Lumbar Vertebral Joint (L2 L3)
Approach	0	Open
Device	A	Interbody Fusion Device
Qualifier	J	Posterior Approach, Anterior Column

INDEX: Fusion, lumbar vertebral 1 joint

Secondary Procedure: Excision of bone for the bone graft **0QB20ZZ**

Character	Code	Explanation
Section	0	Medical and Surgical
Body System	Q	Lower Bones
Root Operation	B	Excision
Body Part	2	Pelvic Bones, Right
Approach	0	Open
Device	Z	No Device
Qualifier	Z	No Qualifier

INDEX: Excision, bone, pelvic, right (Is this a locally harvested bone (not coded) or is it done by separate incision and would be coded)

Rationale: Either of the diagnosis codes for the second or third vertebra fracture could be listed as principal with the second site listed as the secondary diagnosis code. The surgical repairs include the open reduction of the lumbar fractures. The fusion procedure involves the interbody fusion device, bone graft, and interspinous process wiring. ICD-10-PCS coding guideline B3.10c states when an interbody fusion device is used to render the joint immobile (alone or containing other material like bone graft), the procedure is coded with the device value interbody fusion device. The interbody fusion is always placed in the anterior column. The approach can be anterior or posterior. Whether the excision of the bone to use for the fusion is coded separately is the debate. ICD-10-PCS guideline 3.9 states "If an autograft is obtained from a different procedure site in order to complete the objective of the procedure, a separate procedure is coded, except when the seventh character qualifier value in the ICD-10-PCS table fully specifies the site from which the autograft was obtained." The example given in the guideline is "coronary bypass with excision of saphenous vein graft, excision of saphenous vein is coded separately." The author's interpretation is the intent of the guideline of "different procedure site" is meant to state it is code if it was done through a separate incision. The harvesting of pelvic bone is not done through a separate incision so it is not coded. Other coders may interpret it as the site of the pelvic bone is a separate procedure site so it is coded. Coding Clinic has not specifically addressed this example. Site Coding Departments may establish an internal policy on whether to code or not code until clarification reviewed from Coding Clinic for example.

11. **Principal Diagnosis:**   **S36.116A** Laceration, liver, major, initial encounter

     Secondary Diagnoses: **S36.438A** Laceration, jejunum, initial encounter;

                                      S37.011A Hematoma, kidney, see contusion, initial encounter;

                                      S31.129A Laceration, abdominal wall with foreign body, initial encounter;

                                      S41.011A Laceration, shoulder, right, initial encounter;

                                      S81.811A Laceration, leg (lower), right, initial encounter;

                                      T51.0X1A (Table of Drugs and Chemicals) Poisoning, accidental, alcohol, beverage, initial encounter

     Principal Procedure: Repair of liver laceration **0FQ00ZZ**

Character	Code	Explanation
Section	0	Medical and Surgical
Body System	F	Hepatobiliary System and Pancreas
Root Operation	Q	Repair
Body Part	0	Liver
Approach	0	Open
Device	Z	No Device
Qualifier	Z	No Qualifier

INDEX: Repair, liver

     Secondary Procedure: Repair of jejunum laceration **0DQA0ZZ**

Character	Code	Explanation
Section	0	Medical and Surgical
Body System	D	Gastrointestinal System
Root Operation	Q	Repair
Body Part	A	Jejunum
Approach	0	Open
Device	Z	No Device
Qualifier	Z	No Qualifier

INDEX: Repair, jejunum

     Secondary Procedure: Internal examination of the kidney **0TJ50ZZ**

Character	Code	Explanation
Section	0	Medical and Surgical
Body System	T	Urinary System
Root Operation	J	Inspection

Body Part	5	Kidney
Approach	0	Open
Device	Z	No Device
Qualifier	Z	No Qualifier

INDEX: Examination, see Inspection, kidney

Secondary Procedure: Examination of colon for injuries **0DJD0ZZ**

Character	Code	Explanation
Section	0	Medical and Surgical
Body System	D	Gastrointestinal
Root Operation	J	Inspection
Body Part	D	Lower Intestinal Tract
Approach	0	Open
Device	Z	No Device
Qualifier	Z	No Qualifier

INDEX: Examination, see Inspection, intestinal tract/lower

Secondary Procedure: Removal of glass from abdominal wall/fascia **0JC80ZZ**

Character	Code	Explanation
Section	0	Medical and Surgical
Body System	J	Subcutaneous Tissue and Fascia
Root Operation	C	Extirpation
Body Part	8	Subcutaneous Tissue and Fascia, Abdomen
Approach	0	Open
Device	Z	No Device
Qualifier	Z	No Qualifier

INDEX: Extirpation, subcutaneous tissue and fascia, abdomen (glass)

Rationale: The patient had several serious injuries, and the physician should designate the most serious injury if there is any debate. In this scenario it appears the major laceration of the liver would qualify as the principal diagnosis. There is an instructional note at S36 that directs users to code also any associated open wound. Each of the lacerations is coded: abdominal wall with foreign body, shoulder skin, and leg skin. The hematoma of the kidney was diagnosed during the procedure and coded as a secondary diagnosis code. The patient was also treated for the acute alcoholic poisoning. If the blood alcohol level was documented there could have been an additional code. The surgical procedures include repair of the liver and jejunum as well as an inspection of the kidney and colon for additional injuries. Glass was removed from the abdominal wall and fascia. All the procedures were done through a laparotomy or via an open approach.

13. **Principal Diagnosis:**   **S02.651A** Fracture, traumatic, mandible, angle, right, initial encounter

    Secondary Diagnoses: **S02.652A** Fracture, traumatic, mandible, angle, left, initial encounter

        S02.5XXA Fracture, traumatic, tooth, initial encounter;

        S01.81XA Laceration, jaw—See Laceration, head, specified site NEC, initial encounter;

        N39.0 Infection, urinary tract;

        S60.511A Abrasion, hand, right hand, initial encounter

    Principal Procedure: Open reduction/internal fixation mandible, left **0NSV04Z**

Character	Code	Explanation
Section	0	Medical and Surgical
Body System	N	Head and Facial Bones
Root Operation	S	Reposition
Body Part	V	Mandible, Left
Approach	0	Open
Device	4	Internal Fixation Device
Qualifier	Z	No Qualifier

INDEX: Reposition mandible left

Secondary Procedure: Open reduction, internal fixation mandible right **0NST04Z**

Character	Code	Explanation
Section	0	Medical and Surgical
Body System	N	Head and Facial Bones
Root Operation	S	Reposition
Body Part	T	Mandible, Right
Approach	0	Open
Device	4	Internal Fixation Device
Qualifier	Z	No Qualifier

INDEX: Reposition mandible right

Secondary Procedure: Repair of skin laceration on face **0HQ1XZZ**

Character	Code	Explanation
Section	0	Medical and Surgical
Body System	H	Skin and Breast
Root Operation	Q	Repair
Body Part	1	Skin Face
Approach	X	External

Character	Code	Explanation
Device	Z	No Device
Qualifier	Z	No Qualifier

INDEX: Repair skin face

Secondary Procedure: Extraction lower tooth **0CDXXZ0**

Character	Code	Explanation
Section	0	Medical and Surgical
Body System	C	Mouth and Throat
Root Operation	D	Extraction
Body Part	X	Lower Tooth
Approach	X	External
Device	Z	No Device
Qualifier	0	Single

INDEX: Extraction tooth lower

Rationale: The most serious injury appears to be the bilateral fracture of the mandible and either right or left side could be coded as the principal diagnosis with the 7th character of A for the initial encounter. The other injuries were also coded with the 7th character of A for the initial encounter as well. The urinary tract infection was diagnosed as well and not attributed to the surgery as it was present preoperatively in the urinalysis. The procedures performed include two codes for the open reduction of the mandible because the left and right mandibles are separate body parts in ICD-10-PCS. The other procedures for repair of the laceration and extraction of the tooth were coded.

15. **Principal Diagnosis:** S82.852A Fracture, traumatic, ankle, trimalleolar, initial encounter for closed fracture

   Secondary Diagnoses: I69.354 Sequela, infarction, cerebral, hemiplegia;

   E11.9 Diabetes, type 2;

   Z79.84 Long-term drug therapy, oral, antidiabetic

   I25.9 Ischemia, heart;

   N39.0 Infection, urinary

   Principal Procedure: Closed reduction left tibia **0QSHXZZ**

Character	Code	Explanation
Section	0	Medical and Surgical
Body System	Q	Lower Bones
Root Operation	S	Reposition
Body Part	H	Tibia Left
Approach	X	External
Device	Z	No Device
Qualifier	Z	No Qualifier

INDEX: Reposition, tibia, left

Secondary Procedure(s): None indicated by the documentation provided

Rationale: The reason for admission after study was the fracture of the left ankle that required surgical treatment of the tibia. The patient also had medical conditions that were treated, including hemiplegia from a previous cerebral infarction, type 2 diabetes, ischemic heart disease, and a urinary tract infection. Because documentation in the health record identified the use of oral diabetic medication, code Z79.84 was also assigned. The procedure of "reposition" in ICD-10-PCS describes the closed reduction performed to treat the fracture. The application of the cast is included in the fracture care procedure code and not coded separately.

17. **Principal Diagnosis:**   **S72.011A** Fracture, traumatic, femur, subcapital, right, initial encounter for closed fracture

    Secondary Diagnoses: **I10** Hypertension, (essential);

    Principal Procedure: Insertion of internal fixation device without fracture reduction **0QH604Z**

Character	Code	Explanation
Section	0	Medical and Surgical
Body System	Q	Lower Bones
Root Operation	H	Insertion
Body Part	6	Upper Femur Right
Approach	0	Open
Device	4	Internal Fixation Device
Qualifier	Z	No Qualifier

INDEX: Fixation, bone, internal, without fracture reduction, see Insertion. Insertion, femur, upper, right

Secondary Procedure(s): None indicated by the documentation provided

Rationale: A fracture not indicated as open or closed should be coded to closed. The operative report includes "This showed the fracture to be well reduced on its own" so a reposition procedure was not performed. Hypertension is coded because it is a chronic condition still under treatment.

19. **Principal Diagnosis:**   **S42.211P** Malunion, fracture—See Fracture, by site, Fracture traumatic, humerus, upper end, surgical neck, with 7th character of P for subsequent encounter for fracture with malunion, right

    Secondary Diagnoses: **I25.10** Disease, arteriosclerotic, heart—See Disease, heart, ischemic, atherosclerotic;

    N18.9 Insufficiency, renal, chronic;

    E11.9 Diabetes, type 2

    Z79.84, Long-term (current), oral, antidiabetic

    Principal Procedure: Open reduction with internal fixation humeral head right **0PSC04Z**

Character	Code	Explanation
Section	0	Medical and Surgical
Body System	P	Upper Bones
Root Operation	S	Reposition

Body Part	C	Humeral Head Right
Approach	0	Open
Device	4	Internal Fixation Device
Qualifier	Z	No Qualifier

INDEX: Reposition humeral head, right (Body Part Key: neck of humerus = humeral head)

Secondary Procedure: Bone grafting right humerus **0PRCO7Z**

Character	Code	Explanation
Section	0	Medical and Surgical
Body System	P	Upper Bones
Root Operation	R	Replacement
Body Part	C	Humeral Head Right
Approach	0	Open
Device	7	Autologous Tissue Substitute
Qualifier	Z	No Qualifier

INDEX: Graft, see Replacement humeral head, right

Secondary Procedure: Harvesting of bone for bone graft **0QB30ZZ**

Character	Code	Explanation
Section	0	Medical and Surgical
Body System	Q	Lower Bones
Root Operation	B	Excision
Body Part	3	Pelvic Bone Left
Approach	0	Open
Device	Z	No Device
Qualifier	Z	No Qualifier

INDEX: (Harvest) Excision, bone, pelvic bone, left (Body Part Key: iliac crest = pelvic bone)

Rationale: The principal diagnosis, the reason for admission after study, was the malunion of the upper end of the humerus from a previous traumatic fracture. The 7th character of P was chosen from the options to describe a subsequent encounter for fracture care for a fracture with nonunion. The documentation in the health record identifies that oral medication is used to treat the diabetes, so additional code is used from Z79.84. Three procedures are necessary to code: the reposition and internal fixation of the fracture site. The patient's other medical conditions are coded as well.

Chapter 19B

Poisoning by, Adverse Effects, Underdosing, Toxic Effects of Substances, Other Effects of External Causes, Certain Early Complications of Trauma and Complications of Surgical and Medical Care

1. **First-Listed Diagnosis:** **T43.202A** Table of Drugs and Chemicals: Antidepressants, poisoning, intentional, antidepressants, initial encounter

   Secondary Diagnoses: **T42.4X2A** Table of Drugs and Chemicals: Lorazepam, poisoning, intentional initial encounter;

   T51.0X2A Table of Drugs and Chemicals, alcohol, beverage, poisoning, intentional, initial encounter;

   F32.9 Depression

Rationale: Any of the poisoning codes may be listed first. Coding Guideline I.C.19.e states, "Codes in categories T36–T65 are combination codes that include the substance that was taken as well as the intent. No additional external cause code is required for poisonings." The 7th character of A should be used on the poisoning codes to identify it as the initial encounter for care.

3. **Principal Diagnosis:** **T81.41XA**, Infection, postoperative, surgical site, superficial incisional

   Secondary Diagnoses: **L03.311** Cellulitis, abdominal wall;

   B95.62 Infection, bacterial, as cause of disease classified elsewhere, staphylococcus, aureus, methicillin resistant;

   E11.9 Diabetes, type 2

   Z79.84, Long-term drug therapy, oral, antidiabetic

   Principal Procedure: None indicated by the documentation provided

   Secondary Procedure(s): None indicated by the documentation provided

Rationale: Coding Guideline I.C.1.b. states, when there is documentation of a current infection (such as wound infection, stitch abscess, urinary tract infection) due to MRSA, and that infection does not have a combination code that includes the causal organism, assign the appropriate code to identify the condition along with an additional code from Chapter 1 to identify the organism; in this case it would be code B95.62, Methicillin resistant *Staphylococcus aureus* infection because the cause of this disease classified elsewhere is the MRSA infection. The Alphabetic Index entry of "Infection," methicillin, resistant Staphylococcus aureus with code A49.02 is wrong for this exercise as the A code indicates a sepsis or blood stream infection as opposed to the cause of the cellulitis. The 7th character of A is listed on the infection due to surgery to identify it as the initial encounter. The IV antibiotic infusion may or may not be coded and should be based on facility-specific coding guidelines.

5. **First-Listed Diagnosis:** **L29.9** Pruritus

   Secondary Diagnoses: **T36.3X5A** Table of Drugs and Chemicals, azithromycin, adverse effect, initial encounter;

   H66.90 Otitis media, acute

Rationale: This scenario is an example of an adverse effect of the drug azithromycin. The principal diagnosis, the reason for admission after study, was the pruritus caused by the proper use of the azithromycin. The diagnosis of "drug allergy" is found in the Alphabetic Index under allergy, drug, correct substance properly administered—see Table of Drugs and Chemicals, by drug, adverse effect. The drug is identified from the Table of Drugs and Chemicals using the drug name azithromycin with the T code and with the 7th character of A for the initial encounter identifying it as the source of the adverse effect. The patient's other medical conditions that were evaluated and treated during the hospital stay should be coded as secondary diagnoses as well.

7. **First-Listed Diagnosis:** **T82.7XXA** Infection, due to device, implant or graft, electronic, cardiac—or—
Complication, cardiovascular device, electronic, pulse generator, infection, initial

   Secondary Diagnoses: **L03.313** Cellulitis, chest wall;

   Z86.14 History, personal, infection, methicillin resistant Staphylococcus aureus

Rationale: The reason for this outpatient visit is found to be an infection of the chest wall, that is, cellulitis due to the presence of the cardiac pulse generator. There is an instructional note under code T82.7 to use an additional code to identify the infection, which is the cellulitis in this scenario. The 7th character of A is used to identify this as the initial encounter to treat the infection due to the device.

9. **First-Listed Diagnosis:** **T36.8X1A** Table of Drugs and Chemicals, ciprofloxacin, poisoning, accidental, initial encounter;

   Secondary Diagnoses: **R19.7** Diarrhea;

   N39.0 Urinary tract infection;

   B96.20 Infection, Escherichia (E. coli), as cause of disease classified elsewhere or Infection, bacterial, as cause of disease classified elsewhere, Escherichia coli [E. coli]

Rationale: The scenario describes an admission due to an overdose of ciprofloxacin that was identified as an accidental. The code is found on the Table of Drugs and Chemicals with a 7th character of A for the initial encounter for care. The manifestation of the overdose, the diarrhea, is coded separately. The patient's coexisting conditions of urinary tract infection caused by E. coli were also evaluated and treated and coded as secondary diagnoses.

11. **Principal Diagnosis:** **T84.032A** Complication, joint prosthesis, internal, mechanical, loosening, knee, initial;

    Secondary Diagnoses: **G20** Parkinsonism;

    H40.9 Glaucoma

    H54.11 Blindness, one eye, right (category 4), low vision on left (category 1);

    I25.2 Infarction, myocardial, healed or old;

    R94.39 Findings, abnormal, stress test;

    M15.0 Osteoarthrosis, generalized, primary

    Principal Procedure: Replacement tibial component knee **0SRV0J9**

Character	Code	Explanation
Section	0	Medical and Surgical
Body System	S	Lower Joints
Root Operation	R	Replacement
Body Part	V	Knee Joint, Tibial Surface, Right
Approach	0	Open
Device	J	Synthetic Substitute
Qualifier	9	Cemented

INDEX: Replacement, joint, knee, right, tibial surface

Secondary Procedure: Removal tibial surface knee **0SPV0JZ**

Character	Code	Explanation
Section	0	Medical and Surgical
Body System	S	Lower Joints
Root Operation	P	Removal
Body Part	V	Knee Joint, tibial surface
Approach	0	Open
Device	J	Synthetic Substitute
Qualifier	Z	No qualified

INDEX: Removal of device from, joint, knee, right, tibial 0SPV

Rationale: The reason for admission after study, the principal diagnosis, was the mechanical loosening of the tibial surface or component of the knee joint prosthesis. The patient had several medical conditions that were also treated or evaluated during this admission that are coded as secondary diagnoses. The fact the patient is status post total knee replacement does not need to be coded with Z96.651. This would be redundant coding. The patient has a complication of the joint prosthesis (T84.032A); therefore, it is understood the patient had a knee joint replacement in the past. The procedure, called a revision by the physician, is two procedures in ICD-10-PCS. One is the replacement of the tibial surface component prosthesis in the knee with a new device. The second code is the removal of the original device to replace it with another device. The root operation in ICD-10-PCS for revision is correcting a portion of a malfunctioning device or the position of a displaced device, which is not what was done during this surgery.

13. **Principal Diagnosis:**   **T86.49** Complication, transplant, liver, specified type NEC

    Secondary Diagnoses: **D89.810** Disease, graft-versus-host, acute;

    R21 Rash;

    R19.7 Diarrhea;

    R18.8 Ascites

    Principal Procedure: Skin biopsy, chest **0HB5XZX**

Character	Code	Explanation
Section	O	Medical and Surgical
Body System	H	Skin and Breast
Root Operation	B	Excision
Body Part	5	Skin, Chest
Approach	X	External
Device	Z	No Device
Qualifier	X	Diagnostic

INDEX: Biopsy, see Excision with qualifier diagnostic, skin, chest

Secondary Procedure(s): None indicated by the documentation provided

Rationale: The physician describes the cause of this patient's symptoms as due to acute graft-versus-host disease and that this is a complication of his transplanted liver. In ICD-10-CM, codes under category T86 are for use for both complications and rejection of transplanted organs. Two codes are required to fully describe a transplant complication: the appropriate code from category T86 and a secondary code to identify the complication. In this scenario the complication of code D89.810, acute graft-versus-host disease is used. The symptoms vary with this disease, so for this patient each symptom is coded as an additional diagnosis for the rash, diarrhea, and ascites. The biopsy of the skin is a diagnostic procedure of an excision using the qualifier of X to indicate it is a biopsy.

15. **Principal Diagnosis:**   **T40.1X1A** Table of Drugs and Chemicals, heroin, poisoning, accidental (unintentional), initial encounter

    Secondary Diagnosis: **J96.00** Failure, respiratory, acute;

    N17.9 Failure, kidney, acute;

    F11.221 Dependence, drug, opioid, with intoxication with delirium

    Principal Procedure: Mechanical ventilation 72 hours **5A1945Z**

Character	Code	Explanation
Section	5	Extracorporeal Assistance and Performance
Physiological System	A	Physiological Systems
Root Operation	1	Performance
Body System	9	Respiratory
Duration	4	24–96 Consecutive Hours
Function	5	Ventilation
Qualifier	Z	No Qualifier

INDEX: Mechanical Ventilation see Performance, respiratory

Secondary Procedure(s):   Endotracheal intubation **0BH17EZ**

Character	Code	Explanation
Section	0	Medical and Surgical
Physiological System	B	Respiratory System
Root Operation	H	Insertion
Body Part	1	Trachea
Duration	7	Via Natural or Artificial Opening
Function	E	Intraluminal Device, Endotracheal Airway
Qualifier	Z	No Qualifier

INDEX: Insertion of device in, trachea. Intubation, airway – see Insertion of device in, Trachea 0BH1-

Secondary Procedure(s):   None indicated by the documentation provided

Rationale: The reason for admission after study was identified by the physician as the accidental heroin overdose, which should be the principal diagnosis. According to coding guidelines I.C.19.5.b, when coding a poisoning, first assign the appropriate code from category T36–50. The code for the heroin overdose can be located on the Table of Drugs and Chemicals with the intent of accidental included as well as the 7th character of A for the initial encounter for treatment. Use additional codes for all manifestations of the poisoning. The acute respiratory failure is the manifestation of the poisoning. It is the reason the patient had respiratory failure. In addition, the patient was identified as having a heroin or opioid dependency with intoxication delirium and acute renal failure that would qualify as additional diagnoses. The procedure performed was mechanical ventilation, which would be the principal procedure code.

17. **Principal Diagnosis:**   **T82.868A** Complication, graft, vascular, thrombosis, initial encounter

     Secondary Diagnoses: **I12.0** Hypertensive kidney disease with stage 5 chronic kidney disease or end stage renal disease;

           N18.6 Disease, End stage renal;

           N03.9 Glomerulonephritis, chronic;

           Z99.2 Dependence on renal dialysis

     Principal Procedure: Thrombectomy, vein cephalic, right **05CF0ZZ**

Character	Code	Explanation
Section	0	Medical and Surgical
Body System	5	Upper Vein
Root Operation	C	Extirpation
Body Part	F	Cephalic Vein Left
Approach	0	Open
Device	Z	No Device
Qualifier	Z	No Qualifier

INDEX: Thrombectomy, see Extirpation, Vein, Cephalic, Right

Secondary Procedure: Insertion of catheter, internal jugular vein, left **05HN33Z**

Character	Code	Explanation
Section	0	Medical and Surgical
Body System	5	Upper Vein
Root Operation	H	Insertion
Body Part	N	Internal Jugular Vein Left
Approach	3	Percutaneous
Device	3	Infusion Device
Qualifier	Z	No Qualifier

INDEX: Insertion of Device in vein, internal jugular, left

Secondary Procedure: Hemodialysis **5A1D70Z**

Character	Code	Explanation
Section	5	Extracorporeal Assistance and Performance
Physiological Systems	A	Physiological Systems
Root Operation	1	Performance
Body System	D	Urinary
Duration	7	Intermittent, Less than 6 hours Per Day
Function	0	Filtration
Qualifier	Z	No Qualifier

INDEX: Dialysis, hemodialysis – see Performance, urinary 5A1D. Hemodialysis see Performance, urinary 5A1D

Rationale: The reason for the admission was to treat the thrombosis in the renal dialysis site. Using the Index entry of thrombosis, due to device, catheter, dialysis, code T82.868 is located. This code is used for the principal diagnosis with the 7th character of A to identify the initial encounter for care for the thrombosis. The patient's underlying disease, hypertensive kidney disease, ESRD, glomerulonephritis, and dependence on renal dialysis are added as secondary diagnoses. The principal procedure is to remove the thrombus from the cephalic vein by an open approach, which meets the definition of extirpation in ICD-10-PCS. The need for immediate access for dialysis requires the placement of a catheter for infusion in the left internal jugular vein. In ICD-10-PCS this is the root operation of insertion of device into vein as a secondary code. The hemodialysis performed during the hospital stay is coded as another secondary procedure.

Chapter 20

External Causes of Morbidity

1. **External cause code(s):**

   > **Y04.0XXA** Fight, see Assault, fight, initial encounter;
   >
   > **Y92.39** Place of occurrence, stadium;
   >
   > **Y93.82** Activity, spectator at an event;
   >
   > **Y99.8** External cause status, student

   Rationale for selecting the external cause of morbidity codes:

   The event or accident that was the cause of the injury: Fight between spectators that is referred to as an assault by fighting

   This was the initial encounter.

   The place where the event or accident occurred: Sports stadium

   The activity of the patient at the time the event or accident occurred: Patient was a spectator at a sports event

   The status of the patient at the time the event or accident occurred: Patient was a student

3. **External cause code(s):**

   > **V43.52XA** Accident, transport, car, driver, collision, car, traffic, initial encounter
   >
   > **Y92.411** Place of occurrence, highway
   >
   > **Y99.0** External cause status, civilian activity done for income or pay

Rationale for selecting the external cause of morbidity codes:

The event or accident that was the cause of the injury: Transport accident, collision, vehicle with vehicle This would be the initial encounter.

The place where the event or accident occurred: Highway

The activity of the patient at the time the event or accident occurred: No type of activity stated so no code applied

The status of the patient at the time the event or accident occurred: Patient was employed so code as civilian activity done for income or pay

5. **External cause code(s):**

> **W11.XXXA** Fall from ladder, initial encounter
>
> **Y92.017** Place of occurrence, residence, house, single family, yard
>
> **Y93.H9** Activity, maintenance, exterior building
>
> **Y99.8** External cause status, specified NED (unemployed)

Rationale for selecting the external cause of morbidity codes:

The event or accident that was the cause of the injury: Fall from ladder This would be the initial encounter.

The place where the event or accident occurred: Yard at a single-family house

The activity of the patient at the time the event or accident occurred: Washing windows is maintenance on the exterior of a building

The status of the patient at the time the event or accident occurred: Patient was unemployed so code Y99.8 for other specified

7. **External cause code(s):**

> **V95.32XA** Accident, transport, aircraft, occupant, powered craft accident, fixed wing, commercial, forced landing, initial encounter
>
> **Y92.520** Place of occurrence, airport
>
> **Y99.8** External cause status, leisure activity

Rationale for selecting the external cause of morbidity codes:

The event or accident that was the cause of the injury: Transport accident, airplane occupant, forced landing This would be the initial encounter.

The place where the event or accident occurred: Airport

The activity of the patient at the time the event or accident occurred: No activity stated other than occupant of plane that is included in the event code

The status of the patient at the time the event or accident occurred: Leisure activity, flying to vacation

9. **External cause code(s):**

> **W16.032A** Accident, diving, see Fall, into water, in swimming pool, striking wall, initial encounter
>
> **Y92.016** Place of occurrence, swimming pool, private, single-family residence
>
> **Y93.12** Activity, diving
>
> **Y99.8** External cause status, student activity

Rationale for selecting the external cause of morbidity codes:

The event or accident that was the cause of the injury: Diving accident.

This would be the initial encounter.

The place where the event or accident occurred: Swimming pool at single family residence

The activity of the patient at the time the event or accident occurred: Diving

The status of the patient at the time the event or accident occurred: Patient is a student

11. **External cause code(s):**

> **W06.XXXA** Fall from bed, initial encounter
>
> **Y92.230** Place of occurrence, hospital, patient, room
>
> **Y99.8** External cause status, specified NEC (patient)

Rationale for selecting the external cause of morbidity codes:

The event or accident that was the cause of the injury: patient fell out of bed

This would be the initial encounter.

The place where the event or accident occurred: Patient room in a hospital

The activity of the patient at the time the event or accident occurred: There is no stated activity, so not coded

The status of the patient at the time the event or accident occurred: Person was a patient, so other "specified" status

13. **External cause code(s):**

> **X37.1XXA** Tornado, (any injury), initial encounter
>
> **W20.8XXA** Tree, falling on or hitting (accidental) (person), initial encounter
>
> **Y92.017** Place of occurrence, residence, house, single family, yard
>
> **Y99.8** External cause status, leisure activity

Rationale for selecting the external cause of morbidity codes:

The event or accident that was the cause of the injury: two events for this accident: there was a tornado and the patient was struck by a falling tree. There is a note under category W20, Struck by thrown, projected or falling object – Code first any associated cataclysm (X34–X39) or lightning strike (T75.00).

For this reason, the X37.1XXA code is listed first.

This would be the initial encounter.

The place where the event or accident occurred: Single family residence in the yard

The activity of the patient at the time the event or accident occurred: There is no stated activity, so not coded

The status of the patient at the time the event or accident occurred: Person was off work on vacation at home, so status would be leisure

15. **External cause code(s):**

> **W92.XXXA** Exposure, excessive heat, man-made, initial encounter
>
> **Y92.63** Place of occurrence, factory
>
> **Y99.0** External cause status, civilian activity for income or pay

Rationale for selecting the external cause of morbidity codes:

The event or accident that was the cause of the injury: patient was exposed to excessive heat in a steel mill factory (man-made origin) This would be the initial encounter.

The place where the event or accident occurred: Factory

The activity of the patient at the time the event or accident occurred: There is no stated activity nor is there a code for "working"; the fact the patient was at work is captured in the status code and possibly from the place of occurrence of a factory

The status of the patient at the time the event or accident occurred: Patient was at work in a civilian job

17. **External cause code(s):**

> **V00.131A** Accident, skateboard, see Accident, transport, pedestrian, conveyance, skateboard, fall, initial encounter
>
> **Y92.481** Place of occurrence, parking garage, lot
>
> **Y93.51** Activity, skateboarding
>
> **Y99.8** External cause status, student activity

Rationale for selecting the external cause of morbidity codes:

The event or accident that was the cause of the injury: Skateboard accident fall

This is the initial encounter.

The place where the event or accident occurred: Parking lot

The activity of the patient at the time the event or accident occurred: Skateboarding

The status of the patient at the time the event or accident occurred: Patient was a student

19. **External cause code(s):**

> **V00.321A** Fall, involving skis, see Accident, transport, pedestrian, conveyance, skis, fall, initial encounter
>
> **Y92.828** Place of occurrence, mountain
>
> **Y93.23** Activity, skiing, (downhill)
>
> **Y99.8** External cause status, leisure

Rationale for selecting the external cause of morbidity codes:

The event or accident that was the cause of the injury: Fall involving skis, this becomes a transport accident because skis transport a person from place to place

This would be the initial encounter.

The place where the event or accident occurred: Mountain

The activity of the patient at the time the event or accident occurred: Downhill skiing

The status of the patient at the time the event or accident occurred: Patient was spending leisure time as a skier

21. **External cause code(s):**

> **W54.0XXA** Bitten by dog
>
> **Y92.018** Place of occurrence, residence, house, single family, specified (porch)
>
> **Y99.0** External cause status, civilian activity done for income or pay

Rationale for selecting the external cause of morbidity codes:

The event or accident that was the cause of the injury: Bitten by dog was the event. This would be the initial encounter.

The place where the event or accident occurred: Porch on single family house

The activity of the patient at the time the event or accident occurred: There is no activity code available for "delivery of package" or "working."

The status of the patient at the time the event or accident occurred: Patient was an employee, so status is civilian activity done for income or pay

Chapter 21

Factors Influencing Health Status and Contact with Health Services

1. **Principal Diagnosis:**   **Z38.01** Newborn, born in hospital, by cesarean

    Secondary Diagnoses: **P07.03** Low, birthweight, extreme, with weight of, 945 grams;

    P07.26 Immaturity, extreme, gestational age, 27 weeks;

    P22.0 Syndrome, respiratory, distress, newborn

    Principal Procedure: Continuous positive airway pressure **5A09557**

Character	Code	Explanation
Section	5	Extracorporeal or Systemic Assistance and Performance
Physiological System	A	Physiological System
Root Operation	0	Assistance
Body System	9	Respiratory
Duration	5	Greater than 96 Consecutive Hours
Function	5	Ventilation
Qualifier	7	Continuous positive airway pressure

INDEX: Continuous positive airway pressure, greater than 96 consecutive hours 5A09557. CPAP – see Assistance, respiratory, greater than 96 consecutive hours

Secondary Procedure(s): None indicated by the documentation provided

Rationale: An infant born during a current admission requires the newborn category code Z38 to be listed first with any other conditions listed as secondary diagnoses. A note with category P07 states when both birth weight and gestational age of the newborn are available, both should be coded with birth weight sequenced before gestational age. As stated, the patient was placed on CPAP for greater than 96 hours, so it is coded as the principal procedure.

3. **Principal Diagnosis:**   **I10** Hypertension

    Secondary Diagnoses: **Z30.2** Encounter, sterilization, or Multiparity requiring contraceptive management, see Contraception, sterilization (same code)

    Principal Procedure: Fallopian tubal ligation bilateral **0UL74CZ**

Character	Code	Explanation
Section	0	Medical and Surgical
Body System	U	Female Reproductive System
Root Operation	L	Occlusion
Body Part	7	Fallopian Tubes, Bilateral
Approach	4	Percutaneous Endoscopic
Device	C	Extraluminal Device (Falope Rings)
Qualifier	Z	No Qualifier

INDEX: Ligation, see Occlusion, fallopian, tubes, bilateral

Secondary Procedure: None indicated by the documentation provided

Rationale: The reason for admission and principal diagnosis is the hypertension. The secondary diagnoses reflect the request for sterilization due to multiparity. In ICD-10-CM, the multiparity is not coded separately from the code for the encounter for sterilization. The procedure performed is a tubal ligation using Falope rings. Falope rings are placed on the exterior surface of the fallopian tube to accomplish the occlusion.

5. **First-Listed Diagnosis:**   **R26.2** Gait abnormality, walking, difficulty

   Secondary Diagnoses: **Z47.1** Aftercare, following surgery, joint replacement;

   Z96.641 Presence, hip joint implant, right;

   Z79.01 Therapy, drug, long term, anticoagulant;

   Z51.81 Encounter, therapeutic drug level monitoring

Rationale: To explain the home health services provided by the nurse and physical therapists, there could be a variety of codes and in varying sequences for the home health services. The three-day-per-week physical therapy would best be explained by the abnormality of gait code to focus on the reason for the therapy. The nurses serve to draw blood would be explained by the long term (current) use of anticoagulant. All the above may also be described as surgical aftercare.

7. **Principal Diagnosis:**   **Z04.1** Observation (following) accident, transport

   Secondary Diagnoses: **V43.62XA** External Cause: Accident, transport, car occupant, passenger, collision (with), car, initial encounter;

   Y92.411 External Cause: Place of occurrence, street and highway, interstate highway;

   Y99.8 External Cause: Status of External Cause, specified NEC

   Principal Procedure: None indicated by the documentation provided

   Secondary Procedure(s): None indicated by the documentation provided

Rationale: The reason for admission after study was the fact the infant was in a vehicle involved in a serious motor vehicle crash but found to be unhurt. The observation following accident code as principal describes this fact. The external cause codes are optional depending on the hospital's coding guidelines or state-mandated reporting from trauma hospitals.

9. **First-Listed Diagnosis:**   **Z00.111** Newborn, examination, 8 to 28 days old

   Secondary Diagnoses: **L74.0** Prickly heat, Heat, prickly

Rationale: This is a first visit of a 2-week-old infant to the physician's office for a newborn examination with an additional code per the note under code Z00.11 for the abnormal findings of the prickly heat, also known as miliaria rubra.

11. **First-Listed Diagnosis:**   **S60.511D** Abrasion, (right hand), subsequent care;

    Secondary Diagnoses: **S60.512D** Abrasion, left hand, subsequent care;

    W24.0XXD External Cause: Contact with lift, lifting device, subsequent encounter

Rationale: The scenario represents a follow-up visit for a dressing change for the patient's deep abrasions suffered in a work accident that was previously treated. In ICD-10-CM, the original injuries are coded with the 7th character of D for subsequent care. The type of accident is also coded again with an external cause code with the 7th character of D. The 7th characters for the injury and the external cause should match as they are describing the same injury and event. The aftercare Z codes, such as Z48.00 for dressing change, are not used for aftercare of injuries. Instead for aftercare for an injury, assign the injury code with the appropriate 7th character for subsequent encounter.

13. **Principal Diagnosis:** **Z45.09** Admission, adjustment, device, implanted, cardiac

    Secondary Diagnoses: None indicated by the documentation provided

    Principal Procedure: Mitral Valve Replacement **02RG0JZ**

Character	Code	Explanation
Section	0	Medical and Surgical
Body System	2	Heart and Great Vessels
Root Operation	R	Replacement
Body Part	G	Mitral Valve
Approach	0	Open
Device	J	Synthetic Substitute
Qualifier	Z	No Qualifier

INDEX: Replacement, valve, mitral

    Secondary Procedure: Mitral valve removed **02PA0JZ**

Character	Code	Explanation
Section	0	Medical and Surgical
Body System	2	Heart and Great Vessels
Root Operation	P	Removal
Body Part	A	Heart
Approach	0	Open
Device	J	Synthetic Substitute
Qualifier	Z	No Qualifier

INDEX: Removal of device from, heart

Rationale: The reason for admission after study was not to treat a specific disease, but to admit the patient to the hospital to replace the worn out heart valve prosthesis. This is an encounter for specific care for an implanted heart device. In this scenario, there is not cardiac or other disease mentioned specifically, but in another patient, it is highly likely there would have been other secondary diagnoses. In ICD-10-PCS, the replacement of a previously placed device requires two codes: one to remove the previously placed device and another to replace the body part again with the device; in this case, the heart valve. There is no code (Z95.2) added for the presence of the heart valve because of the Excludes1 note under category Z45.

15. **First-Listed Diagnosis:** **Z23** Admission, prophylactic vaccination

    Secondary Diagnoses: **P07.33** Preterm newborn, gestational age, 30 weeks

Rationale: The reason for this office visit was to receive the prophylactic injection of Synagis. There was no disease. A reason for the injection was the fact the infant had been born prematurely. ICD-10-CM coding guideline I.C.16.e: Codes from category P07, Disorders of newborn related to short gestation and low birth weight, not elsewhere classified, are for use for a child or adult who was premature or had a low birth weight as a newborn that is affecting the patient's current health status.

17. **First-Listed Diagnosis:**   **Z94.0** Transplant (status), kidney

    Secondary Diagnoses: **N18.4** Disease, kidney, chronic, stage 4

    Rationale: Given the fact that the patient is being seen in the transplant clinic to monitor her status as a kidney transplant patient, the first-listed code describes the kidney transplant status. The patient's chronic kidney disease present in the other kidney is coded as an additional diagnosis as relevant to her overall medical status.

19. **First-Listed Diagnosis:**   **Z12.5** Screening, neoplasm (malignant), prostate

    Secondary Diagnoses: **Z86.06**. History, (personal) in situ neoplasm, melanoma.

    Rationale: The stated reason for the visit to the primary care physician's office was for a screening examination to rule out prostate cancer. This is a screening visit because the patient has no symptoms of prostate or urinary disease. The main term in the Alphabetic Index is the word "screening" as it is the intent of the patient's visit to the physician. The main term for the personal history of the melanoma in situ is history. The entry in the Index for History, personal, malignant melanoma (skin) would not be appropriate for this patient as this patient's condition was melanoma in situ.

Chapter 22

Advanced Coding Scenarios

1. **Principal Diagnosis:**   **K25.0** Ulcer, gastric *see* Ulcer, stomach, acute, with, hemorrhage

    Secondary Diagnoses: **I16.0** Hypertensive urgency *see* Hypertension, urgency;

    I10 Hypertension;

    I48.11 Fibrillation, atrial, persistent, longstanding

    Z79.01 Long-term drug therapy, anticoagulants

    K70.30 Cirrhosis, micronodular, alcoholic;

    F10.20 Dependence, alcohol;

    Z63.72 Stress, family *see* Disruption, family, due to, drug addiction in family

    Principal Procedure: Gastrectomy, Partial **0DB60ZZ**

Character	Code	Explanation
Section	0	Medical and Surgical
Body System	D	Gastrointestinal System
Root Operation	B	Excision
Body Part	6	Stomach
Approach	0	Open
Device	Z	No Device
Qualifier	Z	No Qualifier

INDEX: Gastrectomy, partial *see* Excision, stomach 0DB6

Secondary Procedure(s):   Bypass, stomach **0D160ZA**

Character	Code	Explanation
Section	0	Medical and Surgical
Body System	D	Gastrointestinal System
Root Operation	1	Bypass
Body Part	6	Stomach
Approach	0	Open
Device	Z	No Device
Qualifier	A	Jejunum

INDEX: Anastomosis – see Bypass, stomach 0D16

Secondary Procedure(s):   Feeding tube insertion **0DHA0UZ**

Character	Code	Explanation
Section	0	Medical and Surgical
Body System	D	Gastrointestinal System
Root Operation	H	Insertion
Body Part	A	Jejunum
Approach	0	Open
Device	U	Feeding Device
Qualifier	Z	No Qualifier

INDEX: Insertion of device in, jejunum 0DHA

Rationale: The condition after study that necessitated admission was the gastric ulcer, which is coded with a combination code to indicate the bleeding. The hypertensive urgency was treated prior to surgery and was coded, noting the instruction that indicates to also assign a code for hypertension. The micronodular cirrhosis found during surgery was determined to be a result of the patient's alcoholism, which were both coded, as was the stressful family situation which contributed to patient's hypertension and ulcer. Three procedures were performed, beginning with a subtotal excision of the stomach followed by a gastrojejunostomy (closure of the proximal end of the duodenum and side-to-side anastomosis of the jejunum to the remaining portion of the stomach). A jejunostomy feeding tube was then placed. ICD-10PCS Root Operation Guideline for multiple procedures states that if during the same operative episode, multiple procedures are coded if multiple root operations with distinct objectives are performed on the same body part (B3.2c). The first procedure performed was a subtotal gastrectomy, which codes to 0DB60ZZ. The root operation Excision is used since only a portion of the stomach (subtotal) was removed. The second procedure performed is the gastrojejunostomy, which codes to 0D160ZA. The root operation Bypass is used because the objective of the gastrojejunostomy is to reroute the content. The ICD-10-PCS Root Operation Guideline for Bypass states that bypass procedures are coded by identifying the body part bypass from and the body part bypassed to. The fourth character body part specifies the body part bypassed from, (Stomach, value 6) and the qualifier specifies the body part bypassed to (Jejunum, value A) (B3.6a). The third procedure performed was the insertion of the feeding tube into the jejunum, which codes to 0DHA0UZ.

3. **Principal Diagnosis:**   **L97.214** Ulcer, lower limb, calf, right, with bone necrosis

    Secondary Diagnoses: **A41.51** Sepsis, Escherichia coli (E. coli);

                                     R65.20 Sepsis, severe;

                                     J96.01 Failure, respiration, respiratory, acute, with, hypoxia;

                                     E05.00 Graves' disease *see* Hyperthyroidism, with, goiter;

                                     G35 Sclerosis, multiple

                                     I10 Hypertension;

                                     H35.81 Cotton Wool Spots (retinal)

    Principal Procedure: Amputation below the knee **0Y6H0Z1**

Character	Code	Explanation
Section	0	Medical and Surgical
Body System	Y	Anatomical Regions, Lower Extremities
Root Operation	6	Detachment
Body Part	H	Lower Leg, Right
Approach	0	Open
Device	Z	No Device
Qualifier	1	High

INDEX: Amputation *see* Detachment, Leg, Lower, Right

Rationale: The chronic skin ulcer of the right calf with bone necrosis codes to L97.214. The patient also had E. coli sepsis (A41.51) with acute respiratory failure. ICD-10-CM Coding Guideline I.C.1.d.1.a states that if a patient has sepsis and associated acute organ dysfunction or multiple organ dysfunction, follow the instructions for coding severe sepsis. ICD-10-CM Coding Guideline I.C.1.d.1.b states the coding of severe sepsis requires a minimum of two codes: first a code for the underlying systemic infection, followed by a code from subcategory R65.2, Severe sepsis. Additional code(s) for the associated organ dysfunction are also required. Following the guidelines, R65.20 (Severe sepsis) and J96.01 (Acute hypoxic respiratory failure) are also coded. Codes should be assigned for each of the patient's additional conditions as well. The code for the below-the-knee amputation is 0Y6H0Z1 with the seventh character (qualifier) being 1 for a High amputation of the lower leg. The definition of *High amputation of the lower leg* is amputation at the proximal portion of the shaft of the tibia and fibula. The operative report specifies that the amputation occurs directly below the tibial tubercle. The tibial tubercle, also known as the tibial tuberosity, is a large oblong elevation on the proximal, anterior aspect of the tibia, just below where the anterior surfaces of the lateral and medial tibial condyles end. Detachment is the correct root operation for all amputation procedures. *Detachment* is defined as cutting off all or a portion of the upper or lower extremities. Per ICD-10-PCS Coding Guideline B6.1b temporary postop wound drains are considered integral to the performance of a procedure and are not coded as devices.

5. **Principal Diagnosis:**   **M51.36** Disease, disc, degenerative *see* Degeneration, Intervertebral Disc, Lumbar region

    Secondary Diagnoses: **I69.910** Sequela, disease, cerebrovascular, cognitive deficits;

                                       E89.0 Hypothyroidism, postirradiation;

                                     Z85.850 History, personal, malignant neoplasm, thyroid;

                                     E11.65 Diabetes, type 2, hyperglycemia;

Principal Procedure: Vertebral Fusion **0SG10AJ**

Character	Code	Explanation
Section	0	Medical and Surgical
Body System	S	Lower Joints
Root Operation	G	Fusion
Body Part	1	Lumbar Vertebral Joints, 2 or more
Approach	0	Open
Device	A	Interbody Fusion Device
Qualifier	J	Posterior Approach, Anterior Column

INDEX: Fusion, Lumbar Vertebral, 2 or more

Secondary Procedure(s): Harvest bone graft **0QB30ZZ**

Character	Code	Explanation
Section	0	Medical and Surgical
Body System	Q	Lower Bones
Root Operation	B	Excision
Body Part	3	Pelvic Bone, Left
Approach	0	Open
Device	Z	No Device
Qualifier	Z	No Qualifier

Rationale: The code for degenerative disc disease of the lumbar region is M51.36. The patient's attention and concentration issues are a result of the CVA and are coded as sequela. Assign the code for postirradiation hypothyroidism and the history of thyroid cancer. Because of her elevated blood sugars, the patient's type 2 diabetes is uncontrolled, and should be coded to hyperglycemic. Spinal fusions are classified by the anatomic portion (column) fused and technique (approach) used. For the anterior column, the body (corpus) of adjacent vertebrae are fused (interbody fusion). The anterior column can be fused using an anterior, lateral or posterior technique. The technique for this procedure was posterior (0SG10AJ) as evidenced by the patient's prone positioning on the table. The laminectomy was not coded separately, as the excision of the lamina is a component of the fusion. Prior to the fusion, the surgeon removes the lamina bones covering the back of the spinal canal to see the nerve roots. During an interbody fusion, once the cages are in place, the surgeon will fix the bones in place using pedicle screws, which hold the vertebrae together and prevents them from moving. The combination of the graft material with pedicle screws holds the spine steady as the interbody fusion heals. The insertion of pedicle screws is not coded. Per ICD-10-PCS Guideline 3.10c, the interbody fusion device takes precedence in coding over the use of autologous bone graft material. The second procedure code is 0QB30ZZ for excising bone from the left iliac crest for the graft material. Whether the excision of the bone to use for the fusion is coded separately is the debate. ICD-10-PCS guideline 3.9 states "If an autograft is obtained from a different procedure site in order to complete the objective of the procedure, a separate procedure is coded, except when the seventh character qualifier value in the ICD-10-PCS table fully specifies the site from which the autograft was obtained." The example given in the guideline is "coronary bypass with excision of saphenous vein graft, excision of saphenous vein is coded separately." The author's interpretation is the intent of the guideline of "different procedure site" is meant to state it was through a separate incision. In this example, the harvesting of pelvic bone is not done through a separate incision so it is not coded. Other coders may interpret it as the site of the pelvic bone is a separate procedure site so it is coded. Coding Clinic has not specifically addressed this example. Internal coding policies may be established to determine if grafts of this type will be coded.

7. **Principal Diagnosis:**   **C34.12** Carcinoma, bronchioalveolar—see Neoplasm, lung malignant (left) upper lobe

     Secondary Diagnoses: **C77.1** Carcinoma, lymph node, mediastinal, malignant secondary

     Z85.72 History, personal, lymphoma (non-Hodgkin);

     Z87.891 Smoker, see Dependence, drug, nicotine but patient had past history (no longer smoking)—see History, tobacco dependence;

     Principal Procedure: Video-assisted thoracoscopic (VATS) left pneumonectomy **0BTL4ZZ**

Character	Code	Explanation
Section	0	Medical and Surgical
Body System	B	Respiratory System
Root Operation	T	Resection
Body Part	L	Lung, left
Approach	4	Percutaneous endoscopic
Device	Z	No Device
Qualifier	Z	No Qualifier

INDEX: Pneumonectomy see Resection, Respiratory System 0BT

Secondary Procedure: Excision of mediastinal lymph nodes **07B74ZZ**

Character	Code	Explanation
Section	0	Medical and Surgical
Body System	7	Lymphatic and Hemic Systems
Root Operation	B	Excision
Body Part	7	Thorax
Approach	4	Percutaneous endoscopic
Device	Z	No Device
Qualifier	Z	No Qualifier

INDEX: Excision, lymphatic, thorax 07B7

Secondary Procedure: Insertion of chest tube for drainage from left pleural cavity **0W9B40Z**

Character	Code	Explanation
Section	0	Medical and Surgical
Body System	W	Anatomical Regions, General